The Invisible Web

The Invisible Web

Gender Patterns in Family Relationships

MARIANNE WALTERS
*Family Therapy Practice Center,
Washington, D.C.*

BETTY CARTER
*Family Institute of Westchester,
Mount Vernon, New York*

PEGGY PAPP
The Ackerman Institute, New York

OLGA SILVERSTEIN
The Ackerman Institute, New York

THE WOMEN'S PROJECT
IN FAMILY THERAPY

The Guilford Press
New York   London

© 1988 The Guilford Press
A Division of Guilford Publications, Inc.
72 Spring Street, New York, NY 10012

Printed in the United States of America

Last digit is print number: 9 8 7 6 5

Library of Congress Cataloging in Publication Data

The Invisible Web.

    Bibliography: p.
    Includes index.
    1. Family psychotherapy. 2. Feminist therapy.
3. Family—Psychological aspects. 4. Sex roles.
I. Walters, Marianne.
RC 488.5.I59 1988   616.89′156   88-30083
ISBN 0-89862-734-6
ISBN 0-89862-482-7 (pbk.)

To Our Mothers

Acknowledgments

AS ALWAYS IN an effort such as this, there are so many people whose lives and work and words have touched our own and made a difference. Our earliest drafts were read and critiqued by Evan Imber-Black, Halcy Bohen, and Rich Simon, whose feedback gave us the encouragement to continue.

We are indebted to our editor, Sheila Friedling, who not only did most competent and sensitive editing, but also raised questions that pushed us to a level we wouldn't have reached without her.

We give special thanks to Fred Silverstein, who hosted, cooked, researched, and cared for us during our endless meetings.

Marianne, Betty,
Peggy, and *Olga*

Family and friends and colleagues—I can name only a few of those who matter in the space allotted me here. Dear friends with whom I have processed every significant life event, including this one, for the past nearly forty years—Zirel Sweezy, Gerry Brittain, and Nonny Majchrzyk. My first supervisor, Dorothy Hankins, who firmly anchored me to social work values. Rae Wiener, who introduced me to family therapy and helped me to integrate it into my own frame of reference. My sister, Barbara, whose feminist consciousness awakened mine. My colleagues at the Family Therapy Practice Center: Halcy Bohen, whose theoretical clarity and clinical judgment have provided a constant source of intellectual renewal; Laurie Leitch, a gifted and compassionate therapist, whose ideas both challenged and expanded my own thinking; Larry Levner, whose enduring commitment to basic human values kept me grounded; Phyllis Jacobson-Kram, who lent perspective to so many difficult clinical dramas. Ed Mumma, Kitty Montie, Rose Tompkins, Otha Wright, Rose McCabe, Fred Brewster, Roz Beroza, Jon Winter, Carol Siegel, Rich Simon, Matthew Sullivan, David Gage, Robert Atkins, Kris Halstead, Carolyn Krol, and Debbie Shore—to name only a few of the faculty, trainees, and associates of the Center whose inquiring minds, and commitment to learning and discovery, inspired me to seek new directions in my own work. My deepest gratitude. And to Blanca Fuertes my great appreciation for the administrative help and support she provided me.

Marianne Walters

My thanks to colleagues at Family Institute of Westchester who read various chapters and gave most helpful feedback: Monica McGoldrick, Evan Imber-Black, Ron Taffel, Judy Stern Peck, and Fredda Herz. Special thanks to Lisa Fine, who cheerfully typed and word-processed material over and over again. And thanks to my husband, Sam, for his willingness to join me in putting these ideas into practice in our own marriage and family.

Betty Carter

I wish to thank my colleagues in the special project at the Ackerman Family Institute, with whom I spent many hours exploring gender issues in the treatment of families and couples: Valerie Clain, Arlene Genatt, Sandra Mann, and Susan Shimmerlik. Their challenging comments and questions stimulated my thinking and shaped my ideas. A special thanks goes to Richard Simon for his insightful critique and valuable feedback on my couples chapter. And, last but not least, I am grateful for the support and encouragement extended to me throughout the long working hours by my mate, Starrett Kennedy.

Peggy Papp

My special thanks to my colleagues at Ackerman who read my material and gave me invaluable feedback: Bob Simon, Virginia Goldner, Peggy Penn, and Marcia Sheinberg. Donald Bloch provided the leadership and freedom to experiment with new clinical models as we struggled to put new paradigms into our work with families. My husband, Fred, endlessly typed and retyped and supported my efforts with patience as well as enthusiasm.

Olga Silverstein

Contents

Marianne Walters

Prologue: Our Experience

The Context

In the beginning it seemed so clear. It was the spring of 1977. De Beauvoir's *The Second Sex* had been out almost fifteen years; Friedan's *The Feminine Mystique* had created the climate for a new awareness of women's concerns within our shared society. All over the country, women in every corner of public and private life were challenging old assumptions and attempting to revise their status in families, in their churches, on their jobs, in their professions. Consciousness raising had been going on for ten years. Journals and popular magazines devoted to women's issues were becoming almost as popular as those devoted to how to get a man. The Equal Rights Amendment was an active issue and a popular cause. Women's political organizations claimed burgeoning memberships. Divorce laws as well as regulations concerning child custody and child support were becoming more egalitarian. Women could finally obtain legal abortions and exercise choice regarding their own reproductive functions. Women were entering the world of work in increasing numbers, often choosing career fields previously denied them. They were changing the demography of the nation by postponing marriage and having children later in life, or not at all. Some women were choosing to be single parents. Others were entering politics. Women could even get credit on their own, purchase a house, or start a small business. Women's writing, and literature about women, were creating new cultural images and domains. Feminist theory had become a field of serious scholarship. And the women's movement was on the public policy agenda.

Within the mental health field there was a beginning awareness, albeit sometimes begrudging, that developmental theory had been

1

based primarily on the experience of men, and that scales of adjustment and maturity were based on male models of behavior. The recognition that the majority of patients were women and that the majority of therapists were men had begun to trouble some of us. Diagnostic categories and theoretical constructs were being analyzed for sex bias by women's study groups and by task forces within the major professional organizations of social workers, psychologists, and psychiatrists. *Towards a New Psychology of Women* by Jean Baker Miller had become a standard text in university psychology courses and women's studies departments, and Chesler's *Women and Madness* had raised some serious questions about the extent to which psychotherapy itself was iatrogenic with respect to women. Her work delineated ways in which the gender bias of the treatment process tended to pathologize women. While most of the theoreticians and teachers in the mental health field were men, their female colleagues were beginning to raise serious doubts as to whether the experience of women growing up in a male-defined culture had been sufficiently represented in either the theory or practice of the field. Women's issues were being addressed more frequently at professional conferences, and feminist therapy was becoming a recognized discipline.

And so, in the beginning it seemed so clear to us that family therapy also needed to address women's issues and to begin to consider the relevance of a feminist perspective to its own theory and practice. It seemed so clear that as I went about organizing the first workshop in family therapy to discuss the changing role of women in families, I didn't even stop to ponder the failure of family therapy leaders to have noticed those changes. It seemed so clear in the beginning, that it never occurred to me that not all family therapists would welcome the discourse on which we were about to embark! Now, in hindsight, it seems highly paradoxical that in a field devoted to the family, there should have been so little attention paid to sex roles in the family, gender-defined functions within families, or the socialization processes, for men and women, that create the culture of marriage, of child rearing, and of the family.

The family as a social system is gender-based. It exists to structure the relations and organize the social lives of the two sexes that inhabit the planet; to accomplish in an orderly fashion the functions of procreation, protecting and rearing the young, and assuring social continuity between the generations. Of course, it also has an economic base, which is also gender-based. If men were to be free to explore, or to make discoveries, or to develop new societies, or to go to work in offices, they needed someone to manage the households in which they would reside with their offspring, and to tend to the daily necessities of life. So how could it be that family therapists were not deeply conscious of gender socialization? How could the field have ignored sex-role stereotyping in family formation?

In hindsight it would appear that systems theory itself—at least as applied to family therapy—blurred the vision of our theorists. The self-contained principles of systems theory gave its adherents permission to claim neutrality for themselves, as well as for family members, by describing families as governed only by laws that exist within the family system itself. Understanding human behavior, motivation, symptomatology, growth and development through the organizing principles of systems theory was indeed a breakthrough for mental health professionals. But it seemed to have become a prison of sorts, suspended in its own space, barricaded behind a wall created by its own inner logic. Yet all human systems inhabit an open space in which multiple subsystems interact, creating a broad context of experience. No context could be more pertinent to the understanding of all family systems than that of gender. There is no "neutral" context within which human systems exist.

So, in the beginning our purpose seemed so clear—so clear that none of us was fully prepared for the complexities, the struggle, and conflict that were engendered when we, as women therapists, declared our committment to exploring the issues and experiences of women in families, and to understanding the implications of a patriarchal culture for the mental health of women as well as for our own clinical work.

Where We Were When We Began

Having returned from a year of teaching at the Tavistock Clinic in London, I was working at the Philadelphia Child Guidance Clinic where I saw families, and administered, supervised, and taught in a variety of training programs in family therapy. Though I was glad to be back in my "own shop," the year in London had been thrilling. The critical debate and intellectual exchange among people in the mental health field was broader in scope and generally more erudite than at home, and I felt challenged to continue to sharpen my own critical thinking. At the same time, the field there seemed hopelessly burdened with traditional therapy techniques and analytic formulations I had long since abandoned. The contradiction was troubling. Back home some of the women therapists were concerned about the opposite contradiction—advanced therapy techniques that "worked," but little openness to critical discussion of theory and basic concepts. Here one was to "do," not think; there one was to think with more rigor than one was expected to do. Surely there had to be some middle ground.

These women therapists wanted to take a critical look at some of the theoretical assumptions of family therapy, particularly as these assumptions influenced their roles as women working with families. They were concerned about implicit sexist messages in much of family practice, and wanted to evaluate their own work from a feminist perspective. I was asked to lead a study group focused on women's issues in families and the role of women as family therapists. This proved to be a challenging and difficult task. There were no precedents, no support within the agency, and no network outside of it, feminist therapists having rejected family therapy some years earlier. Although at the time no serious field of study, or area of practice within the humanities, was not engaged in considering the implications of feminism in relation to its own theory, a feminist critique of family therapy was dismissed as "nonsystemic," and clearly made most family therapists uncomfortable. Our study group practically had to go underground. We brought each other tapes and critically dissected our interventions to elicit women's issues for ourselves as well as for our clients. As the only "senior" staff person in the group, I was concerned that we would be isolated and realized the importance of networking with women family therapists outside of the Clinic.

I had met Peggy Papp some years before when she did a presentation in Philadelphia of her family sculpting. We met, started to talk, had dinner, talked some more, and have been friends and colleagues ever since. Later we asked Peggy to spend one day a week at the Clinic supervising an extern training group. Although by the spring of 1977 Peggy was no longer commuting to Philadelphia to teach, we began to meet to discuss the possibility of forming a network of family therapists committed to women's issues. Despite hectic schedules, we began to set aside time to share some of our own personal and professional struggles as women, in a field dominated by men.

Peggy had been on the staff of the Ackerman Institute since the mid-sixties. Along with Virginia Satir, she was one of the first women to achieve prominence in the field of family therapy. Her early years as an actress were background to a broad range of improvisational skills that she used in her therapy as well as in the development of innovative techniques. Peggy initially became attracted to family therapy after viewing one of Nathan Ackerman's tapes at the New York City welfare department; it was the impetus that sent her back to school for her master's degree. Later she joined the staff of the Institute and trained initially with Ackerman himself. In 1970 Peggy was a field placement supervisor for the Hunter College School of Social Work when she was blessed with two of the best and brightest students ever to pass through those hallowed halls: Olga Silverstein and Elizabeth (Betty) Carter!

In 1973 Peggy Papp and Betty Carter co-founded, with Tom Fogarty and Phil Guerin, the Center for Family Learning in New Rochelle, New York; and the following year Peggy and Olga Silverstein began the Brief Therapy Project at the Ackerman Institute, putting together an experimental treatment program that was to serve as a prototype for other such programs. While Peggy lectures and gives workshops all over the world, the Project was the place where she struggled with new ideas and innovations in method and technique.

Betty Carter became the first woman in this country to found and direct a family therapy training institute. That occurred in 1977, following a split at the Center for Family Learning, which Betty had helped to establish and develop. In 1980 I followed suit, founding The Family Therapy Practice Center in Washington, D.C. Since then, two or three other training institutes have been headed by women—out of almost 300 family therapy training centers around the country! Over 70 percent of the trainees in these institutes are women. Does that give you pause? Betty Carter and a group of colleagues founded the Family Institute of Westchester without benefit of the "old boy" network in the field, and none of us were sure at the time that a female-headed institution would be able to survive. Her process of developing friendship networks of support, creating alternatives for effective leadership, and establishing women role-models, set precedents for other women leaders. We have spent many fruitful hours together as training institute directors, solving problems ranging from organizational structures, to staff relationships, to funding, to how to share the load.

Olga Silverstein and Peggy Papp have been collaborating in their clinical work, supervision, and training since the mid-seventies. Olga's own history is mirror to the changes that women have forged in their lives during the past twenty years. The daughter of immigrants, Olga married young, and after thirty years as a housewife and mother she applied to the Columbia School of Social Work to do graduate work. She was refused admission on the grounds that she was "too old" to make a contribution to the field. She was fifty at the time. It turned out to be a fortunate turn-down. At the Hunter College Graduate School of Social Work she met Betty Carter, and both had second-year field placements at the Ackerman Institute. Olga's life experience was quickly translated into clinical wisdom and expertise, and soon after she joined the staff at the Ackerman she was teaching, supervising, and mentoring younger therapists.

Olga and I share some social and cultural traditions that shaped our view of the world. Both daughters of Jewish immigrants, we were raised in an atmosphere of social consciousness and political protest to which we became committed and often active participants. When the women's movement came along it seemed a natural extension of the various movements for social change that we had witnessed over the years. But we both soon realized that, for us, this was different. Here was a consciousness that directly affected the way we conducted our lives, entered into relationships, reared our children, experienced ourselves as women. It had the potential to transform, not just reform, the substance and conditions of our own lives. For Peggy there was the legacy of pioneer forebears who settled the West and of parents who lived by traditions forged from the experience of those who, excluded from the social mainstream, sought out their own territory. Feminism was another avenue for the expression of her personal struggle for independence, and her search for new ways to center her own life and extract its meaning. Betty's father had built his life around the conviction that society needed to create opportunity for its disadvantaged members. He convinced businesses to hire the handicapped and developed training programs to enable people with special needs to enter the world of work. Understanding the special needs of any group of people who had been denied access to opportunity and instrumentality was second nature for Betty, and feminism did not seem far from the ethical concerns of her family.

When the four of us met together the first time in the summer of 1977 to discuss ways to bring women's issues and feminist consciousness into the mainstream of family therapy, we were struck with how much the women's movement had already begun to affect our lives and our thinking. Surely this must be happening to many of our colleagues. Betty's reading of Friedan had laid to rest much of the traditional thinking of her Irish Catholic upbringing, and Peggy was examining some of her own choices and personal development through the prism of women's consciousness. Olga was restructuring some aspects of her family life as she and her husband shared a feminist "awakening" and a rethinking of old roles. And I was involved in the heady challenge of making it on my own with three children, grateful to the women's movement for having made this choice possible.

All of us were experiencing a new freedom to take leadership in our field and to assume a more "public" presence, and we were also struggling with the personal implications of such moves. Since I had initiated our coming together I knew I needed to have a plan for keeping us together. Here were four extremely busy professional women functioning as therapists, teachers, supervisors, administrators, program heads; rearing children, managing households, dealing with marriages and divorces, caring for aging parents; maintaining friendships, arranging family gatherings, and organizing family transitions—four women of diverse backgrounds who shared a profession and, now, a common cause. It was exciting. I suggested we begin by doing a workshop together exploring the situations faced by women as family therapists, using our own tapes and clinical material to illustrate some of the critical professional issues and dilemmas. It was agreed. And so we began our work together.

The Women's Project in Family Therapy

We presented for the first time as a group in December 1978. Our workshop, entitled "Women as Family Therapists," was held in Philadelphia. Prior to the workshop we met several times to prepare our material, and initiated informally what was to become the structure of our collaborative style. Each of us took responsibility for a subject area with which we particularly identified, or a clinical piece with which we felt most familiar. At our meetings we would try to identify the women's issues in our cases and presentations and discuss ways of addressing them. Then each of us, separately, would prepare a presentation from the perspective of our own style and methodological orientation.

That first workshop was a definite high for us. The participants not only gave us enthusiastic feedback; they were insistent that the need to continue bringing women's issues into family therapy was a pressing one. Women in the audience spoke, some for the first time in a large group setting, about their own concerns. They raised issues ranging from women therapists' use of authority to how to restructure service delivery systems in behalf of women. Some women described their experience of sexism in their agencies of practice, or in their family therapy training programs. Most important, there was general agreement that the distinct voice of women in mental health, in social agencies, as therapists, as clients, within family systems, had not been heard amid the many current librettos of family therapy, and that this workshop was "a first" in raising that voice.

In pursuing the concerns of women as family therapists during that workshop, we found ourselves confronting issues ranging from social policy and service delivery systems to a therapist's use of self. We found that we, as well as our audience, raised more questions as we rounded each corner, and that we had few answers. We discovered our own lack of familiarity with new theories of female development, or with research on the economic and social consequences of woman's traditional role in the family. There was much to learn and much to be done. Were we the ones to do it? Should we make this inquiry a priority in our already overextended personal and professional lives? Were we prepared to challenge some of the theoretical assumptions and practices of family therapy? How would we begin to organize and structure such a project? And what should our role be in it? After the exhilaration of challenge, discovery, and broad-based support that we experienced in our first workshop came that period of collective self-exploration and self-doubt that "tries (wo)men's souls."

We made four major decisions: (1) We would continue to collaborate around the issues of women in families and in family therapy. (2) We would call ourselves "The Women's Project in Family Therapy."

(3) We would conduct another workshop outside our centers of practice, and sponsored solely by the Women's Project. (4) We liked working together and found our collegial relationship to be both intellectually stimulating and professionally nurturing.

For the purpose of presentations as well as the conduct of our own meetings, I became the chairperson, and The Family Therapy Practice Center in Washington the administrative arm of the Project. We made it a rule that if any one of us had strong objections to any activity, procedure, or policy, or to any idea, theory, or approach, we would all respect the right of individual veto. We agreed to strive to achieve consensus on theory pertaining to women in families and women's issues, and to avoid such efforts with respect to our methodological differences. Out of this agreement, and the experience of our first workshop, we evolved a clear format for our continued collaboration: We would work together to develop a theoretical framework for the analysis of women's isues as well as a feminist perspective in family therapy, and we would work separately to illustrate or present this feminist perspective within our own individual techniques and approaches. We all felt sure that we did not want to develop a membership organization. We wanted the Project to serve as a vehicle for the introduction of women's issues and feminist theory into the mainstream of family therapy, and we wanted to involve an ever broader constituency of therapists concerned about and committed to the subject. To this end we began to prepare a series of workshops.

At this point, we still had the illusion that the Women's Project would be a small but important addition to our already strained schedules. Yet, without realizing it, we had embarked on the most complex, stormy, and rewarding journey of our professional lives. We had tapped into a responsive chord in women in the field.

In March 1978 we presented a workshop on women's issues in family therapy at the annual meeting of the American Orthopsychiatric Association. We had not expected the large turnout we had for this meeting, and we were stimulated and encouraged by the mutually respectful, active, and informed participation of many who attended. In June of that year the first two articles on feminist approaches in family therapy appeared in family therapy journals: Rachel Hare Mustin's "A Feminist Approach to Family Therapy" in *Family Process*, and Hare-Mustin's article with her colleague, Hines, on "Ethical Concerns in Family Therapy," which appeared in the *Journal of Marriage and Family Therapy*.

Our first workshop series, in 1979, was designed around the title "The Dilemma of Women in Families." As we grappled with this broad topic in developing our ideas and our presentations, we realized we would need to narrow our focus. We decided to organize our thinking around the roles and relationships of women within the structure of the family, focusing on a particular relationship, in order to explore it as fully as possible. Out of this effort came our next public presentation, "Mothers and Daughters." Five or six hundred people came to our first workshop on this topic, which was held in New York in the spring of 1980. Therapists brought their mothers, or their daughters, and several generations of women therapists were represented in the audience. Process, politics, personal and clinical experience, methodology, and theory were examined with respect to the relationship between mothers and daughters. Using the larger context of gender socialization to examine relationships, instead of an exclusively internal family system, provided us with the necessary tool to experiment with clinical revisions and adaptations.

We repeated our workshop on "Mothers and Daughters" in various parts of the country and in England in 1981–82, culminating in a weeklong woman's residential seminar/workshop/symposium held in the Berkshires in the summer of 1983. The following year we prepared and presented workshops on "Mothers and Sons, Fathers and Daughters" and published two monographs containing representative presentations from these workshops. We were networking with other women family therapists here and abroad, lending our support and what input we could to the work of younger women therapists who were developing critical theory, writing, and doing research in the field of feminism and family therapy, and mentoring gifted women therapists in our training programs. Our own friendship and respect for each other was deepening, and despite our competitive natures it was clear that we were genuinely enjoying and sharing our individual successes as well as our collective efforts in the field. With a sense of the inevitable we knew that there had to be a new task at hand.

This Book: Our Process

And so we found in our work together a book to be written, and during the summer of 1984 we started to map it out. Needless to say, since that time we have changed our course many times and navigated through a number of stormy seas. As we got together during the summer of 1986 in one of our seemingly endless writing sessions, we talked of what had kept us going, and how it was that the quality of our collaboration had grown, and even improved, through five years of workshops, meetings, presentations, and administrative wrangling—in addition to two years of writing, editing, rewriting, and yet more meetings. Clearly, a major factor was the significance all of us attached to the subject we were exploring, the compelling motivation to bring women's consciousness and women's experience to bear on the theory and practice of family therapy. Even when there were hurt feelings, misunderstandings, disappointments, and the competing demands of per-

sonal and professional priorities—even when we felt like simply walking away from the endless pressure—we would return to the task at
hand because it was an agenda we could not escape.

Moreover, the growing sense of connectedness and of a deepening
friendship kept us going and became a commitment that none of us were
willing to risk and all of us wanted to sustain. Looking back on it, we felt
sure we could not have maintained the collegial rapport and personal
friendship that evolved during our years of collaboration had we not
been, from the beginning, a group of peers, professionally as well as
personally. It might not have worked if there had been a large disparity
between us in terms of experience or authority in the field; or if there had
been considerable age differences, or unequal levels of professional at-
tainment. As peers and teachers, our collaboration became one of the few
arenas where we could be endlessly contradicted and challenged. From
the beginning, the Women's Project had been a place where we vigorously debated our ideas. This turned out to be a good training ground for
the even more rigorous ideological and clinical debates that took place
during our book writing. Even as we argued, and despite some strong
disagreements, our commitment to one another grew.

Our structure and style of collaboration changed in writing the
book. We each drafted a "working paper" that we used as the basis for
discussion, searching out core ideas and themes and discarding others.
Then each of us wrote a chapter; we then met and, reading the chapter
aloud, the four of us went over each other's work. Often our personal
encounters would trigger an issue we wanted to put in the book, or
would sharpen an idea that we had been going over while working on
the chapter materials. And conversely, we would find ourselves relating to the material at hand with personal anecdotes and memories, and
would stop reading a chapter to tell family stories and recount illustra-
tive experiences. Gradually the personal experience became part of the
work, and the work part of the personal, so that there was a sense of
enrichment and integration.

Of course, this process mirrored one of the main themes of our
book: the integration of reason and emotion, of the personal and the
"political," of the relational and the instrumental. Over and over again
we found ourselves informed in our work by our own processes of
learning and relating, by our personal experiences. And over and over
again we found our personal experience transformed by what we were
thinking. The process of reading our work aloud to each other, and
opening ourselves up to criticism, challenge, and disagreement, put us
in a context of intense proximity requiring both trust and respect for
our individual differences.

The business of determining authorship for this book is an example
of our process. In the beginning, in the interest of being "democratic," I
suggested we author it alphabetically, to which we all agreed. (Betty
Carter was delighted!) But I began to hate the idea and regret that we all

had so readily agreed to it. (Carter, Papp, *et al.* in the "bibs" did not appeal to me!) It rankled that I had initiated the Women's Project but would end up last author on its book. But how could I say this to the others without appearing pushy and mean-spirited and competitive? At one of our meetings I even half-jokingly suggested that our names appear in a circle, with no beginning or end. Luckily, no one took me up on it!

I knew I needed to talk about this with the others, but I was amazed at my reticence to do so. Then, at one of our meetings Olga and I, almost simultaneously, said we wanted to discuss authorship. Obviously, it had been bothering her too (since we were the ones most adversely affected by an alphabetical listing). And we both, independently, had come up with the same solution—to have collective authorship, that is, The Women's Project as the author of this book. Betty and Peggy readily agreed. In this supportive atmosphere we could talk about my conflict in terms of the generalized dilemma for women in being at once accommodating and assertive, relational and yet self-defined. This event served to illustrate the degree to which women are socialized to avoid behaviors that seem aggressive, and to shy away from affirming the need for recognition of their contributions lest this be experienced by others as self-serving. Although I thought I had finally become comfortable with saying what I wanted, I realized the struggle was not over for me, the sense of entitlement not yet achieved. In this way individual feelings about an interpersonal process could be, and were, used to inform us all.

Some months later, when the book was nearly complete, we reviewed this decision and decided that an organizational authorship was inappropriate. My colleagues felt that, as the originator of the Women's Project, I should be first author, and that their authorship should be in alphabetical sequence. For me, that recognition, from these particular women, will remain the more enduring experience than that of the authorship sequence itself.

I think one of the most difficult things for us in writing this book was to refrain from getting into the sociology of women's issues as our own awareness, and growing familiarity with feminist theory and the women's movement, was deepened. When we started our work together in the Women's Project, it was for us the beginning of a gradual evolution and deepening feminist consciousness, and we were motivated to share, through this book, some of what we had learned. We needed to continually remind ourselves that we are not social theorists writing about women's issues in general, or even as they applied to the general field of mental health. The fact that we are primarily clinicians, fundamentally committed to a family therapy approach in our clinical work and in our teaching, had to be the foundation on which we would build our case for a feminist perspective in family therapy.

Our book is focused on women's relationships in the family. We have made no effort to exhaust the subject. We are well aware that huge chunks of that experience have been left out. For example, we have not included chapters specifically devoted to sisters or grand-mothers. We have attempted to raise some of the issues, some of the common scenarios, and some of the consequences of gender socialization for relationships within the family. There is no question that gendered constructs within the family raise many issues and have many consequences for men; but that is not the focus of this book and we will rarely address those issues. You will note in our cases, however, the positive consequences of feminist interventions for men in families. Each issue we discuss, and each relationship we explore, has its implications at some level for our mates, and for our male colleagues. But these are not the focus of our book.

The material of this book is designed to have clinical application. The introductory essay in each chapter will, it is hoped, provide a context for looking at family problems, client interactions, and clinical interventions from a feminist perspective. To facilitate this process we have each contributed a case to each chapter. At no time did we attempt to arrive at consensus regarding our individual theoretical orientations and clinical styles, which, from the beginning and throughout our collaboration, have been diverse and distinct: Betty Carter presents a transgenerational model of family therapy with roots in Bowen systems theory; Olga Silverstein practices an evolved inter-generational systemic method with roots in the Milan, Bowen, and Milton Erickson schools; Peggy Papp practices a systemic/strategic method with roots in MRI, Milan, and Milton Erickson; and I offer a model of therapy that has evolved from structural theory to concepts of context and competence as parameters of change.

None of us would approach any one case in the same way as the author of that particular case. There are many cases in this book. Each represents a woman's issue or feminist intervention. And each illustrates the particular methodology and style of the reporting therapist. It is one of the tenets of our work together not to let our differences interfere with our commitment to apply a feminist perspective to the repertoire of techniques and interventions typical of the various clinical orientations that the four of us represent. During the many workshops that preceded the writing of this book we took special care not to allow our theoretical differences to get in the way of our developing a new basis for consensus and connection.

As you read this book, you will find one or the other of the theoretical orientations more familiar and more congenial to your own way of thinking and working. We ask you to try to distinguish between the feminist points we are making, on which we agree, and the theoretical orientations or methodological differences, on which we diverge. In other words, try not to throw out a feminist point that has been made because it is presented within a method with which you are not familiar or with which you do not agree.

part one

Some Redefinitions

1

Toward a Feminist Perspective in Family Therapy

THE PRESENT PARADIGMS of family therapy are based on the value system of the American family of the forties and fifties and lag sadly behind the social changes already in full swing.

Major changes in family structure and functioning are now well-established in our society. Women in ever larger numbers not only work outside the home but can no longer choose to stay at home as the two-paycheck family has become an economic necessity in working-class families and an expectation in the upwardly mobile middle class. The increase in divorce and remarriage has resulted in an enormous increase in new family forms, with mothers raising children alone and remarried couples struggling to integrate his children and her children with ex-spouses and complicated networks of extended kin. There is increasing incidence of serial, live-in relationships, with postponement of marriage and childbearing into the middle years. There has been an increased awareness by women of their own sexuality and their power over their own bodies, as well as a revision of sexual expectations on the part of both sexes. Of central significance in all of these changes is the recognition of a woman's right to control reproduction.

With regard to these changes in the family, and in women's roles in the family, family therapy theory lags behind the culture as a whole. It is now imperative that there be new approaches in family therapy built on new assumptions about what constitutes a viable family.

There were three phases in the evolution of our feminist perspective on family therapy. *Phase I* was our process of defining a common feminist frame of reference while preserving our clinical diversity and differences. *Phase II* could be described as the phase of exploration and critique in which we examined systems theory and the absence of gender in its formulations, and in the process became aware of sexist social constructs, sex-role function in families, and sexist attitudes in our own field. In this phase, we focused clinically on what to avoid in our practice. *Phase III* is current and ongoing. It is the process of developing nonsexist and feminist systemic interventions and revising and adapting traditional systemic interventions to take gender into account. These alternative interventions incorporate a sensitivity to the experience of women as different from that of men.

Phase I: Defining a Feminist Framework

In the very beginning of our work together, we made no attempt to discuss the theory and methods of family therapy. We knew that there were theoretical and methodological differences among us, and we were concerned, in the beginning, that direct debate about our four different methods would divide us. We had no terminology or jargon that was mutually acceptable, so we couldn't couch our discussions in terms of triangles, cybernetic cycles, hierarchies and boundaries, family of origin, or any of the other comfortable terms of family therapy discourse.

What we had in common was our friendship, our respect for each other's work, and our commitment to focus attention on the experience of women, which we felt had been neglected or distorted in the family therapy field. Without thinking or talking about it, we automatically adopted a nonhierarchical structure and a collective, consensus-seeking process in our discussions. And since we couldn't communicate fruitfully from *within* our various methods, we started trying to talk and to think *beyond* these methods.

Our discussion then focused on the social, cultural, or political implications and origins of any clinical intervention or conceptualization. We asked ourselves: Would this technique or this formulation simply reflect gender stereotypes, or would it challenge or counteract such stereotypes? What are the social or cultural roots of a particular concept? What is the metamessage conveyed to each gender by a specific intervention? How does the metamessage of a technique vary with the gender of the therapist? Will this intervention support a sexist situation, or will it offer an alternative?

In our discussions, then, we began with a clinical situation, or with our own personal life situations, and then took the discussion up two levels to the social system, bypassing the level of family therapy theory and method with its constraints on our thinking. We were defining a shared viewpoint, a value system, that would be strong enough to permit us to break through our commitments to our various methodologies. It was quite a bit later in our process that we came to value our differences for the wide range of clinical choices and directions they offer. In the beginning, we tried to avoid direct discussions of these differences while we worked out a place to stand together.

In Phase I, then, we agreed on a working definition of "feminism" and outlined two general principles to guide our further critique of the family therapy field. Feminism, we agreed, is a humanistic framework or world view concerned with the roles, rules, and functions that organize male-female interactions. Feminism seeks to include the experience of women in all formulations of human experience, and to eliminate the dominance of male assumptions. Feminism does not blame individual men for the patriarchal social system that exists, but seeks to understand and change the socialization process that keeps men and women thinking and acting within a sexist, male-dominated framework.

The central operating principles of our revisions of family therapy derive from this feminist perspective. First, no systems formulation can be gender-free. Formulations that purport to be gender-free or "neutral" are in fact sexist because they reproduce the social pretense that there is equality between men and women. Women, in fact, are disadvantaged in our society, and a failure to acknowledge this fact doubly disadvantages them. Second, all interventions need to take gender into account by recognizing the different socialization processes of women and men, with special attention to the way in which these socialization processes disadvantage women. We need to recognize that each gender hears a different meaning in the same clinical intervention and accordingly feels either blamed or supported by an identical therapeutic stance.

Phase II: An Examination of Systems Theory and How It Is Used to Disadvantage Women

During this phase we pursued an examination of family systems theory and explored the ways that it is used to disadvantage women. In our discussions we outlined the concepts that were shared assumptions in the major schools of family therapy. We then tried to determine whether a given concept was itself sexist, whether it lent itself to sexist assumptions, and/or was widely abused by family therapists to the disadvantage of women. As our thinking progressed in this direction, and we became aware of the sexist ramifications of certain clinical interventions, we stopped using them.

It was at this point that each of us began to question her own clinical certitude and to watch and listen more carefully to each other. It is an error to assume that because we are women, we were automatically aware of the ways in which women's position in the social structure is maintained. It was difficult for us to unearth the ways that sexism had "naturally" become part of the family therapy field, and of our own professional practice. The fact that the four of us are successful in this field, and that we have good careers going despite any sexist disadvantages that might have been in force, did not make it easier for us to see the sexism in our work. It is true that we were not putting jobs at risk by taking a new position. But what made it especially hard for us were our many years of life experience, as well as professional experience, in doing things a certain way, of feeling confident and competent at what we did, and reluctant to de-skill or unsettle ourselves too much. It is quite possible that had we realized at the outset the degree of change—personally and professionally—that we were setting into motion for ourselves, we might never have begun. Certainly, if we had realized the amount of anger and personal criticism to which we would be subjected by colleagues, we might have had second thoughts about setting forth on this new course. But these stormy reactions were in the future, and it was chiefly our own "resistance" that we struggled with as we began to critique the assumptions of family theory and therapy.

We agreed that unless the underlying patriarchal assumptions about family are explicitly addressed and/or taken into account in family therapy formulations and interventions, they will be understood by clients to be implicitly accepted. This is why we believe that there is no such thing as "gender neutrality." "Neutrality" means leaving the prevailing patriarchal assumptions implicit, unchallenged, and in place.

The Patriarchal Assumptions

The prevailing patriarchal model of family is grounded in a number of assumptions we have long taken for granted. Basic to patriarchal family organization is the concept of *role complementarity*, with instrumental tasks such as earning money through work the province of the male, and emotional tasks such as nurturing, building, and maintaining relationships, and child rearing the province of the female. In this model, the organization of power is based on male hierarchy.

In contrast to this organization is our feminist model of family, which is characterized by *role symmetry*, in which each sex engages in both instrumental and expressive tasks, in both work and nurturing. This model reflects an egalitarian approach to power between male and female, and a more democratic and consensual approach to parental management of children.

Although many people acknowledge that the feminist model of family would be more humanistically fulfilling for both sexes, it is clear that men would have to give up power, which involves status and often money, to gain less tangible rewards, and that they are often unwilling to do so. It is also difficult for some women to give up the idea that they should be financially supported by men and that they need a man to make their lives successful—economically, socially, and emotionally.

The systemic view of male-female and intergenerational relationships is that they are *interdependent*. Ideally, maturity in this context would be defined as *autonomy with connectedness*. This ideal is in contrast to the patriarchal splitting of these attributes, assigning "autonomy" (actually separateness) to males, and assigning "connectedness" (actually dependency) to females. In effect, such splitting leads us to mistake separateness or disconnectedness for autonomy, a valued sign of maturity, while "connectedness" is equated with dependency, a sign of immaturity, and thus devalued.

A major conceptual error is to assume that traits such as "autonomy" or "dependency" are intrinsic to the person of men or women rather than assigned to them by a patriarchal society on the basis of gender. Thus men are assigned "autonomy" with both the power and emotional disconnectedness that goes with it, while women are assigned "dependency" with both the emotional connectedness and the powerlessness that goes with it. Although being disconnected and being dependent both have drawbacks, it is clearly a far more serious threat to survival to be dependent.

Currently, we are living in a period of social transition in which the rigidity of the traditional patriarchal family structure has been challenged, and changes have been introduced within that system. Most of these changes, however, are behavioral and have been in the direction of women entering the work force and shouldering permanently a portion of the economic burden of the family. There has been no significant shift in men's focus toward family life, nor any real change in the basic attitudes of most men and women about the organization of family life—although there are more isolated cases of shared roles than there used to be. Economic, social and legal institutions in our society do not support changes that would enable women to work more outside of the home, and men to work more inside, by providing practical child-care arrangements and giving economic priority and social status to the work of child rearing.

In spite of unequal opportunity and unequal pay, and the lack of social supports, women are working more outside the home, some out of necessity, others for the freedom of choice and fulfillment it gives them. Whatever the reasons, now women have gained for themselves the freedom to work full-time at two jobs—career and family— and have lost the legal and social expectation that they, and their children, would be financially supported by men. The shift that is needed to complete this change in a direction that would benefit the entire family is for men to assume co-responsibility for child care, sharing financially and by participation, and to give up the idea that the main focus of their energy must be devoted to outside work. Such a shift, of course, would entail a loss of status, money, and power for men.

Family Systems Concepts

When we analyze how family therapy interventions emerged from the patriarchal assumptions about male-female roles and family organization, we must consider the impact of the leading family systems concepts. Following is a review of the field's main concepts and how they are widely abused to the disadvantage of women. We start with the basic concept of fusion.

Fusion and Distance Are Opposite Sides
of the Same Coin

Our feminist view of the concept of fusion or "enmeshment"—the merging and reactive distancing that occurs in couples and throughout family relationships—acknowledges that the roles traditionally assigned to the sexes color the way in which each sex manifests its "immaturity." Thus it is often the female who shows the symptoms of dependency: seeking approval, avoiding conflict, placating, leaning too much on others, and acting incompetent. Males manifest exactly the same degree of immaturity in a different way: through emotional isolation, unavailability, seeming indifference, withdrawing, withholding from others, and fear of vulnerability. When either of these sets of symptoms show in the oppostie sex (that is, men with dependency symptoms or distant behavior in women), it is doubly pathologized by therapists.

There are several ways in which the concept of fusion is misused in the practice of family therapy. First and foremost, fusion is misunderstood to apply only to the *close* relationships in the family, which invariably include females, while the related function of the distant male is ignored or overlooked. In effect, the terms "close" and "overclose" are often used to discredit the genuine intimacy and positive engagement of mothers and children. Certainly, our jargon could provide a better word to designate emotional entanglement or negative involvement.

Because of the central role assigned to women in marriage maintenance and child rearing, women are usually the ones who raise the important emotional issues in the family. In therapy, instead of validating women's concerns, therapists frequently label them automatically as "overconcerns" or emotional "pursuing," as if *raising* the issue, or the *manner* of raising the issue, were the issue. In this way, therapists devalue the active, connecting role of women in families. Therapists also tend to focus first on the part of the problem involving the wife or mother, because women will tolerate being blamed or held responsible in this way.

Thus, there is often an initial and negative focus on relationships perceived as "enmeshed," as well as a courting of the distant male in a positive or placating fashion that leaves the impression that the wife/ mother is to *blame* for a dysfunctional relationship, or she alone is responsible for bringing about change. This bias is treated as a *neutral* principle of good practice, and is reflected in training slogans such as the following:

1. Never pursue a distancer in treatment.
2. Always intervene first with the overfunctioner or the overresponsible one.
3. The enmeshed relationship has to be loosened *before* the distancer can move in.
4. Begin with the one who is most available to change.

Such teaching slogans ignore or deny the fact that terms such as "distancer," "overfunctioner," "enmeshed," and the like almost always refer to specific, predictable genders carrying out socially mandated tasks, and are not neutral terms describing dysfunctional positions. This terminology is linked with the clinical assumption that if only the wife/mother will "back off" or "let go," then the "distancer" will move in, which really does imply that the engaging partner is blocking the distant one, and so is to blame for problems in the family. In fact, the "distancer" does not move in automatically, and needs attention and assistance to do so. And the close-in partner (usually the woman) is correct in fearing a vacuum if she "lets go" or "backs off." Such practice techniques also disrespect men since they suggest that men are unable to be available for emotional engagement in therapy or in the family, and should not be challenged or confronted lest they flee or collapse. Above all, it should be noted that although these techniques were developed because they "work," they generally "work" to restore an unbalanced system to its previous patriarchal balance, with the old hierarchies and boundaries in place. Thus it is not really these techniques that are the problem, but the outmoded and sexist paradigm of family to which they refer.

Reciprocity

The concept of reciprocity states that everyone involved in a problem plays a part in the maintenance of that problem by reinforcing the behavior of the other. Common examples given are the nagging mother and the dawdling child, or the battering husband and the battered wife. However, this concept as it is taught fails to explain that "playing a part" does not mean "playing an *equal* part." A two-month-old baby can be said to "play a part" in being abused by crying, for instance, since it can be argued that child abuse would not occur if the child were not there, or did not cry. But it is clear that the parts played by the child and the abusing parent are not equal in force. The child is not responsible for the abuse, does not have equal power, or responsibility, or equal options, or equal ability to change the cycle. Neither does the battered wife, the incest victim, the dawdling child, or anyone who is overpowered by someone of greater size, strength, age, or position of influence.

Clearly the two examples given above of reciprocal behaviors present two situations at opposite ends of any spectrum of significance. Nagging mothers and battering husbands have little in common except when we are considering them within a closed belief system that views all interpersonal interactions as equally reciprocal. Unfortunately, even putting these two situations side by side as examples of the same process—as will often be found in our family therapy literature—lends itself to a blurring of any clinical evaluation. Reciprocity is a useful conceptual tool, but also one that can organize us to think clinically as if all behaviors are not only similarly constructed, but are of the same order of significance.

Questioning by the therapist that purports to be "neutral," "circular," or "systemic" in fact often implies one-sided responsibility or blame—for example: "What do you do to get your husband angry?"; "How does your mother get your father going?"; or "How do you help your husband to drink?" A way of focusing on the systemic factors that may contribute to the maintenance of the problematic pattern, without ignoring individual responsibility for behavior or the social context, would be to ask questions such as: "What do you do when your husband gets angry?"; "What do you do when your parents are fighting?"; or "What do you do when your husband drinks?" Such questioning acknowledges both the interactional features of any familial interchange, and the individual responsibility of each family member for his or her own behavior.

Complementarity

Balance is an attribute of a system requiring that the different roles, behaviors, and emotions of individuals within the system exist in dynamic equilibrium. A balanced system may typically include polarized roles such as good kid-bad kid; distancer-pursuer; worker-nurturer.

However, our perspective would regard polarization as a poor way to achieve balance, requiring, as it does, lopsided individuals to maintain equilibrium within the system. Polarized roles reflect the priority of a balanced system over the needs of the individuals in it. Instead, it is potentially more liberating for each individual within the system to achieve some *internal* balance of complementary traits and functions.

Complementarity has to do with the inductive nature of interactional patterns: that is, how the behaviors of one person induce the other into behaviors that complement them, and vice versa. This concept, in addition to roles and functions, refers to emotional characteristics such as upset and calm, effusive and withdrawn, volatile and stable, talkative and quiet, generous and withholding, and so forth.

The need to maintain complementarity or balance in the family is used as a reason to assign roles to women that complement the roles chosen by men. In this way, women perform those tasks that men prefer not to do, for example, housework and child care, and do not compete in those areas that men select as their domains, namely achievement, work, finances, and the like.

Systems therapy discriminates against women by seeking balance and equilibrium for the family system as a unit, without addressing the unequal access of each individual to choice of role. The pretense that men and women are genderless cogs in the system prevents us from noticing that women are held more responsible than men for making it work, in the family and in family therapy, and that the "complementary" roles, tasks, and rewards of the stable system are allocated by gender, unequally, to its male and female members. But the social context lends meanings and images to those complementary behaviors and roles. So, for example, the talkative woman "chatters," the silent man "runs deep"; the anxious mother "hovers," the distant father is "preoccupied." And so on. These socially constructed images and associations carry with them positive and negative connotations. None of us, client or therapist, can escape them.

The theory of complementarity includes both contingent responses (in that one behavior induces another) and derivative responses (in that it is reactive and responsive to another's behavior). A certain parity is implied in that definition—but with different implications for men and women. For women, who are defined culturally as contingent on male behavior, such ideas act to keep them in the same psychological place. Men, who see themselves as self-defined, will have their context for new behavior expanded by calling attention to the impact of relationships on their behavior.

The concept of complementarity is a useful therapy construct, a practical way of creating change. The problem is that practitioners using such concepts can begin to believe that they reflect reality. For the idea of complementarity in human interaction to be other than a hypothetical construct, it would need to reflect the social, economic, and political structures within which the family system exists. There can be no true complementarity in human relationships if the antecedents of those relationships are skewed in terms of access to social, legal, political, and economic opportunity and power. Thus, to believe in circularity and complementarity in human relations, we must assume some basis of parity. If such a basis does not in fact exist, then we are dealing with a hypothetical abstraction that does not take into account the social origins of those relationships. We are in fact responding to a relational system at a point in time (when "it" enters therapy) as though it had no precedents in larger social constructs. This victimizes the member of that system who entered the relationship in the less powerful position; that is, we must recognize that although it takes two to tango, if one is to lead and the other to follow, then their steps are not equally interdependent.

Hierarchy

Hierarchy is a structural concept ranking the relative power and authority of the individuals and subsystems in the family, and indicating the boundaries between them. When applied rigidly, or in a sexist manner, the concept of hierarchy disadvantages women and children who will always end up on the bottom of any authoritarian ranking. As taught and practiced in family therapy, the concept of heirarchy often does not leave room for the female style of decision making in a more consensual or collective way, or for exerting authority (with children, for example) more through relationship than through explicit use of power.

Boundaries

Linked to the structural concept of hierarchy, the concept of boundaries prescribes appropriate separateness between individual family members, and between generations. It also draws a line around the nuclear family as a whole. In this view, a well-organized family has clearly delineated boundaries that define "appropriate" closeness and distance in relationships.

This concept is most often abused through clinical applications that fail to recognize a different female understanding of relatedness. For example, in the therapy room, when mother speaks for others when attempting to explain family problems to the therapist, her behavior is often defined as "intrusive" or "controlling," and she may be blocked by the therapist in some way. The implication is that mother's talking is causing the others to be silent, and that it is an intrusion into their space; on the other hand, silence is seldom defined as "controlling" or as creating a vacuum that the mother tries to fill.

Triangles

Unlike a threesome, which may be a functional group, "triangle" is a term used to describe dysfunction, as in the detouring of the conflict of a twosome through a third party. As tension rises, the three members move toward and away from each other in predictable moves designed to reduce tension and avoid direct exposure of the basic conflict, which might divide the original twosome.

It is common to conceptualize family emotional relationships as a triangle whose interactions are then predictable. There are several pitfalls in this abstract way of thinking about human relationships. Triangles provide no differential explanation of gender-related behavior, such as an explanation of why mothers are most often found on the so-called "overclose" or "fused" leg of the triangle and fathers in the distant position. Furthermore, describing emotional problems primarily in terms of triangles defines the problems as *inside* the family system alone and ignores their direct connection to the larger social system. For example, a triangle that conceptualizes a husband in the distant position, with his mother and his wife on the conflictual, "overclose" end, would require the conventional intervention of moving the wife closer to her husband, and putting the husband in charge of setting boundaries with his mother. If the therapist understands such a triangle as a case of a "controlling" or "over-responsible" wife fighting her husband's mother for primacy with him, and/or a mother who can't "let go" of her son, interventions will probably not be delivered in a way that will preserve the self-esteem of either wife or mother-in-law. The feminist therapist will see this triangle as a case of two women bumping into each other as each tries to carry out her family responsibilities in the face of the man's withdrawal. The interventions will then be delivered in a way that explicitly respects the women's views of their roles, and then challenges the husband to engage more fully in his relationship with each of them.

Function of the Symptom

Systems theory focuses on how families function within the closed systems they have organized. Within these self-contained family units, all behaviors, including symptoms, have a stabilizing function; that is, they maintain those patterns of personal interaction that establish equilibrium. In this view, the symptom may be seen as a *necessary* means of regulating the larger system. This conceptualization of how the family is organized purports to be value free, genderless, and egalitarian. In its concern with maintaining the overall system as the balanced sum of its parts, it focuses on patterns needed to provide internal stability, and ignores the broader social and cultural context in which the family itself exists.

A feminist view of the role of the symptom in stabilizing the system would consider the impact of gender when formulating interventions. The paradoxical prescription of the symptom often lends itself to mother-blaming—for example, "If Johnny were to leave home, mother would be lonely, since father is away at work." Although father's distancing is included in this formulation, the implication is that mother's holding on to her son is the primary problem. It is not that it is intrinsically harmful to prescribe a symptom, but that the therapist's wording of the prescription itself should not reinforce a negative view of the mother's role or behavior.

Phase III: Devising Feminist Interventions

Phase III is the current and ongoing phase of our work—the revision and adaptation of conventional systemic interventions to take gender into account.

This is the most challenging phase since it involves creating guidelines for putting our feminist perspective into clinical practice. What follows is meant to be only a beginning and certainly does not cover all of the possibilities. The process of self-examination entailed in looking so critically at one's own work, as well as that of esteemed colleagues, is painful and difficult. It is easier to recognize errors than to develop new techniques. We are sure that other examples and interventions will occur to you.

The work of this phase focuses on: (1) articulating feminist formulations and techniques, and (2) suggesting feminist adaptations and revisions of traditional interventions. Please keep in mind that we are not formulating a new method, but rather presenting an outline of clinical guidelines informed by the feminist perspective in which gender is an organizing principle. The basis of a feminist intervention is a feminist conceptualization of the problem.

Toward a Feminist Family Therapy: Some Guidelines

(1) *Identification of the gender message and social constructs that condition behavior and sex roles.*

Gender themes are not merely "content," which may or may not be problematic in a given family. Rather, gender is seen as an essential wellspring of all behavior, and one of the chief connecting links between a culture and its members. We demonstrate this in four different methodologies, unbraiding the gender issues from the more abstract systems theories that we use as the basis of our work, identifying common abuses and oversights regarding gender, and then re-braiding an appreciation of gender into the work, with interventions that address gender, explicitly and implicitly.

(2) *Recognition of the real limitations of female access to social and economic resources.*

Women's actual limited social and economic options and socially mandated shame are always factors in her handling of situations. For example, a woman may stay with or return to an abusing husband because, economically, she may not have other options. A mother may deny knowledge of father-daughter or sibling incest because of the shameful consequences of disclosure for herself and her family. A woman may keep a rape secret rather than subject herself to the humiliation that comes with public disclosure. Or a woman may remain in an unsatisfactory marriage because her options outside of the marriage, emotionally and financially, are so limited. A therapist who understands the position of women in such situations will refrain from "blaming the victim" for causing or staying in them, and will not push women precipitously into actions that would leave them alone and unsupported.

In situations of incest and other violence, systemic formulations that do not take these factors into account lend themselves to a "blaming of the victim" by the presumption of neutrality.

Every ethical therapist must ask her- or himself how it is possible to conduct therapy with a divorcing woman without addressing the fact that her income may well plunge to poverty level. She may have difficulty in actually collecting whatever child-support payments she is granted. She will certainly not be awarded half of the couple's actual assets, and she may well lose her children if she angers her husband to the point where he goes to court to request custody of them.

(3) *An awareness of sexist thinking that constricts the options of women to direct their own lives.*

Sexist thinking, which is pervasive in families and in family therapy, embodies ideas such as: the belief that women need men to support, direct, and validate them; the denial of women's right to control over their own bodies; the belief that women are illogical and overly emotional, and that competent and self-determined behavior is unattractive and "unfeminine."

These are universal beliefs that shape individual consciousness and self-definition. The consciousness and identity of women, regardless of race, class, or individual differences, is conditioned by such attitudes and circumstances. This frame of reference will enable therapists to connect the behaviors of women to experiences and conditions outside of the family, where their behaviors can be seen as less pathological.

The differences between the way in which men and women have been socialized to experience danger in attachment and autonomy is graphically illustrated in a study of college students done by Pollack and Gilligan (1982). The students were asked to respond to images and stories of violence that appeared on a Thematic Apperception Test. Men experienced danger as arising from close personal affiliations more than from the struggle for achievement and success. Women, on the other hand, perceived danger in impersonal, achievement situations such as competition in the world of work. Men described danger in terms of intimacy, entrapment, and betrayal—being caught in a smothering relationship or humiliated by rejection and deceit. Women saw danger in isolation and alienation—being deprived of personal relationships or set apart by success. The authors concluded that men experience danger in connection and women experience danger in separation. This socially generated dichotomy lays the groundwork for the many complex problems that arise in male-female relationships.

(4) *Acknowledgment that women have been socialized to assume primary responsibility for family relationships.*

It is not unusual to expect a woman to facilitate the relationships in a family. The expectation, indeed the demand, that she do so may be covert. That she complies to the extent that she does is then often seen as her pathological need to serve, or control, or to remain central. It is not surprising, then, that when things are not going well she will try harder to make things "right," and will accept blame for whatever goes wrong.

(5) *Recognition of the dilemmas and conflicts of childbearing and child rearing in our society.*

Becoming a mother immediately sets up conflict for women between the responsibilities of child rearing, for which they are assigned primary responsibility and any other activities women may choose or need to perform, such as working, having a career, travel, social events, or creative avocations. Therapists need to take this unavoidable role conflict and overload into account when assessing a mother's functioning with her children.

(6) *An awareness of patterns that split the women in families as they seek to acquire power through relationships with men.*

In a male-dominated society a woman's power is derivative, and she must affiliate with men in order to acquire it. Common patterns that emerge in families as women seek to achieve this aim include the following: (1) Women detour conflict away from men either because it's too dangerous to confront them directly, or in order to protect men. (2) Women in families compete with each other for the "best" way to maintain emotional well-being in the family, since this is designated as their primary province. (3) Since women are acculturated to move *toward* emotional problems and not away from them, the legendary conflict between mother and daughter and stepmother and stepdaughter, wife and mother-in-law, and even much of the tension between sisters, can be understood in this way.

(7) *Affirmation of values and behaviors characteristic of women, such as connectedness, nurturing, and emotionality.*
While in our society intimacy and attachment are considered positive aspects of personal relationships, at the same time our culture bombards us with other messages that contradict this view, and therapists often characterize these attachment traits in terms such as "intrusive," "controlling," "overinvolved," or "hysterical."

(8) *Recognition and support for possibilities for women outside of marriage and the family.*
Some therapists believe that there is something wrong with a woman if she has not been able to form a satisfactory relationship with a man, and will proceed to analyze her "fear of commitment," examine her "unreal expectations," explore the origins of her "hostility toward men," or probe her "problem with intimacy." This conveys to the woman that once she overcomes her "neurotic problem" she will find a suitable man and live happily ever after, and that this is properly her major goal.
Women need to maintain a network of relationships in which they feel useful and appreciated. Whether the form that such a network takes is conventional or experimental is of little importance. A woman's relational skills can flourish in the workplace, the family, or in any type of friendly or romantic relationship.

(9) *Recognition of the basic principle that no intervention is gender-free and that every intervention will have a different and special meaning for each sex.*
There must be commitment to the principle that therapy is a political act and cannot be separated from the social issues in which the family is embedded.

Conclusion

The essence of feminist clinical work lies in the therapist's attitudes toward gender and her or his sensitivity to the differential impact of all interventions. The changes wrought in our work from "thinking gender" have been profound. This is the edge that cuts across all methodology and schools and is adaptable within a broad range of clinical and theoretical frameworks. Of course, a feminist approach does not include lecturing, scolding, blaming, haranguing, or proselytizing.

Good clinical work must include a recognition of the central fact of a client's gender socialization. Surely, as you read our clinical cases, you will spot feminist interventions that we have failed to list here, or sexist interventions that we weren't aware of. We hope our guidelines will be helpful as you put your own clinical work under scrutiny and begin to formulate your own guidelines.

Marianne Walters
Betty Carter
Peggy Papp
Olga Silverstein

part two

Family Relationships

2

Marianne Walters

Mothers and Daughters

**To my daughters, Lisa, Pamela, and Suzanna, with whom
I shared my life when they were growing up and who,
now that they have wonderfully achieved their own
adulthood, so generously share their lives with me.**

> *We are together my child and I, sisters really, against
> whatever denies us all that we are . . ."*
> Alice Walker

THE PATHWAYS OF a woman's life are mirrored in the mother-
daughter relationship. Coming together in the familiar processes of
giving birth, raising the children, nurturing the family, and caring for
the aged, mothers and daughters are "intimate partners" within the
confines of their shared private life. The knowing that a mother has in
being parent to her daughter is deeply personal, embedded in an
awareness of what is necessary for both of them in order to be able to
care for others and to be taken care of. It is a knowing from within,
based not so much on the explicit as on the implicit, on that which is
experienced, and on learning that is inductive and intuitive.

The Bonds of Intimacy and Familiarity

Mothers and daughters share a world of the everyday and the familiar.
And they are bound together in the function of producing and nurturing the next generation. They are expected to provide continuity between the families within which they reside; to bridge the formation of

the new family to the families of origin from which it emerged. Daughters are expected to seek a mate and then to perform family functions and services as their mothers before them have done, thus binding the new family to the old. Mothers are expected to care for the young and daughters to look after the aged, and both to expect that from each other. Mothers may worship their sons, but they depend on their daughters for personal and familial needs. The familial parameters of the mother-daughter relationship renders it crucial to generational continuity and to the transmission of the values, morals, and mores of the prevailing culture from generation to generation.

If mother is the cornerstone of family life, the mother-daughter relationship is the brick and mortar that holds it together. The "everyday" aspects of family life—its routines and rituals, household chores and housekeeping tasks, shopping for and preparing the meals, doctor's appointments and health care, vacations and social calendars, buying clothes and maintaining appearances—encircle the relationship of mothers and their daughters. While boys are *assigned* household tasks, mothers will *include* their daughters in household and homemaking activities, and will expect them to begin to know what needs doing. So when sons leave their clothes about the house it is annoying, maybe even infuriating to their mothers—but then "boys will be boys." When daughters leave their clothes about, it is also annoying and even infuriating, but it will be assigned more meaning, as an act *between* them. When a son can't learn to boil an egg, his mother will reassure herself that he will eventually get himself a wife to boil his eggs! When a daughter can't learn to boil an egg, mother will be fearful that her daughter lacks those skills she needs to get a husband and to take care of him properly.

The bonds of shared responsibility for family life are strong indeed. They create a special kind of attachment built on the intimacy of that which is private and personal. Childbirth and child rearing occupy a compelling emotional centrality in the lives of mothers and daughters, drawing them together around experiences that are difficult to articulate and that are understood in highly subjective ways. Over the centuries the most diverse cultures have mystified the experience of childbirth and of maternal love so that mothers have shared these experiences with their daughters in a world of half-light, shadowy and obscured by myth. Although contemporary social theorists have attempted to demystify the experiences of birth and maternity, Erich Fromm, writing in the late '50s and early '60s, and influencing a generation of mothers whose daughters are still reproducing, wrote: "Mother's love is bliss, is peace, it need not be acquired, it need not be deserved. . . . Mother is the home we come from, she is nature, soil, the ocean. . . . Motherly love . . . is unconditional affirmation of the child's life and his needs. . . . Mother love . . . makes the child feel it is good to have been born; it instills in the child the *love of life*, and not only the wish to remain alive . . . the happiness in being alive" (Fromm, 1956, pp. 33–41). What a legacy for mothers to leave their daughters!

Because society expects a mother to raise her daughter to, in turn, become a wife and mother, their relationship is largely defined within the confines and the life space of the intrafamilial. In contrast, raising a son is not primarily about raising a father nor even a husband, although this may be part of parental expectation. Rather, it is about raising a man, a worker, a person of public pursuit and individual achievement, an autonomous individual. Raising a daughter is primarily about relationships, caretaking, homemaking, attachments and affiliation, private and interpersonal achievements. Mothers are the family gatekeepers, responsible for the emotional well-being of the family and for protecting its members against the *psychic* dangers of the outside world. Fathers are responsible for the economic well being of the family and for protecting it against the *physical* dangers of the outside world. So mother's job is to affiliate their daughters with intrafamilial life and to affiliate their sons with the extrafamilial.

Thus, the relationship between mothers and daughters is often conceptualized within a context that is distinct and separate from the larger world outside of the family, indeed even viewed as not functional within that larger world. Furthermore, since the activities of private and family life are artificially separated from the extrafamilial, or public life, they are often treated and defined as trivial and subordinate, rather than as integral to the dominant and more "significant" activities of the society at large. From this perspective, the mother-daughter relationship can be understood as one constructed in contradiction. It is powerful because it is so intensely personal and yet vulnerable precisely because it lacks definition outside of the immediately personal and familial. It is framed in activities that are subordinate to the activities of men and their broader social and economic domain. What makes it so powerful and rich also renders it vulnerable to the vicissitudes of a patriarchal value system.

Carroll Smith-Rosenberg, a historian, studied the diaries and letters of women, including mothers and daughters, from 35 families during a period ranging from the 1760s to the 1880s. She found in these letters between women a "female world," separate from the world of male concerns, a world in which women were of primary importance in each other's lives. She describes "an intimate mother-daughter relationship . . . at the heart of this female world" and a "clear apprenticeship system" within the family where daughters learned from their mothers the domestic arts and child-rearing practices. "Daughters were born into a female world. . . . As long as the mother's domestic role remained relatively stable . . . daughters tended to accept their mother's world and to turn automatically to other women for support mother's world and to turn automatically to other women for support and intimacy." Smith-Rosenberg notes "the absence of that mother-daughter hostility today considered almost inevitable to an adolescent's struggle for autonomy" and suggests that "it is possible that taboos against female aggression . . . were sufficiently strong to repress even that between mothers and their adolescent daughters. Yet these letters seem so alive, and the interest of daughters in their mother's affairs so vital and genuine, that it is difficult to interpret their closeness exclusively in terms of repression and denial" (1975, pp. 1-29).

The confluence of the growing absence of this female world after the turn of the century and the early efforts of women to liberate themselves during the 1920s and early 1930s led to a weakening of that earlier mother-daughter tie. With the advent of Freud and the psychologizing that followed, the bonding of women, according to Adrienne Rich (1977), could "be tolerated between schoolgirls as 'crushes,' but were regarded as regressive and neurotic if they persisted into later life" (p. 237). This carried, of course, a particular "truth" for mothers and daughters. As Rich writes: "Before sisterhood, there was the knowledge—transitory, fragmented, perhaps, but original and crucial—of mother-and-daughterhood. This cathexis between mother and daughter—essential, distorted, misused—is the great unwritten story. . . . The materials are here for the deepest mutuality and the most painful estrangement" (p. 226).

The Binds of Intimacy and Familiarity

Mother-daughter relationships are endangered in the world beyond the family by the very familiarity and intimacy that characterize them within the family. This is a disturbing contradiction. Although in our society intimacy, familiarity, and attachment are considered positive aspects of personal relationships, our culture bombards us simultaneously with other messages about these interpersonal characteristics. We learn that "familiarity breeds contempt," that social status is built not on human but on economic achievement, that power is based on hierarchy rather than mutuality, that intimacy is associated with sexuality, not necessarily attachment, and that autonomy is equated with separation from the family, most particularly from the mother. To be "tied to mother's apron strings" is to be infantilized, unable to function independently in the outside world. Yet a daughter will some day need to wear that "apron."

As these contradictory messages and value systems are internalized by mothers and daughters, they inevitably engender conflict within and between mothers and daughters. Both the conscious and people, are constructed and framed by the messages we encounter in the cultural and social context within which we live. In our culture women are regarded and portrayed largely in terms of their relation to men, not to each other. From Miss to Mrs., from shoemaker's daughter to doctor's wife, women are identified with the men in (or *not* in) their lives. Spinster has a different ring to it than bachelor. It doesn't conjure up images of an "about town" life-style, or even of personal choice; instead it evokes images of rejection and a constricted life. When a daughter marries, it is her father who accompanies her "down the aisle" and "gives her away" to another man who promises to take care of her. And during this crucial ceremony of transition, her mother (quite literally) stands aside. Typically, the daughter will assume her husband's name (although the women's movement has made it possible for women to choose to keep their "maiden" name or combine it with their mate's surname). But the daughter's title will change from Miss to Mrs., both of which identify her connection to a man; the man continues to be called Mr., whether he is attached or unattached to a woman. Such social structures, institutionalized expectations and messages, multiplied tenfold, as profoundly condition the way mothers and their daughters experience each other as their particular psychological makeup and personal life circumstances.

Indeed, the very concept of the individual self for women is a recent development and still on the drawing boards. Those identified as leaders, authorities, providers, heroes, and even achievers are ascribed primarily male characteristics. Relationships, social roles, and individual behavior are gender-defined, with *primary* significance being assigned to the extrafamilial, the work domain and the public sphere of activities and functions associated with men. Women are considered significant basically in terms of their roles as wife and mother within the private, inner, and *secondary* world of the family. While social and psychological norms render family life crucial and central to the emotional well-being, and individual achievement, of its members, at the same time such norms suggest the family has a destructive potential to diminish the personal effectiveness of those members who remain too close to it. What a bind for mothers who must prepare their daughters for family functioning; and for daughters, who must break away if they are to achieve a self beyond the family.

As women are entering the world of work and public purpose in ever increasing numbers, they are continuing to search for definitions and images of the individual, autonomous self that include and encompass intimacy and familiarity, caretaking and family. Unfortunately, even within the women's movement this search for an identity that is both expressive and instrumental has sometimes engendered increased tension between the generations, and rejection of family-identified women/mothers by their daughters. This is not surprising in a society where the relationship of mothers and daughters simply does not pay off in the marketplace. Autonomy and occupation are the milestones of adult life and they are accessed through the father. Fathers entitle; mothers entwine. If daughters remain too closely identified with their mothers they run the risk of being labeled undifferentiated and dependent. As long as power rests with father, daughters will, at some level, be angry with their mothers for not possessing it. And, conversely, mothers who experience themselves as not possessing power in their own lives will be threatened by their daughter's attempts to achieve it. Few daughters would be willing to lay claim to themselves as individuated, self-determined individuals without having gone through the ritual of liberating themselves from mother bondage. And very few daughters who have achieved success or power outside of the family would attribute it to their mothers.

The feminist movement and feminist writings have changed this state of affairs somewhat. More contemporary daughters, conscious of women's issues and the need for more positive female images, are seeking to identify with their mothers in more mutually affirming ways; to explore their mother's lives in the effort to find positive meaning there for their own lives. But we still have no mother-daughter equivalent of being "a chip off the old block" and of "following in his father's footsteps," with the meaning these metaphors convey of the value and personal potential in being identified with the same-sex parent. Fathers and their sons bond in the outside world as well as within the family. Popular images of father and son running the farm together, father handing the business over to the son, or son carrying on the father's political crusade as his enemies close in on him, all support and encourage such identification. Mother-daughter bonding, still primarily rooted in the intrafamilial and obscured by social contradictions and dichotomous messages, is rendered redundant in the world of power and privilege outside the family.

Small wonder then that the very familiarity, the intimacy, the special knowing that a mother feels for her daughter is so often tinged with regrets and a sense of "less than." Harvard psychologist Carol Gilligan (1982) has written about the significance of attachment and intimacy in the human life cycle:

> The elusive mystery of woman's development is in its recognition of the continuing importance of attachment in the human life cycle. Woman's place in man's life cycle is to protect this recognition while the developmental litany intones the celebration of separation, autonomy, individuation and natural rights. . . . The life cycle itself arises from an alternation between the world of women and that of men. Only when life cycle theorists divide their attention and begin to live with women as they have lived

with men will their vision encompass the experience of both sexes and their theories become correspondingly more fertile. . . . When assertion no longer seems dangerous, the concept of relationships changes from a bond of continuing dependence to a dynamic of continuing interdependence. (p. 23)

Mother Blaming

The psychology of the mother-daughter relationship is framed, described, and explained in the prevailing terms of male-identified analytic, psychosocial, or systemic theories, where "mother bashing" has been a popular sport for years! Only the code words within each theoretical framework differ—hysterical, overinvolved, enmeshed, intrusive, clutching, clinging, dependent, needy, smothering, selfless, selfish, covert, overemotional, unreasonable, and so on and on. While mother is reified, mystified, and idealized she is, at the same time, blamed for any emotional ills that may befall her children. She can never do enough for her children and is always in danger of doing too much. The myth of the perfect mother and the myth of the demon mother are forever competing with one another. Mother may be placed on a pedestal, but her feet are leaden with clay.

Too much mother love can lead to symbiosis, too little to maternal deprivation. In fact, the idealized mother and the demonized mother are two sides of the same coin. Both concepts mystify motherhood; both concepts are dehumanizing and as such serve to hinder mothers from taking charge of their own maternity. Neither idols nor demons are real, or accessible, or able to possess and construct their own reality. Such images are larger than life; they cast shadows that no human form can fit. Both the idealization and the demonization of mothers keeps them in a place where failure is assured.

In a study conducted in 1985, the researchers Caplan and Hall-McCorquodale noted that "the authors of the 125 articles read for this study attributed to mothers a total of 72 different kinds of psychopathology" (pp. 345–353). Mother blaming can be quite explicit, or it can come in a variety of implicit forms, which become part of the culture of our profession. It can appear quite "innocently" in our language, our humor, what we choose to emphasize or make significant, what we value, our attitudes, the way we describe things, our metaphors and messages, our behavior with clients, or who we choose to move for change. Further, mother blaming can unconsciously become part of our conceptual and intellectual tradition. Unless we consciously struggle to identify and reject mother-blaming ideas and attitudes, they will become internalized as part of our repertoire of professional beliefs and behaviors, as surely as they are internalized by every mother's daughter.

And therein lies the dilemma. If mothers are blamed by the "experts" for the emotional and psychological problems of their children, can daughters be far behind? How is it possible for daughters to escape blaming their mothers for whatever goes wrong in their lives when this view is supported by popular cultural images, and codified by social and psychological theorists? Denied a system of support for positive identification with the same-sex parent, daughters will be inducted into a socially constructed continuum of generational struggle and conflict with their mothers. This hardly seems auspicious for the mental health of either mothers or daughters.

Perhaps not since *The Generation of Vipers* (1955) has mother blaming been so elegantly expressed or more persuasively argued in pseudopsychological terms than in Nancy Friday's book *My Mother, Myself* (1977). In this best-selling book (more than 3 million copies in print), mother blaming is treated as psychological truth. Friday's analysis, descriptions, and narrative are characterized by such statements as: "Unless we have separated from mother long before marriage, it is almost impossible to set up a healthy relationship with a man" (p.69); or "How father responds to his daughter's adolescence can determine which way we go: *toward men and our own identity*, or back to mother and the symbiotic tie" (*italics mine*) (p. 169); or (quoting Dr. Shaefer) "Woman's *desire* to subordinate themselves to the man is the pattern of dependency learned from the mother" (*italics mine*) (p. 345); or "Mothers raise their daughters as fools because they believe in the divinity of innocence. Sexually, all mothers are Catholics. They pray for their daughter's innocence while simultaneously praying for a man for their untutored unblemished daughters" (p. 286). (No wonder Jewish mothers weren't thrilled about this book!); or "No two people have such an opportunity for support and identification, and yet no human relationship is so mutually limiting" (p. 40). This book, which Friday incongruously dedicated to her mother, is infused with a belief system that assumes a dangerously incapacitating effect of mothers on their daughters—sexually infantilizing while covertly competitive; restraining and overprotective; denying the self and constricting autonomous behavior. Dependence, sexual dysfunction, ambivalence about men, fear of success, envy, anger, and every other conceivable torment that can befall a woman flows from mother to daughter. (Only the last four pages offer a glimpse of some positive mother images). If they are to escape the debilitating effect of "symbiotic" bonding, Friday asserts, daughters must devote themselves to "separation" from their mothers (of course, while pursuing a man).

Like so many others before and since, Friday strongly criticizes mothers for behaving in the ways, and performing those tasks, that society has mandated. Friday analyzes the mother-daughter relationship in patriarchal terms; her value system is male-identified. In the process, Friday grossly overstates the case; wishing for the perfect mother, she finds her wanting and ends up demonizing her—not unlike her predecessor, Philip Wylie. She makes the common error of those social and psychological theorists who take the conceptual leap from mother as the primary source of all infantile gratification to mother as the primary source of all developmental trauma; from the notion of infantile bonding to that of adult bondage; from ideas of attachment to the loss of autonomy. These are the terms of a belief system and an epistomology that perpetuates a legacy of struggle and conflict for mothers and daughters.

I am concerned that Friday's book is considered a "woman's" book, avidly read during the last decade by young women who were searching for a new sense of identity. What a paradox for womankind that these daughters need to deny their mothers in order to affirm themselves. Or perhaps this is not so paradoxical; perhaps it is yet another example of the pervasive influence of patriarchal thinking on all of us. It is, of course, terribly difficult not to identify with the source of power, with dominant social values and themes, even though they may be, at some level, oppressive. We have seen examples of this throughout history.

Double Binds

Family therapy and systems thinking have not escaped the fallout from these paradigms. Although in systems theory the family is viewed not as a composite of discrete individuals but as a set of relations rooted in patterns and feedback loops of mutual expectation, in practice it is impossible not to assign names to those discrete individuals whose set of relations form patterns and feedback loops. And these names have a set of gender expectations, roles, values and attitudes attached to them: wife, mother, father, husband, sister, brother, mother-in-law, father-in-law, grandfather, grandmother, and so on. Thus, for instance, when Bateson (1972) elaborated the family pattern (double-bind) within which schizophrenia is most likely to occur, he distinguished three traits of the schizophrenic family system as follows (p. 212, *italics mine*):

1. A child whose *mother* becomes anxious and withdraws if the child responds to her as a loving *mother*.
2. A *mother* who cannot accept her own feelings of anxiety and hostility toward her child and who denies them by overtly expressing love to persuade the child to respond to her as a loving *mother*, and to withdraw from him if he does not.
3. An absence of anyone (father, sibling) in the family, such as a strong and insightful father, who can intervene, between the *mother* and the child in the relationship.

Is it possible to read this description of the double-bind pattern and continue to think in some unbiased, neutral fashion about family patterns or "a set of relations"?

While much has been said of the double bind with which mothers engage their children, little attention has been paid to the double binds that few mothers can escape in relating to and rearing their daughters. Mothers must pledge their allegiance either to the dogma of selflessness or of selfishness, to the ideology of accommodation and subordination or to the ambivalence of self-assertion and self-definition.

The knowledge a mother has about what is expected of women, about what is socially acceptable, and about the implicit rules that govern the life of women in a male-centered world cannot help but distort many of the messages imparted to her daughter. How does a mother encourage autonomy in her daughter when such behavior could jeopardize her ultimate security? How are mothers to say "be sure" when they themselves are warned to "never let him know you can do it better"? Dorothy Parker's axiom that "men don't make passes at girls who wear glasses" spoke to a generation of women of the dilemma in growing up female: women who think don't attract men. A recent *Newsweek* article described the power of a president's wife as the "warm embrace, cold stare, or worried brow" with which she can "affect her husband's mind or mood"! And where was she supposed to have left *her* mind?

So mothers raising daughters do so within a set of socially constructed double binds. A mother wants her daughter to be able to define her own needs as an adult, independent self, but she will be plagued by doubts, knowing that it is not wise for her daughter to become too autonomous, and that she must learn dependent ways. A mother wants her daughter to be forthright, open, and honest, yet knows that she must learn to practice artifice, coyness, and mild deception. She wants her to be able to manage for herself, but not too well; to have a career or work, but not to achieve too much; to be her own person and yet to allow herself to be owned. She wants to build her daughter's self-confidence, but still wants her to be aware of the need to attract; she wants her to be able to speak for herself—but not too loudly; to care for herself—but first for others; to be able to nurture, but selflessly. She should have a positive self-image, but must learn to use it to reflect others. She wants her daughter to be assertive, but to know how to hide her assertiveness. She may admire the developing mind of her daughter, but wants to make sure her intelligence will not threaten prospective mates. She should be a good student, but not the best. She can be athletic, but not too competitive. A daughter should be private and discreet, but popular and sought after. She should dress properly, but be seductive. She must learn to care for her appearance but never appear too made up. And she must learn how to covertly seek the mate by whom she wishes to be sought.

Mother/Woman

Perhaps the penultimate double bind encapsulating the mother-daughter relationship is the age-old dichotomy between "woman" and "mother." When Friday wrote of "acting like a woman instead of a mother," she was voicing, in one simple sentence, all the ingrained attitudes, stereotypes and biases that presume a split, and distinction, between the person of mother and the person of woman. Mother is not a woman, she is MOTHER. The images of mother are universal. Woman, however, comes in a variety of individual shapes and sizes, not necessarily determined by her intrafamilial functioning. One is the image of the nurturer and caretaker; the other is of the sexual and self-directed person.

The mother-woman dichotomy is most explicitly evident and especially debilitating to women in the area of their sexuality. From the ideal of immaculate conception and the virgin mother, on the one hand, to sexual woman as tramp or vamp (taken from the word *vampire*, meaning bloodsucking), on the other, images of sexual woman have been divorced from those of mother. Seldom do we encounter in literature, film, or the popular media, mothers whose sexuality is explored and treated as part of the womanness they bring into motherhood. And when mothers do present themselves as sexual to their daughters, it is usually to advise them on how to protect themselves, rather than on how to be self-directed and achieve satisfaction in their sex lives. Within this context, mothers can be seen to deny their own sexuality and constrain that of their daughters in order to prepare them properly for motherhood. Mothers fear that to empower their daughters sexually, they may endanger their maternity.

There is no clear way in which a mother can be a fully sexual person to her daughter. A mother may teach her daughter that sex is good and pleasurable, a natural extension of love and relationship. She can talk to her of enjoying sex, of the sharing and the passion to be experienced in fulfilling her sexuality. But this must always be tinged with caution and prohibition. Not to caution her daughter would constitute gross neglect as a parent. She needs to caution her daughter about the sometimes devastating consequences of pregnancy outside of marriage. She must advise her on what to do if a man accosts her on the street. She needs to find a way to tell her about the fact that many women are raped; and if this is too painful to discuss with her daughter, she will need to contend with feeling anxious about not having brought it up. She must counsel her on how to conduct herself if a man exposes himself to her on the street, or if a man tries to "pick her up," or if men make sexual remarks about her as she's walking to school. If her daughter is buxom, or particularly pretty, she will have to teach her how to deal with the "cat-calls" and sexual innuendos from the guys lounging in front of the drug store, or the construction workers on the new building site. These are all experiences shared by mothers and daughters as sexual women.

Small wonder that a mother's messages to her daughter about sex are mixed. Empowering her daughter sexually can be dangerous; cautioning her will be inhibiting. Protectiveness will be viewed as repression, permissiveness as irresponsible. For the daughter, taking charge of her own sexuality is too aggressive; being cautious and careful, too submissive. A mother may resort to teaching her daughter how to use sex to manipulate and feign power. She may prohibit overt sexual behavior while covertly encouraging her to be seductive. She may warn her daughter about promiscuity while secretly admiring—even envying—her ability to attract men. Whichever way she goes, the message will be, must be, mixed. The trick will be to get the mix just right.

By contrast, fathers can own their sexuality and openly encourage their son's sexuality. Father can talk freely of his sexual exploits (albeit premarital) and even advise his son to "sow wild oats" before being tied down in marital bliss. Mother, on the other hand, cannot own her premarital exploits since she is presumed to have been a virgin before submitting to her marital vows. And it is difficult to encourage her daughter's sexuality when at the same time she is fearful that she may become pregnant outside of marriage. It is a very different matter to warn your son against getting a girl pregnant and warning your daughter not to allow herself to become pregnant. The latter sets up a cautionary, protective, vulnerable edge to any sexual discourse between mothers and their daughters.

It seems strange to me that a mother's caution, conflict, and ambivalence about empowering her daughter sexually has been understood almost exclusively as the mother's "problem"—the expression of her own sexual negation and repression, her sexual "lack" inflicted on her daughter. For not only is a mother caught in the cultural dichotomy of woman/mother, and the biological bind of the unwanted pregnancy, she is witness to the real dangers that all women face in a world where sexual violence continues to be a reality. A mother does not have to have been raped or sexually harrassed to know that these are realities that threaten the safety of her daughter. These realities become part of the consciousness mothers have in raising their daughters. To be other than anxious about her daughter's sexuality would seem to constitute poor reality testing. And if she is anxious, protective, and restraining of her daughter's sexuality, there will surely be repercussions for her own sense of sexual viability and power.

And so the dysfunctional cycle of struggle and conflict between them is constructed: mother *must* restrain and caution her daughter about her sexuality and in the process will herself feel constricted in the presentation of her sexual self. Daughter will resent her mother's constraints and will become critical of her. Mother will feel less sure, less in control, and thus more anxious; mother's "message" to her daughter will become more "mixed." Daughter will begin to blame her mother for any sexual problems she experiences. Mother will feel guilty and defensive. Now daughter will see the only pathway to her own sexuality in the rejection of the mother's sexual "inadequacy" and "inhibition." Mother will stand blamed for repressing her daughter's sexuality. And all of this is supported by a culture that is ambivalent about female sexuality, and within which mother and woman are not yet seen as an integrated whole.

Reasonable Emotions

Such dichotomies and contradictions obscure the relationship of mothers and daughters as surely as their shared familial functioning shapes it. In Western intellectual tradition the split between reason and emotion, the polarizing of intuitive and analytic modes of thought, is yet another way in which women, and their relationships with each other, are compromised. For example, the knowing that springs from involvement, from the familiarity of shared experience, from intimacy and the intuitive sense of connections, is not, in our society, assigned significance as a tool of intellectual pursuit or cognitive experience. Instead it is put in the back pocket of "emotional" thinking, which translated means thinking that is clouded by our feelings, by induction, by too much proximity to our subject. Emotional or intuitive thought is considered the antithesis of the objective, scientific, and rational. It is also "less than." The former is biased, ambiguous, unstructured, amorphous—and associated with the feminine. The latter is neutral, disciplined, structured, substantive—and associated with the masculine. In this context the entire sphere of knowledge that derives from subjective experience, including maternal sensibility, is devalued. Such knowing is discredited when measured against the tough, pragmatic requirements of the "real world," the "marketplace" of economic, intellectual, or public pursuits. This polarization creates a conflictual and ambivalent environment for mothers who will need to deny their (devalued) intuition in order to confirm their (valued) rationality.

Intuition and analysis, reason and emotion commingle in most interpersonal interactions. In defining these modalities as separate and distinct, as better or worse, as more or less significant, as primary or secondary, we end up with a consciousness that negates the emotional and affirms the analytic. And when these polarities are then assigned a gender—as in the emotional woman and the rational man—the prospect for our achieving an unbiased view of our clients is certainly dimmed. I think we need to be cautious about the "objectification" of our "subjects" by any systemic interpretation, intervention, strategy, or maneuver that, however subtly, suggests this bias. Suffice it to say that in the world of therapy the emotional gets treated; the rational gets discussed!

Jerome Bruner in *The Process of Education* (1960) has this to say about intuitive as compared to analytic thinking:

> Intuition implies the act of grasping the meaning, significance, or structure of a problem or situation without explicit reliance on the analytic apparatus of one's craft. . . . The intuitive mode . . . yields hypothesis quickly . . . hits on combinations of ideas before their worth is known. . . . Intuition by itself yields a tentative ordering of a body of knowledge [that] aids principally by giving us a basis for moving ahead in our testing of reality. . . . In contrast to analytic thinking, intuitive thinking characteristically does not advance in careful, well-defined steps . . . it tends to [be] . . . based . . . on an implicit perception of the total problem. . . . Intuitive thinking rests on familiarity with the domain of knowledge involved, and with its structure. . . . The complimentary nature of intuitive and analytic thinking should . . . be recognized. Through intuitive thinking the individual may often arrive at a solution to problems which he would not achieve at all, or at best more slowly, through analytic thinking. . . . The formalism of school learning has somehow devalued intuition. . . . It may be of the first importance to establish an intuitive understanding of materials before we expose [children] to more traditional and formal modes. (pp. 58-60)

Bruner does not dichotomize emotion and reason, the intuitive and the analytic, but contrasts them in order to arrive at a cognitive synthesis. He describes the effectiveness of intuitive thinking as resting on familiarity with the subject, a sense of the connectedness of things, and the development of the self-confidence needed to take a conceptual leap with a limited set of cues. This seems to me a notion of major significance for family therapy. If we are to avoid implicitly devaluing women, we need to explicitly validate intuitive thought, and emotional reason, by incorporating these cognitive processes in our work and in our intellectual traditions. Yet family therapy seems to be moving more toward the formalism of formulas, the construction of opposites, the mediated rather than the immediate, the task rather than the process, the directive rather than the interactional. Surely we must understand that reason and emotion, intuition and analytic thinking, the creative leap and logical progression are *not* dichotomous ways of perceiving and exploring our world. There can be no reason without emotion, or emotion without reason. They inform each other. Intuition advances analysis and analysis enhances the intuitive. The creative leap furthers the pursuit of logic and logic creates a context in which the creative leap can occur. To dichotomize these modes of being and of understanding, to assign primary and secondary significance to one modality as opposed to the other, in our gender-defined society will lead to a referencing that devalues women and their relationships.

A Feminist Reframing

My thesis throughout this discussion has been, clearly, that in dichotomizing, and then prioritizing, the values assigned to the intra- and extrafamilial, to reason and emotion, mother and woman, attachment and autonomy, public and private, work and family, the epistemology of patriarchy has inhibited the realization of the creative power and energy in the intimate, personal, and familial connectedness of mothers and daughters. The conflict mothers and daughters may experience living in a male-dominant society has been turned inward, locking them in struggle with each other, blaming each other for whatever goes wrong in their lives. This struggle has become part of their legacy, an ongoing prophecy to be fulfilled. Of course, I don't think this is an accident. If women were to be realized and powerful through each other rather than through their association with or entitlement by men, the very foundation of the system of patriarchy would be challenged. If women were to experience validation through identification with their commonality, their personal self-esteem would be less contingent. And if women were to become more conscious of their collective experience, they would be less vulnerable to the messages that keep them subordinate.

The mother-daughter conflict we so often see in our offices is part of that process of women dividing in order to join more successfully with men. It is, in fact, the prototype of that kind of division. Many of the psychosexual theories of our profession, from Oedipal and Electra to overinvolved and smothering, have perpetuated the conflict between mothers and daughters. So it seems to me to be particularly important to revise our conceptualization of the mother-daughter relationship to include the social as well as the family context that structures it, and that predicts the inevitability of struggle and conflict. The conflict needs to be depathologized, the struggle reframed, and the relationship itself empowered.

References to gendered social messages by the therapist, where appropriate, can be used to validate, interpret, and/or reframe behaviors. Thus, I might connect an interaction between a mother and daughter to the way we're taught things should be: "Women learn early on that their job in the family is to smooth things out, so maybe talking for your daughter is a way to try to keep her and her dad from getting into a fight." Or I refer to popular images, myths, or fashions about mothers (wives, daughters, women): "Aren't all stepmothers wicked?"; "Aren't girls supposed to be overemotional?"; "Have you ever seen a TV soap where a strong, smart woman was *really* happy?" Or I will talk about the experiences of other mothers and daughters, including my own: "When my middle daughter was 14 she had a similar reaction, and I thought it would drive me crazy; now at 22 she sees things so differently." And I will universalize the particular: "What mother hasn't worried about her daughter dating?"; "What daughter hasn't felt, at times, that her mother doesn't trust her?" In addition, I will often explain my comments by explicitly referring to social conditioning: "Our society expects mothers to worry and then, unfortunately, sometimes penalizes them for doing so"; "Daughters hear that they can't grow up until they cut those apron strings, and unfortunately they think that also means cutting off the person wearing the apron." And so on. Such references are important because they highlight conditions and experiences that have been subsumed under the largely male-oriented and male-defined generalization of "human experience." As a result, the social and psychological experiences of women, of mothers and daughters, have been either neglected as the subject of investigation, have remained invisible, or have been interpreted within a masculine frame of reference.

Of course, making generalizations about women's experiences, or a collective consciousness, can be dangerous, leading to pejorative stereotypes (such as found in racial slurs), and we need to guard against this. And, of course, the specifics of such experience is as varied and as different as there are variations and differences among people and within racial, ethnic, and class divisions. Yet there are universal conditions that shape individual consciousness and self-definition. Ranging from the implicit message of the teacher who expects more intellectually from the boys than the girls in her class, to the explicit message contained in the fact that women college graduates, on the average, earn less than male high-school dropouts, the consciousness and identity of women, regardless of race, class, or individual differences, is conditioned by such attitudes and circumstances. This commonality is a frame of reference that can connect mothers and daughters not only to each other and to other women, but also to conditions and experiences outside of the family that, paradoxically, will render their intrafamilial issues and conficts less threatening. This is particularly true for a relationship so largely fashioned within the confines of the family.

Mothers and daughters learn early in their journey together that they should anticipate interpersonal conflict and pain in the injunctions to bond at birth and to "separate" when the daughter enters young adulthood. For mothers and their young daughters the relationship is less complicated by gender-defined mixed messages or the need to prepare daughters for feminized roles and functions. But when her daughter enters adolescence, the conflictual goals and messages the mother needs to transmit, in fact begin to undermine her own self-esteem at a crucial junction in her own life. When her daughter enters adolescence the mother is usually entering midlife—a time of evaluation and renewal, of regrets and possibilities. Self-assertion for the mother may mean risking loss emotionally, maritally, socially. Yet this is the very time she is required to be more assertive with her daughter. She needs to provide protection and direction at a time when she is questioning her own direction, and feels least protected. She needs to help her daughter, as well as herself, weigh the price of strength against the cost of dependence.

So at a time when a mother must appear most powerful, she is most vulnerable to her daughter's overt pressures to disengage as well as her covert messages to hold on and protect. The decreasing options for authority experienced by all parents as their children become young adults is thus compounded for mothers and their daughters as mothers begin to feel less in charge. Closeness with her daughter arouses fears of dependence on her already overloaded self. Moreover, failure or success in the function of mothering is being tested by the very person who must in turn by prepared to assume that function. Her daughter's moves for autonomy are experienced, and often labeled, as oppositional and critical, and a cycle of conflict is initiated. It is difficult to view, much less experience, the behavior of an adolescent or young adult daughter as ambivalent experimentation with personal power, judgment, and choice.

The perspective of a feminist therapist might suggest a framework that would enable mothers to view their daughters as they mature as not so much struggling to free themselves from the maternal bonds that constrict them, but rather moving toward a self-determined, powerful, autonomous position of their own. In this way the conflict could be viewed as the product of two people seeking alternative ways to bond at different life stages. By putting the picture in this frame we arrive at different implications, perceptions and psychological "truths." The young adult daughter is experiencing a new and frightening sense of her own power, a beginning trust in her own judgment and capacity to make choices; she is not simply being angry and oppositional. The adult mother is seeking new ground, a way to stay connected to her daughter without fear that their intimacy will burden either of them. They are both in the process of restructuring a relationship, not "splitting" from it; and in restructuring their relationship they will need to find ways to acknowledge their *sameness* in order to be comfortable with their differences. The daughter will need to know *more* about the context and content of her mother's life—not less; the mother will need to explore her own sources for knowing and understanding her daughter's developmental issues. The daughter seeks affirmation in the mirror of her mother, an image that will confirm her own. She is challenging her mother to be assertive and self-directed. The mother seeks validation of her success as mother especially from her daughter, who will share her life experience.

If therapists can free themselves of the mythology of separation as autonomy, and from their romance with law and order in the family, they can turn some of their attention to the business of providing mothers and daughters with alternative ways to attach. Mothers and adolescent daughters need to feel functional in relation to each other, not just in setting and abiding by family rules, or by letting go and leaving home, but by engaging in the ongoing process of exploring new means through which they can expand and enhance the quality of life for each other.

Two women writers have expressed, in one-liners, the two faces of mothering daughters: the poignancy of shared experiences tinged with a guilty belief that they are responsible for whatever happens to their daughters.

> What's come over our daughters that they don't like essence of violet anymore?
>
> Colette

> I don't know what I did but I know I did it . . .
> Marsha Norman, *'Night Mother*

Mothers and Daughters in Therapy

Underlying all of the following clinical examples of our work with mothers and daughters is the conviction that the quality of this relationship is central to the development of woman and so needs, in a variety of ways, to be validated and affirmed. Our mutual clinical purpose is one of eliciting and enhancing the positive power of the relationship as a counterpoint to the prevailing view of daughters caught in an endless struggle to escape from overinvolved, pathologizing mothers.

Yet none of us are Pollyannas and we are all well aware that some mothers can be destructive, others punitive, and still others sadly dependent on their daughters. Olga discusses the work of reconstructing a mother-daughter relationship that has become so oppressive and debilitating to the daughter that she had effected a complete cutoff and was devoting herself to a therapy of "separation." Her discussion illustrates the ways in which the larger belief system of the therapist interfaces with her methodology and her choice of interventions. Peggy describes her work with a mother and daughter whose relationship is constricted by unresolved marital issues. Directing her interventions initially toward empowering the mother—as a woman and wife as well as mother—she expands the field within which the mother and daughter can negotiate their interaction and improve their understanding of each other. She demonstrates interventions that enable the daughter to become part of the process of empowering her mother. And Betty's case features the story of a daughter who describes the generational triangles, and triangulated struggles, that have organized her own relationship with her mother, in a scenario that attaches us to familiar themes and images. The moves of the daughter to break the dysfunctional cycles that have blocked both mother and daughter from realizing the positive potential in their relationship are orchestrated in a therapy clearly designed to release that potential.

My case illustrates the particular crises of adolescence confronted in the evolving relationship between mothers and daughters. The crisis abounds in mixed messages for both mother and daughter, but like all crises presents a unique opportunity for change. The discussion covers the entire course of therapy, some seven or eight months, with excerpts from selected family sessions.

The frame of reference guiding my work with this family is presented in my discussion of a "feminist reframing." Throughout my work with the family, my interventions were directed toward restructuring the relationship between the mother and her two daughters by focusing on areas where attachment and positive communication could be successfully achieved. I was particularly intent on highlighting competent behaviors that occurred *within* the therapy sessions by turning them into experiences of competence that could be shared by mother and daughters. The transcripts illustrate my preferred style— the use of process during sessions in ways that provide immediacy, provoke thought, and encourage a sense of the familiar.

This was a family that defined itself as vulnerable and chaotic. And indeed the symptoms presented by the youngest daughter were severe, having required hospitalization just prior to beginning therapy with me. The mother presented herself as ineffectual, confused, and hopeless, and the anger, verbal abuse, and outright rejection experienced by mother and daughter seemed a formidable barrier to efforts at positive reframing. What was particularly helpful to me in working with the family was the larger gender context that I could use to interpret and depathologize their behaviors. It offered all of them a frame of reference outside of their family—a referencing to which they could attach and then return to the family fray with improved self-esteem.

cases

Marianne Walters

Caught in the Muddle

The Presenting Problem

A divorced woman in her late thirties came to see me with her two teenage daughters. Sally, the mother, is a nurse and loves her work, though her irregular hours make household planning and management difficult. Joan, her 14-year-old, had just come home from a 3-month stint in a residential treatment center. Betty, her 17-year-old, is finishing her last year of high school. Sally has had individual therapy; she and her ex-husband had been in couple therapy before their divorce; and she and the girls had been through family therapy sessions before and during Joan's hospitalization. The summer of Joan's entry into residential treatment was preceded by difficult, highly charged behavior that was traumatic for the whole family: Joan was expelled from school for drug abuse, academic failure, and truanting; she refused to conform to rules and limits at home; she constantly fought with mother, sister, and father; she was acting out sexually; and she was verbally abusive to her family and to school authorities. "Out of control, angry, low self-esteem, but very bright," wrote the therapists at the hospital.

Our first meeting lasted a couple of hours. Sally was wan and soft-spoken. She seemed to cower against the verbal onslaught from both girls. Betty, attractive, articulate, and emotional, sat between mother and Joan, interceding for each and attempting to orchestrate the proceedings. Joan, punk and pudgy, was clearly disapproving of everything, and lashed out fearlessly at everyone (including me), muttering a litany of profanity.

Sally, the mother, presented herself as the problem—an evaluation with which the whole family and several previous therapists agreed. My initial effort was to challenge this perspective and offer a new one. That proved to be no easy task, so organized was everyone (including Sally) around mother's failures.

The Initial Interview

SALLY: (*Talking softly, slowly, weighing her words*) Greg, my husband, had always been the disciplinarian. I guess I was the rescuer, in the middle, and I found it hard to have much authority over the children. I could never get it just right, so I vacillated a lot. We were married for 17 years. But even after the divorce, I remained in the same position—always pulled in different directions. When things are going fine at home, I can relax a little. But when we differ, all hell breaks loose . . . it goes berserk, out of control—we lock horns. (*The girls begin to giggle and make fun of mom's use of the expression "lock horns."*)

THERAPIST: I can see, Sally, that one thing your girls do is make you feel ill at ease about what you say, and the way you say it, as if you are being silly. In fact, I think they're uncomfortable here . . . which is natural; but they react by making fun of you. I wonder— maybe they just don't understand your metaphor. Joan, what do you think mom meant by "lock horns"? (*I say "your girls" deliberately throughout our session to emphasize connectedness between the girls and mom.*)

JOAN: How the fuck would I know?

THERAPIST: Well, let's see . . . rams, male sheep, fight by banging their heads against each other . . . it's pretty awful . . . they have horns on their heads and sometimes they lock horns when they are really going after each other, and then neither one can move. Come to think of it, that is really a terrific analogy for how it is for you all, Sally. Do you understand it better, Joan?

JOAN: (*Grunt, mumble, squirm*)

THERAPIST: Well, Sally, in so many ways, your family has been undergoing change and upheavals with people needing to make lots of adjustments—the divorce, your job, Joan's hospitalization. Joan, you said when we began here today that you were happy to be out of the "looney bin," but not happy to be home. What do you think needs to be worked out for it to be better for you at home?

JOAN: (*Angrily*) Nothing, nothing, nothing—nothing's wrong . . . anyway, you can't fucking change people . . .

THERAPIST: Oh, Sally . . . it's so hard for Joan to believe that anything she does really matters . . . so she thrashes around, and fusses and cusses . . . and I guess you'd say, acts sort of childish for a kid with so much savvy. Well, Joanie, if you can't change others, do you believe that people can change themselves?

JOAN: Yeah, yeah . . . and I've changed a lot already.

THERAPIST: I believe that . . . and it looks like your mom is agreeing with you. Now . . . in relation to your family . . . would you say that the arguing . . . and locking horns . . . is one of the things that needs to be worked out?

JOAN: (*Mumble, grunt, squirm—but looking at me for the first time*) Yeah, yeah . . . I guess so.

BETTY: (*Interrupting—with great intensity*) You shouldn't be asking her . . . it's mom you should ask. She should tell us what needs to be changed.

THERAPIST: That's interesting advice. Joan, does your sister help you out a lot like this?

JOAN: Yeah, we talk . . . she knows how it is with mom.

BETTY: I know how to get on her good side or her bad side, I've learned her ways. I mean, we're like more on each other's level.

THERAPIST: When you said, "Mommy should tell us," Betty, I wasn't sure who you were taking care of? Was it Mother or Joan?

BETTY: (*Getting more distraught*) Both, because at times we're told that we have to take more responsibility and then that we have no rights in the household; therefore we can't say what should or shouldn't happen. So you can't start handing her [Joan] the authority and then expect my mom to . . . we've been fighting about that ever since Joan went into therapy at all . . . who has the authority in the family, who makes the decisions . . . it's all messed up . . . and . . .

THERAPIST: My goodness, Betty, you've described it so well. So, you believed I was turning over the authority in the family to Joan by wanting to know what she believed.

Isn't it a bitch, Sally, the way authority and responsibility and who believes what get all mixed up in a family? So, Betty, you jumped in to give mom support and I suspect also to get Joanie off the hot seat. I think you were being kind, and trying to see that things are fair for both members of your family. What a responsible daughter you've raised, Sally. It's impressive. But also—I wonder—I suspect Betty, that you feel pulled in different directions . . . caught very much in the middle of a lot that goes on in the family . . . much like your mom does. Well, Sally . . . so you believe—and maybe that's why Betty believes—that the main problem is that the kids don't know who's in charge?

SALLY: (*Dejected*) Yes, at least partly. I so often feel so unsure about being in charge . . . where . . . how . . . when . . .

JOAN: The problem is that she doesn't show that she's in charge.

BETTY: Yeah—she's given authority to all three of us.

THERAPIST: Isn't it extraordinary what happens, Sally . . . how the girls jump right in? They're saving, they're blaming—they want to be in charge, they want you to be in charge. It's confusing and yet it's caring and . . . I can see how it gets the way you described . . . that you're locking horns. So you end up talking *at* each other—not *with* each other.

SALLY: Yeah . . . that's how it goes. And the latest thing is that they have been acting goofy, and embarrassing, and in a rather rude manner when the man I'm dating comes around, and I'm having a hard time stopping that.

JOAN: (*Mumbling*) We wouldn't if he wasn't such a turkey . . .

BETTY: (*To Joan*) Be quiet.

THERAPIST: There she goes again, helping out. Do you see what I mean, Sally? Betty, for some reason, feels the need to help you out and to save her sister . . .

BETTY: (*Getting really worked up*) That's the way it's been . . . I would protect her (Joan), mom would protect me, dad used to protect mom. Now Bob (mom's male friend) protects her. If I'm not there to protect her (Joan) maybe something worse would have happened.

THERAPIST: I think that's maybe too great a burden for you, Betty. Besides, I don't think your mom needs your help as much as you think she needs it.

BETTY: (*Adamant*) No . . . it's not a burden. I want the responsibility of protecting and caring for someone. Are you saying that's bad, to take on the protection for others?

THERAPIST: No, I'm not saying that . . . in fact, I think that's a wonderful way to be. (*Turning to Sally*) And, obviously, you have daughters who are caring and loving along with all the crap they give you. And it's lovely that Betty wants to be useful, to take care of people, much like you do. And I can see that you love that part of Betty and want to facilitate it. Perhaps that's why it's hard for you to let her know she's taking on too much at her age . . . helping you make decisions, protecting her sister, deciding how things should go in the family. It gets confusing—on the one hand you want to support the way Betty cares and protects . . . on the other hand you know it's often inappropriate and gets in the way of your being in charge . . . so you're caught in the muddle again . . .

SALLY: (*Becoming more energized*) Yeah, it feels good, then it gets out of hand . . . and in the end, it all makes me feel like I can't do it right . . .

JOAN: I don't think it's bad . . . what Betty does.

BETTY: (*Very agitated*) You can tell me it's wrong, but it's not something that's going to change. It's not a burden; it's my choice. I'm sorry if I say something you don't like . . . maybe it's not right— anyway, Joan can oppose me, mom can oppose me, but I don't feel that an outsider can tell me what's wrong.

SALLY: I think you're getting yourself all worked up and should calm down.

BETTY: We didn't want to come here in the first place, and we'll go home and discuss how we're probably not coming back. This is not how I pictured it. You just talk to mom—we can't express our feelings . . . we probably won't come again.

THERAPIST: Sally, you can see how hard Betty tries . . . how hard she works to take care of everyone just as you do when you intercede between them or with outsiders. She's so like you. And then she feels pulled apart. Why she even thinks the therapy you choose will be a joint decision, that she needs to help you with this.

SALLY: It feels so good to see how it can be different . . . like how we're talking here. At home it's a constant battle and I basically don't want to do battle. I want everything to be nice and happy. I'm sure the kids are not any happier with the way it is than I am.

JOAN: (On the verge of tears) But, Mommy, it's just like you gave up on being a mother . . . you didn't want any responsibility. I could come home any time I wanted . . . you didn't say there was anything wrong with it, and then all of a sudden you say, "You're going away to school whether you like it or not—go, get in the car and leave" . . . You let us act any way we want—and then, when it suits you, you say "stop." Well, that's not my idea of a happy family.

THERAPIST: Sally, you have two very severe critics here.

SALLY: The problem is, I agree with them right now.

THERAPIST: You're right, exactly . . . That is the problem . . . that you agree with your critics, you forget what you've done, and do, well. That's how you block your own effectiveness. And you and your kids have gotten into a way of being together—the dance of the locked horns. Whenever you begin to get it together, they remind you of what you didn't do—and you listen and get back into step!

SALLY: Yes, that's just how it happens, just how it feels. It's true . . . as soon as things seem to improve something happens and we're locked in a dead heap again.

THERAPIST: So, Sally—what else is new? Like every other mother you blame yourself for anything that goes wrong in the family—and your kids follow your lead. They take their cues from you. It might just be that they listen to you a lot more than you think. Maybe you just have to be more clear in your own head about what you're *really* saying to them.

In this exchange, centering on Betty's position in the family, I view her caretaking efforts as congruent with role models for women in families, not as functioning out of mother's parenting failures or triangulations with father. This conceptual frame allows me to be free to validate Betty's "parenting" behaviors even while indicating how they get in the way in the family. It also allows me to emphasize "sameness" and connectedness in a family while challenging the credibility gap concerning mother's ability to be in charge. Sally needed help in understanding her own choices so she could experience being effective in taking leadership. To do this she would first need to help Betty out of the middle.

So now the work moved to challenging and supporting mother to engage in dialogue, in the session, with Betty; to define those areas where she welcomes her caretaking behaviors and those where she does not. This was a painstaking effort since Sally had never thought about the issue in this way before. There were numerous false starts, defensiveness, arguing. The scenario needed to be framed and re-framed many times. When Betty got angry, Sally wanted to give up. I wouldn't let her. Joanie cried and mumbled several times, "Why are you on her case (Betty's)? What about me?" As Sally was more clear with Betty she became energized, and began to reach into her own knowledge of her daughter to suggest ways, outside of the family, in which Betty could put her caretaking skills to good use.

Later I asked the girls to wait downstairs and Sally and I talked.

SALLY: Boy, I feel shaky . . . exhausted. That was like a marathon. Sometimes I see a constant battle stretching ahead of me. I remember the way it was—with Greg being effective, but a dictator. God, the disciplining, the yelling. And it's hard for me to see an in-between. It's so good to sort some things out like this and yet it all just sometimes seems so overwhelming.

THERAPIST: Yes, it's hard; but it won't need to be a pitched battle for life! You'll have the peace you want so much. Sometimes people have to fight for it in ways that seem alien. Your girls are smart—they know you're battle weary and that you fear acting like a dictator.

SALLY: Yeah, I hate it. It's not me. But I think it's what they need. I just don't know how—I just can't give it to them.

THERAPIST: It's not the preferred way for many women, many mothers. I guess women tune in more to working things through, to what goes on between people. They listen a lot, weigh the sides, the issues. But I don't think you want peace at any price!

SALLY: No—no, I sure don't. The price is getting fearsome. What we did today was good. I'm just not sure I can hold on to it.

THERAPIST: Well, Sally, maybe begin with just not being such a good listener for a few weeks. Your girls know you believe you should listen and that kids need to be heard. But if you hear too much, your own thoughts get muddled. Mine do. So maybe you need to hear less so your own thoughts are more clear, and then your own voice can become stronger. Tell you what, Sally—I think you can lay the groundwork by letting your daughters know that you know that much of what's gone down in the past has been lousy, and that you've forgiven yourself and are ready to move on!

In this initial interview the therapeutic intention was to empower the mother by providing a context in which she perceives that she has, and can exercise, choice in conducting her life with her children.

To do this, past "failures" need to be understood differently. Thus, it is not that mom can't take charge, it's that she's battle-averse and consequently chooses to facilitate rather than restrain. The mother's past choices have to be validated before change, built on self-esteem and self-determination, can occur. The therapeutic assumptions here are that mother has given up power on behalf of peace, that there are positive values in her uncertainty, and that even the most dysfunctional interactions among the members of this family encompass intimacy and caring.

The themes developed in the initial interview continued throughout the therapy: Joan's rebelliousness is framed as childishness and later as conflict about growing up, rather than as opposition. Betty's caretaking is framed as lovingly misdirected rather than the problem of a parentified child. And mother's difficulty in taking control is framed as the result of personal constraints and conflicting choices rather than poor parenting skills. The proposition that the family brings to therapy—that Joan is out of control, that mom can't take charge, and that Betty is playing the parent—is countered with the proposition that they are all so tuned into each other and that mom listens so well that she has trouble finding her own voice.

But all this "wisdom" does not make for immediate change. Although Sally was far more energized in the second session, and began by describing how pleasant it was during a visit from her sister when everyone got along well, Joan quickly threw a "temper tantrum."

Session 2

JOAN: Well, it wasn't pleasant for me! We still get penalized because of the way *you* brought us up. Why are we getting all this shit for being the way we are, when it's your fault . . . by giving in to us and letting us pull you in . . . so why are we getting blamed for that and why is this our problem? It's your problem, you're the one who did it, not us. We didn't ask you to be a pushover; we took advantage, but you let us . . . like Don (*their previous therapist*) told me. It's like now she's (*indicating me*) putting all the blame on us. Shit—just like when you and Betty were talking here last week.

SALLY: Joan, that's not how it was . . . I just wanted Betty to get it out . . . get her feelings out, like you're doing now.

THERAPIST: Sally, you want the kids to express their concerns; that's evident, and it's good. But . . . let me ask you . . . have you heard any of this before?

SALLY: I guess so. Yes, she's said these things before.

THERAPIST: How often?

SALLY: I don't know.

THERAPIST: Oh, I think you do. Once, twice, three times?

SALLY: More like twenty times.

THERAPIST: Do you think it is important for Joanie to say the same thing over and over again?

SALLY: I don't know. I'm not sure.

JOAN: (*To therapist*) You interrupted me . . . that makes me god-damn mad!

THERAPIST: I am sorry, Joan, for interrupting, but this is an important thing for your mom and me to get clear. (*To Sally*) I think this is a hard, but a really major decision for you to make. How many times do you think Joan has to say the same thing in order for her to get her feelings out? You keep listening and Joan keeps throwing you questions that don't have answers. But you can help Joan with questions for which you do have answers . . . like how to manage school better, how to get along at home, how to deal with rules. You really need to put an end to these rhetorical questions . . . and find your own voice.

JOAN: Okay . . . sure . . . go ahead . . . put an end to why I'm so hurt!

SALLY: What you say makes such sense . . . I guess I'm so unaware of it happening when it happens and so I can be sucked into it, and it can be real painful. And I don't want to be a dictator.

THERAPIST: Would you buy being maybe . . . a director? . . . at least for the time being . . . while you get things straightened out?

SALLY: It's not a bad idea—I certainly have a talented cast.

Later Betty makes a last ditch effort to "go-between" and maintain the status quo in the family.

BETTY: Just answer this mom, yes or no. Do you want *any* help with the decisions and responsibilities? If not . . . I'll stop completely. Fine. I will. No more . . .

JOAN: I hate this . . .

SALLY: I don't think it has to be all or nothing.

BETTY: I can't be any other way . . . my personality does not allow me . . .

SALLY: Betty, we're here to find a middle ground . . . for you, for me . . .

BETTY: (*In tears*) I can't be a middle person . . . I've tried my whole life . . .

SALLY: (*Firmly*) I think you can, honey.

THERAPIST: I agree . . . and I believe you can help her achieve that—even if it's not her style.

JOAN: (*Furious with me*) Just because it's your style doesn't make it right, you know!

BETTY: Mom, I'm sorry . . . Joanie said it in a bad way . . . I can say it in a good way. She said it, like angry . . . all I want to know is, was I wrong this summer when everything went berserk? I worked five nights a week . . . you hardly ever saw me. Was I wrong to help? I feel like I'm damned if I do and damned if I don't.

SALLY: This summer was something that just fell apart all around us . . . there was no foundation, no structure . . . and that's what we're trying to solve at this point . . . so we never get into such a bad muddle again . . . I'm sick of it.

JOAN: I'm sick of you . . .

BETTY: Oh, shut up. I'm fed up with you, too . . .

JOAN: You make me sick, too . . . you can't shut me up . . . you're not my mother!

BETTY: I know I'm not—I just want you to shut up from my own point of view.

SALLY: Well, that's better. I know you're furious, Joanie. And that you want to help, Betty . . . or that you don't want to even hear it . . . but it's happening, and you can hear it and know it's between Joan and me; and leave it alone. I'll try and help you know when to stay out.

This exchange provided an opportunity to highlight and affirm Sally's taking charge in the family without losing control or acting like a dictator. I asked Betty to come and sit by me. When she hesitated, Sally backed me up and Betty reluctantly complied. While Sally talked to Joan, making clear to her that the therapy would continue and laying out some expectations for her behavior in family sessions, I tried to engage Betty. To no avail—she was having none of me. Her attention was rooted on her mom and Joan. As things became more heated between Sally and Joan, Betty started to cry. Sally immediately let up on Joan and leaned over to comfort Betty. When I interrupted and pointed out the sequence of their interactions, it had a visible impact on Sally. She seemed momentarily stunned. Then she "got it"—not just for herself, but with a real sense of the meaning of this experience for the whole family. She returned to Joan, handing Betty some tissues as she did so.

Betty became pensive and withdrew, seemingly preoccupied with her own thoughts. She still wouldn't talk with me. Joan calmed down, but mostly pouted while Sally talked with her. Again, at the end of the session, Sally and I talked alone to debrief and to demonstrate Sally's authority in the family and our interacting as adults, apart from the young people. Of course, Sally's preferred behavior in such a situation was to explore, indeed obsess over, why she hadn't observed these family patterns of interaction before, how they triggered each other, and how she always got sucked in. I suggested she would have plenty of time to "put herself down" after things were more settled with the kids, and I promised to join her in this favorite sport for as long as she wanted after she had acted on what she understood now. Then we'd be free to really dwell on why she hadn't understood it all before!

Session 3

In the week prior to this session there was a crisis. Joan stayed out all night and mom called the police; she came home late the next morning of her own accord. Betty slept through the night, worried with mom the next morning, but came to the session unaware of what had transpired between Sally and Joan around this transgression. She was curious, but stayed out of it, and could even accept some ribbing about her curiosity.

SALLY: Joanie and I seem to be in constant struggle. I feel like a jailer. I asked her not to go out the other night. Then she asks if she can just walk down to the corner with some friends and disappears . . . for the whole night. She knows what the consequences are of her doing such things . . . it's happened before . . . but she does them anyway . . . and then I have to act like a prison warden. I was so furious at her for not obeying.

THERAPIST: That's terrific!

SALLY: (*Taken aback*) What's terrific?

THERAPIST: Your being furious instead of saddened and hopeless about Joanie's behavior . . . you sound stronger—more sure. Before, you talked about Joanie as if she wasn't *able* to get it together. Now you talk more like you believe she knows how to . . . but won't. It's sort of like the difference between being sick and being disobedient. When you thought Joan just maybe couldn't manage, couldn't be any different, you panicked, she got hospitalized, you felt sad, and you both felt failed. Now you see her more as disobedient—a refusenik—and you're just plain pissed!

SALLY: (*In a defiant manner*) You know—I tell you what, Marianne. The fact is, Joan has a good home. I think I'm a—well, basically, a good parent. I know there are problems. There has been a lot of chaos and change. I understand that. I don't even know what Joan is feeling now . . . she won't tell me. And that's okay. But whatever it is, it doesn't warrant this kind of behavior. I don't deserve it. It doesn't have to be this way.

JOAN: You bet it doesn't . . . you don't need to be so . . .

THERAPIST: (*Interrupting*) I do agree with you, Sally. I guess that somewhere along the way you learned that being clear or getting tough was like a dictator, certainly not like a woman, or a mother, and setting rules—disciplining—like being a jailer. Such ways offended your sense of justice and fairness . . . maybe even your image of how to be loving. You wanted peaceful coexistence . . . but clearly not at any price. I think you'll have much less difficulty being in charge when it no longer makes you feel mean-spirited. When you can see it, even the conflict that goes with it, as caring—competent. You might think of it as sort of like a nursing regimen you would set up to help one of your patients with a backache.

JOAN: Oh, so now I'm a backache!

SALLY: Oh, honey—more like a pain in the . . . ! (*They both start to laugh*).

Much of this third session was devoted to a long and difficult exchange between mom and Joan regarding a rather complex set of consequences Sally had devised to deal with Joan's "overnight." Betty asked permission to wait downstairs for a while and do her homework. When she returned at the end of the hour for a discussion of some general family planning—schedules, assignments, and the like—Sally let her know how pleased she was that she had absented herself so appropriately.

Subsequent Sessions

The next several sessions were devoted largely to issues of family organization and Joan's behavior at school. There was a lot of the usual jockeying for position and concern with those monumental questions that confront every normal American family with teenagers. Who's going to wash dishes Tuesday night? Why does laundry have to be done every week? Why don't towels belong on the bathroom floor?

Why does vacuuming have to be done "your" way? What constitutes an appropriate length of time for a telephone call from the girlfriend with whom you just walked home from school? Where is it written that beds should be made every day? Why can't a person watch TV and write a term paper at the same time unless she's stupid?

It was tough going. Schedules went up on refrigerator doors. Alarm clocks were installed in each bedroom, weekly household assignments posted by the hall phone. Joan's behavior at school was even tougher. She broke the rules of her probationary status. Mom went to bat for her, helping her to renegotiate with the school and at the same time setting up with the school a rigorous system of checks and balances. When the young people strayed off task, complaining about too much structure and not enough flexibility, their complaints were framed as a necessary frustration in healing a breach of trust between them.

A few weeks before Christmas both girls ganged up on Sally, complaining about the inclusion of her boyfriend in their holiday plans. They pulled out all stops, raising again the specter of past failures.

JOAN: You got divorced from your husband, we didn't get divorced from the family.

BETTY: It's not family anymore . . . it's family and outsider.

JOAN: Why do we have to suffer just because you and Dad couldn't get it together?

BETTY: And now we're forced to be with someone we don't even like, just because you want him there.

JOAN: It's going to be a lousy Christmas.

Mom almost backed down in the face of this onslaught, but with suggestions, coaching, and support she managed to hold her ground and not get pulled into being defensive about the past. She included her boyfriend in the family holidays and it all went okay. Later, I saw Sally alone for several sessions to talk about some issues in her own personal and professional life and to review the main themes and general direction of our work together.

Perhaps the real turning point occurred when Sally was planning a ski trip with her male friend and wanted her ex-husband to provide some backup care for the girls while she was gone. This precipitated a major battle between them. The father complained that he thought Joan was getting worse, not better, and began to insist that she be hospitalized again. He refused to accept any responsibility for the children's supervision while Sally was gone unless he were given more say in determining Joan's psychiatric needs. Sally was distraught.

I saw the parents together. Greg, the father, was pleasant, but absolutely adamant about enforcing his requirements. He felt Joanie was in very bad shape and her living arrangement unhealthy. He thought he might have to sue for custody, and that they surely needed a psychiatric evaluation. I encouraged Greg to pursue, on his own, whatever course of action he deemed appropriate for his daughter —in fact asserting it was not only his right but his responsibility, given his very serious concerns for her welfare. I also strongly advised Sally to make her plans for the care of her daughters while she was away without requiring or depending on the services of their father.

Throughout this session with both parents, I refused to enter with them into any negotiation, stating that it seemed to me that they had parted with good reason and that trying to reconcile their differences would only serve to make each feel more angry, defensive, and beleaguered. I told them I believed that it would be best for Joan if each of her parents would be true to his or her own beliefs and concerns, and not try to convince the other parent to accommodate or to agree. I assured them that children could very well survive strong differences between their parents.

Joan's father did not follow up on any of the courses of action he had insisted were vital to her welfare. He called me a few weeks later to say he had decided to just bide his time and see how things went, but wanted me to know how much he had appreciated my support. Sally, through her network of friends and colleagues, organized the care and supervision she needed for the girls while she was away.

The week that Sally was away went well. Everyone felt quite good about it, and at our next session the girls kidded around and even boasted about their part in managing it, and managing each other, in mom's absence. Of course, they had to take a few pot-shots at Sally in the process—how they could do this and that better without her interference—but Sally didn't, for the most part, get sucked in. Joan made a stab at starting up something with her mom by saying things had really deteriorated since Sally's return. But Sally responded merely by stating she disagreed, although that didn't mean she wasn't really proud of them for doing so well in her absence.

The important change was in Sally's ability to let go of the cycle of self-blame and guilt concerning the problems with her daughters, Joan in particular, which kept her comparing herself to their father and feeling she could not manage without his input and support. She told me that in some ways she had gotten more satisfaction from making her own arrangements for the trip than from the trip itself. Most important, she was beginning to enjoy her daughters again.

Conclusion

For the rest of the school year I saw different members of the family on an "as needed" basis, seldom all together. Betty was involved in the senior play and her preparations for college. She came in a couple of times to talk about whether to live at home her freshman year, or on campus, and to discuss career choice. She thought she might like to be a social worker! Joan came in to discuss altercations at school, problems with teachers, and study habits. Sally came in to solve some problems when she got into tight situations with Joan. She also used me to work out some personal decisions, particularly concerning her relationship with her male friend.

I saw them all together for the last time just before Betty's graduation. They were delightful. Betty had decided to live on campus and the girls allowed that they might miss each other. Joanie mused that maybe now she'd have the chance to be "the good girl." Betty noted that she used "positive reinforcement" on herself by turning her body away whenever mom and Joanie had a fight. Joan suggested mom had been a "pushover" before because she was "scared," and they all cracked up when she added that maybe mom needed to go back to being a little more scared these days!

The following year Sally called me a few times, particularly to discuss school problems with Joan. In the second semester we worked together to arrange a more appropriate school placement and to get Joanie into a tutoring program to make up for some of the work she'd lost when she was truanting.

In the late spring Sally came to see me. She had been offered a job with significant career advancement, and had decided to move out West. She had ended the relationship with her male friend. She wanted reassurance that moving would not be harmful to Joanie as well as help in discussing arrangements with Greg in relation to her move.

Sally and Joan moved in the summer, and Betty spent her school vacation with them. I received a letter from Sally about six weeks into the next school year. It was going much better for Joan academically; she seemed to be using the move to make a "fresh start"—no drugs, no acting out, no truanting. At home they still fought a lot and still disagreed about "almost everything." But when they "made up" it was great!

I received a postcard from Joanie just after Christmas. She was skiing with friends in Utah. She was having a great time. She ended with, "It's cold enough to freeze the tits off a boar hog. Wish you were here." I wonder how she meant that?

Betty Carter

"I Can't Believe You Thought My Going to See Uncle S. Meant I Didn't Love You."

I chose this particular case because it demonstrates so well a common dilemma in which women are caught in the parental triangle in such a way that they idealize their fathers and devalue their mothers, and thus themselves.

Parental Triangles and Cutoff

The client, Anne, a 30-year-old female doctoral student, is the oldest of three daughters. She had had a lifetime of conflict and uproar with her mother, who had cut off from *her* mother (Anne's grandmother), and so the pattern went back as far as anyone knew. All of these women, including the client, had experienced warm, idealized relationships with their fathers. The mother-daughter relationships, then, are conceptualized in this model as embedded in intense triangles, with daughter caught in an alliance with father against mother, acting out his negativity toward mother and receiving the brunt of mother's alienated, emotionally isolated wrath. This mother-daughter-father triangle interlocks with the triangle composed of grandmother, mother, and daughter, in which grandmother and granddaughter soon discover the camaraderie of having a common "enemy," leaving mother "odd man out" in both triangles.

In this family, the process of triangulation had intensified over generations to the point where total cutoff was used more and more often in an attempt to manage the anxiety provoked by these relationship patterns. When she first came to see me, Anne reported her mother's cutoffs with her mother, her brother (Anne's uncle), and a secret ex-spouse. Anne's father was extremely distant from his parents, and "out of touch" with his brother. Anne herself was not in communication with an ex-spouse and was on the verge of dropping contact with her mother.

I do not believe that dropping contact with one's mother can be construed as part of "individuation" or "differentiation" or "autonomy." On the contrary, an inability to remain connected with the members of one's family, especially one's mother, is a sign of the failure to acknowledge the interdependency basic to the human condition. Therapy that supports such a basic cutoff or tries to "go around it" fails to grasp the central feature of maturity: *autonomy in the context of attachment.* It can easily happen that the intensity that leads to cutting off significant family relationships seems to block a person's flow of ideas about *how* to reconnect without needing to blame or be defensive. That, one would hope, is where the therapist comes in.

How to Reconnect

Since it takes two to maintain a cutoff, Anne was coached to handle her end of the relationship differently. In order to break the cycle of cutoffs, she was taught not to take her mother's actions so personally, but to see them in the context of the family's transgenerational emotional process. This is far easier said than done, especially regarding mothers. In order not to take your mother's actions too personally, it is necessary to see her as a human being rather than as a "mother." Human beings have their own needs and their own lives to lead; "mothers" exist in our mythology only for others. A crucial aspect of bettering relations with the client's mother involved changing her "alliance" with father into a separate personal relationship with him.

The task for the therapist in this and similar situations is to avoid joining the client in reacting to mother's cold, rejecting behavior and to continue to interpret that behavior as a concomitant of forces in the larger family systems in which it is embedded. I have found with clients and therapists alike that while some outrageous behavior may be accepted from most family members as part of life, our mythology of motherhood proclaims that no sane mother ever rejects her child, and we tend to react punitively when such rejection occurs.

The following report was written by the client when I asked her permission to include her story in this book.

Client's Report of Her Therapy

I come from a line of daughters who have had trouble getting along with their mothers that goes back at least three generations. I know that my maternal grandmother got along terribly with her mother, from what my mother has told me, with much uproar and arguing between the two of them. I did not have contact with my grandmother on my mother's side (let's call her Grandma S.), after my childhood, as my mother cut off from her rather completely when I was about 8 and she died about ten years ago.

I remember Grandma S. much differently and more positively than my mother does. She stayed with my family for several months a few times when I was young, and I recall that she liked to spoil me, that she took my side in my disagreements with mom (which were numerous), and I enjoyed doing things with her.

My mother found most of this pretty annoying, I'm sure, but then, the triangle with the three of us was just one aspect of a long history of problems between them.

As awful as Grandma S. seemed to my mother, Grandpa S. seemed wonderful to her. A good, kind, patient, saint of a man (according to mom), he and my mother got along very well. I tended to think, over the years, of my father in much the same way that my mother thought of her father—as a man burdened unfairly in life by having such an obnoxious wife.

After lots of arguing with my mother when I was a child, I became a teenager, which made matters worse. I was fairly shy outside the house during this time, but not at all too shy to stir up trouble when I was home. I blamed all of this, of course, on mom, and literally counted the days during most of high school until I could leave home.

The great day finally arrived, and I left for college. I was not so shy in college, and managed to do just about every rebellious thing that kids were doing in the late '60s and early '70s. My pattern with my parents during these years was one of bad arguments, cutoffs on my part, and then great emotional reconciliations, which were sooner or later followed by the next argument.

All of this did not leave me particularly well prepared, as the end of college neared, to take care of myself. Being rebellious had taken priority over preparing for a career. Therefore, I decided to get married, and became involved with Fred, who had graduated a year ahead of me and who showed promise of doing well in life. We enjoyed many things about each other, but fought easily and early in the relationship. We both felt quite ambivalent about becoming engaged, but went through with the marriage despite our misgivings. My parents hated Fred, who was arrogant with them. Several months after the marriage, I got very angry at my family and cut off from them completely, thus following in my mother's footsteps.

My marriage to Fred was stormy and relatively brief. I initiated a separation after about a year, not thinking that such a step could be permanent. Fred and I did not live together again, although we remained involved, arguing and reconciling, for another two years. When I realized that the marriage would end, I became very distraught. A long-time woman friend contacted my parents at this point and told them about my situation. They got in touch with me, and offered to have me live with them again. I didn't find this plan very appealing, so I got a job, found an apartment to share with a female roommate, and began therapy.

At the suggestion of my first therapist, I reconnected with my family and started gathering information about them. This included getting in touch with the brother my mother had cut off twenty years before, but I felt unable to tell my mother that I had done so. The anxiety I felt about this secret, which engulfed me like a white noise, made it almost impossible to be with them. At the end of one wild, conflictual visit home, my therapist suggested I shift to someone who specialized in family-of-origin coaching, which is how I got to Betty Carter.

Therapist's Comment

The family history of cutoffs plus the client's own stormy involvement in the pattern of cutoff and reconciliation with her parents and husband bespeak a relationship system of great intensity and volatility. The cutoffs are an attempt to gain freedom or autonomy in a relationship in which there are no mechanisms to handle difference or conflict. In actuality, the need to cut off from family in order to pursue one's own agenda indicates great dependency, rather than autonomy, but the cutoffs temporarily reduce anxiety and are experienced as a resolution. Actually, though, cutoffs intensify emotional reactivity and trigger recurring bouts of justification whenever brought into awareness. Thus, the client's contacting the brother her mother had not spoken to for twenty years was totally against the system's deepest rules and should have been preceded by other smaller moves of attachment and differentiation before being undertaken. Now that contact had been initiated, however prematurely, it had to be dealt with, since keeping it a secret was intolerable. However, it was clear to me that revealing the reconnection would create a major family crisis.

One can more easily make changes in the emotional structure of a family system when the system is in a state of flux, for example, in times of crisis or major life cycle events. My contact with good old Uncle S., which had created a secret that prevented any contact with my family, could be used to provide the impetus, in my family system and particularly in my relationship with my mother, to get things moving. Such a crisis would provide an opportunity for me to behave differently with mom, and in doing so, to establish a different, better kind of relationship with her and the rest of the family.

The plan that Betty Carter and I developed was as follows: without attacking mom or being defensive, I was to tell her calmly that I'd seen her brother. (Of course, handling interpersonal conflict without attacks or defensiveness would be totally new for me.) I did this in a brief letter that was also more friendly than I had been lately.

I didn't hear anything for over a week, and did not know my father had written me a furious, enraged letter. At Betty's suggestion, I called, and got his reaction on the telephone: other things I had done in the past were trivial compared to this. Uncle S. was their mortal enemy, and I had made mom suffer a severe attack of one of her illnesses. My instinctive reaction to this response was to become very angry. But because the plan developed in therapy had predicted the family reaction as a possible response, I was able to do something different. As planned, I expressed enormous upset and concern about my mom and her health, dramatically repeating how awful all this was, my worst fears realized, and so on. In response to everything my father told me, I exaggerated, expressing concern about the "terrible situation." When I got off the phone I felt a little giggly; this way of reacting felt very new and strange. But it was a relief not to be overwhelmed with anger and depression.

When I got the letter from my father, I wrote back to mom, with Betty's help, expressing much concern about her and this terrible situation, "the last thing I had intended." I also said I just could never seem to get the family rules straight, even though I tried. This letter was meant to indicate that they would not be able to control me, but at the same time I cared about them and felt concern.

Mom did not answer the letter. In fact, after this letter, she returned letters I sent to her unopened. My letters to her always reiterated some variation of my basic position, with greatest emphasis on my care and concern about her, and my dismay at the terrible situation between the two of us. I sent her a Christmas present that year; she had it returned to "sender." She continued to be sick on and off.

Therapist's Comment

Mother's return of the client's letters unopened signaled her profound level of hurt and her entrenchment in the pattern of cutoff. I advised the client that her mother was settled in for the long haul and that we should do likewise. Since interaction was conducted by mail and phone at lengthy intervals, we agreed to meet monthly or as needed. In our meetings, I continued to direct the client's thinking toward seeing the long-standing family patterns and away from dwelling on personal emotional reactivity.

Over the next year, I continued to meet with Betty monthly. According to plan, I wrote to my sisters, talked with my father on the phone, and sent my mother letters, which she never answered. I always expressed much concern about mom when I spoke with dad, and his anger relented to some extent. Mom, however, had dug in her heels, and seemed immovable. (Recall that she had had a lot of practice in family cutoffs with her other relatives.)

I continued to work on my relationship with dad. Instead of focusing on my problems with my mother in conversations with him, I began to ask him about himself and his work, and to tell him in more detail about my life and studies. About a year of this produced very satisfying results in terms of a more personal relationship between us. I learned, during this time, to recognize how extremely guarded dad was with mom, shielding her (and, of course, himself) from difficult emotions on the grounds that such feelings would harm her health. In the midst of this phase, my 27-year-old sister moved into her own apartment for the first time. This was the first positive sign I had had that the family system might be opening up somewhat due to my efforts.

Therapist's Comment

The client had always had warm feelings toward her father. Until now, however, she had not realized that their relationship was often an unspoken alliance that revolved around the question of how to deal with mother rather than a personal exchange between them. During this year, the client worked at changing her relationship with her father. As she continued to stay connected in a friendly way with all family members in spite of her mother's anger and disapproval, her younger sisters began to move on in their own lives.

The client's relationship with her two sisters had been chiefly determined by the triangle of father-mother-daughters, with the women fighting with each other and dad in the distant position. The client, the family rebel, was "daddy's girl," and from that position fought her mother and two younger sisters. The more conflict there was between the client and her mother, the more her younger sisters moved protectively toward mother and felt negative and angry at their oldest sister for "causing mother so much pain." Thus, the relationship among the sisters was totally determined by loyalty issues concerning their parents. The more dad remained in the distant position, the more the parental battle was fought by mother and daughters. As the client began to understand the dynamics of this family triangle, she was able not to take her sister's hostility so personally and to start trying to develop with each of them, by mail and by telephone, a person-to-person relationship that was not based on attacking or defending their parents. Also, as the client's new positive attitude toward mother came through to the younger sisters, they felt released from their protective role toward their mother and thus able to

respond more positively to their oldest sister and to put more
flexibility into their own relationship with both parents. Their
sister's reconnection then provided enough space and freedom for
them to focus more on their own lives.

I continued to write my mother. She did not write back, until
finally, after almost two years, one terse note acknowledged flowers I
sent on Mother's Day. I felt hopeful that now perhaps the great freeze
would begin to thaw, but she did not respond to further letters. At
Betty's suggestion, I began sending postcards rather than letters with
the hope that she would not be able to resist the temptation to read
them. But still she did not respond. Several months later, she had an
operation.

After many months of no further change, Betty suggested that a
visit might move things in a positive direction, and we began to plan
the trip. Now I needed somewhat more frequent therapy sessions.

The plan had two main stages. First, I had to get my foot in the
door, and somehow begin speaking to my mother. Second, I had to
address the issue over which she had cut me off—my defiance of her
rule against contact with Uncle S.

Therapist's Comment

*The content of the final conflict that leads to cutoff invariably
gets flash-frozen at that point and will reemerge as fresh as ever
at any attempt to reconnect. It is thus important to prepare a
client to deal with the specific content issues of the original
conflict in a way that won't lead to a more profound split, but
rather will further the goal of the client's differentiation. The
content issue here concerned the client's contacting her cutoff
Uncle S.*

Even looking back on it, the plan we evolved seems a bit auda-
cious and I felt terrified but also amused and challenged, naturally,
with a fair amount of anxiety underlying everything. I planned to stay
in a hotel, supposedly in the city on business. When I arrived, I would
buy a plant or some flowers, and leave them at the front door with a
note addressed to "Dear Family." The note would say something to the
effect that I was in town for work and did not at all want to bother
them since I knew that I was *persona non grata*. However, I had been
overwhelmed by the desire to come by since I was so close, thinking
perhaps that I might catch sight of one of them going in or out of the
house.

Two things could happen at this point: either no one would see me
or someone might open the door at the moment I was there. If the latter

happened (which seemed less likely) I would ask very quietly, in a sort of whisper, if I could come in and take a tiny peek at mom for just an instant. I would then proceed to Stage 2 of our plan.

If no one saw me, I would then go back to my hotel and wait to see how they would respond. Betty and I thought of three possible responses to the note and plant. One: nothing. In this case, I was to interpret such a response as ambivalence, and return to the house the next day to try to get to Stage 2. Two: my father might call me on the phone (I would leave my number on the note), grudgingly saying that I could come over if I must. Three: dad might call, enraged, accusing me of trying to kill my mother. If that happened, I was not to try to go over there again on this visit, since their message that they could not tolerate any attempt at change would be clear. However, I was to react to my father with upset, astonishment, and bewilderment that they could be so angry because I had just left a little plant.

Therapist's Comment

A major move in a family should be somewhat consistent with family style—so they don't call the police—but yet be unpredictable enough to be recognized as new information. In this family, the drama of the long silences and the returned letters, as well as the general tendency to make "much ado about nothing," is matched in the reconnection plan. The detailed planning and execution of a nonhostile, not hurtful, nondefensive move puts the client thoroughly in charge of herself in the midst of the predicted family emotional reactivity so that she can emerge a bit more autonomous instead of again feeling victimized.

As it happened, no one did see me when I left the plant and the note. I was relieved; I had to summon up a lot of courage just to go to the house, and I preferred to take the tasks one by one if possible. I went back to the hotel and waited.

By the next morning no one had called, so I put the next part of the plan into action. I went back to the house and rang the doorbell. My youngest sister answered the door, and (in my best stage whisper) I asked if I could see my mom, just for a minute or two; I didn't want to upset her, but was so close and just wanted to take this chance that she might let me look at her for a moment. My sister was clearly not thrilled with this development, but said she'd go tell mom I was there. My mother came to the door, looking pale and much thinner than the last time I'd seen her. She invited me in.

There I was! It was time for Stage 2, which Betty and I had also planned quite thoroughly. We sat down, with my sister Sue staying around almost as a guard for mom.

I did not have to bring up Uncle S. (which I would have done if mom didn't); she began talking about my contact with him almost immediately, as if several years had not elapsed, asking me why I had done it. I understood the futility of arguing about my reasons with her, and instead planned to keep the focus on our relationship. I had written a list of many nonhostile responses to her questions, which Betty and I had predicted, and I had spent time memorizing the list so that anxiety wouldn't paralyze my mind and tongue. Some of my responses expressed what I thought were her interpretations of what I had done (for example, "I know you think I meant to hurt you," "I know you didn't like it"). Some stated the fact that I felt sorry she'd been so upset and hurt (but never that I was sorry I'd done what I'd done). Still others stated my feelings toward her (for example, "It's terrible I've never convinced you I love you," "*I can't believe you thought my going to see Uncle S. meant I didn't love you*"—this last response being the one I ended up saying the most, and the one that fit best). In this conversation, I also talked regretfully about what a terrible child and teenager I had been.

Therapist's Comment

The response that fit best unlocked the intergenerational pattern: mother, in a beleaguered, isolated position, with her husband placating her, her oldest daughter defying her, and her own mother criticizing her, felt her family didn't love her. No wonder she was sometimes cold, often angry, and chronically ill. As often happens, when the right key turns, it unlocks the entire relationship pattern, and those involved find themselves talking about more than the specific conflictual incident. Notice that the crucial response addressed the toxic issue openly, did not blame mother nor defend daughter, and referred to the basic relationship issue— that mother and daughter were unsure of each other's love.

My mother was fairly emotional through all of this, and so was I, although, for a change, neither of us yelled or cried. However, Sue, observing the exchange, noticed that I had not responded directly to any of mom's questions about the reason I had gone to see my uncle. She finally asked me, "But why did you go to see Uncle S.?" I replied with another of my prepared responses, and she gave up.

After about forty-five minutes, I didn't think we could say much more about the same things, and the discussion wound down. I said I didn't want to make her sick by upsetting her, so maybe I should leave. She asked me to stay for lunch. Sue decided to do some things she needed to do and no longer stood guard over mom.

I spent the rest of the day there. Pam, who called just after lunch, certainly sounded surprised to hear my voice on the phone, and to learn that I had arrived without causing World War III. My father called later in the afternoon to check on mom, concerned that she might feel upset or sick because of the flowers and my note of yesterday. He too sounded quite surprised that I had been there for several hours and nothing dire had happened. He worriedly warned me not to mention Uncle S., whatever else I did. I enjoyed saying quite casually, "Oh, we talked about that already." I asked my mother where my flowers were and she looked guilty. Sue told me that they were in the trash in the garage, but she had put them there very carefully. We rescued them and put them into a pretty vase. Dad came home, and my sister Pam came over, and we all ate dinner together. My plan had succeeded.

I visited a couple more times during that trip. I maintained my pretext that I also had work that needed to be done. I then returned home to New York very pleased about what had happened.

Since then, I have visited my family three times, at about six-month intervals and I stay in touch regularly on the phone and by letter. In general, my anxiety is lower these days, and in many ways I feel more self-confident. I am pleased with my career, which is developing nicely (in such contrast to the doubts and disorganization that I felt about my work in the past). I broke off a fairly serious relationship with a man many months ago because I did not want to marry him. I seem to have higher standards for myself in all areas and am far less prone to blame myself for everything that goes wrong around me. Life is far from perfect, but I am very glad to have been able to make the changes I've made.

Some other time, I'll tell you what I did when the family announced that my sister Pam was getting married, my grandmother (father's mother) was not invited, and I was not to let her know.

Peggy Papp

"Go for It, Mom!"

It is difficult for a mother to bestow a legacy of competence and self-confidence on a daughter when she herself feels in a subservient position to her husband. The quality of her mothering will always be partially determined by the relational context in which she mothers. The following case illustrates the way in which the relationship between a mother and daughter is affected by the unresolved issues of power and autonomy in the marital relationship. The teenage daughter is caught up in fighting mother's battles with father, which mother avoids fighting for fear of breaking up the family. This results in both mother and daughter sacrificing their relationship as well as their individual independence and autonomy for the sake of family unity. Through therapy, the power in the marital relationship is rebalanced, freeing mother to provide a role model for her daughter of a strong independent woman.

Exploring the Problem

The Drayton family sought therapy because the parents were having difficulty controlling their 14-year-old daughter, Vicki, who was truanting from school, running away from home, and frequenting bars until all hours of the night. For the past five years, she had been starting school with her classmates but then gradually truanting more and more as the year progressed until she would finally be expelled. All the family members attended therapy sessions, including Vicki's older brother, Alex, and her younger brother, Greg.

During the first session, father, a big, impressive-looking man in his mid-40s, was the spokesman for the family, enumerating all of Vicki's misdemeanors in a weary and exasperated tone of voice. He said he and his wife had tried everything—pleading, lecturing, reasoning, placating, even forcibly dragging Vicki to school—all to no avail. They were at the end of their rope. "This causes great turmoil in the family and if it happens again I don't know how this family can survive. It divides us all and surfaces issues that were resolved years ago." However, when questioned further he would not divulge what those old issues were and told the therapist in no uncertain terms, "If you have the impression there is difficulty between my wife and me, there is not. We are very allied and jointly agree on decisions."

Father then attacked Vicki, and they became embroiled in a heated argument. All the open fighting was between Vicki and her father while mother and the two brothers sat listening. They argued with intense passion, and father said he found it difficult to control himself in the face of what he felt was Vicki's deliberately provocative behavior. Recently, at home, he had become frightened when he found himself striking out at her physically. Mother had rushed in to stop him.

Although father stated he and mother were in agreement on how to handle Vicki, mother dropped certain hints that led me to believe that was not always the case. With some encouragement from me, mother began to express some of her disagreements with father. She objected to his violent way of trying to deal with the situation. Although she had allowed her husband to coerce her into helping him drag Vicki to school, her heart was not in it and she deeply resented his pressure. Father accused mother of undermining his disciplinary efforts by giving Vicki "tacit approval." Mother denied this, saying, "You have a take-charge personality. You are a big executive used to controlling your environment and having a lot of power. But we found out we can't force her." Father replied vehemently, "She has to be forced or she can't live with us. If she doesn't obey the basic rules, we can't survive as a family." The father believed Vicki had chosen to defy them concerning education because this was an area of prime importance to him. He wanted Vicki placed in a residential treatment center, but mother objected and threatened to leave the marriage if he followed through on that plan.

In her relationship with Vicki, mother alternated between trying to rescue her from father's harshness and making abortive attempts to control her rebellious behavior. This resulted in the mother's taking a supplicating position with Vicki, begging, pleading, and placating. Vicki took advantage of her mother's vacillation by reneging on agreements and making inappropriate demands. Mother and daughter ended up relating "through" father rather than "with" each other. As a result their relationship was filled with confusion and conflict.

As I explored further the disagreement between the parents, mother began to complain that her wishes on other issues were not respected at home. She had wanted to work but had deferred to her husband's objections. And for the first time she expressed her resentment over having to move from one city to another so that he could live near his father. It became evident that mother resented feeling overpowered by her husband and fought him covertly by protecting Vicki rather than herself from his arbitrariness. Father reacted to mother's lack of cooperation by taking his anger out on Vicki, whom he saw as her accomplice.

Therapeutic Goals

It was clear that Vicki was fighting mother's unfought battles with father by rebelling against authority both inside and outside the family. I saw my therapeutic goals in terms of helping mother to assert herself with father and to provide a role model of a strong, independent woman who did not need her daughter to fight her battles for her. This would also enable father to relate to Vicki on his own terms rather than as an accomplice of mother.

This case was seen in the Brief Therapy Project at the Ackerman Family Institute at a time when our major method of working with families was through the use of the therapeutic debate. The debate takes place between two or sometimes three therapists in front of the family. Each therapist assumes a different position in relation to the issue of change in the family. The purpose of the debate is to connect the symptomatic behavior of the identified parent to specific interactions in the family that serve to maintain the behavior. The debate makes explicit the covert patterns that mitigate against change. As the family becomes involved in the debate, the family members begin to accept the reference points of the therapists. In so doing, they perceive the problem and consequently the solution to the problem, differently.

The Therapeutic Debate

In the following sequence, the first therapist took a position for stability, respecting the family's way of solving its problem through Vicki's symptom and outlining the consequences of change. This therapist argued that no individual could change unilaterally because all were governed by the central rules of the system. The other two therapists disagreed that the system was all-powerful and acted as advocates for change, one supporting the parents in the direction of change, the other supporting Vicki.

THERAPIST 1 [Stanley Siegel] (*Stability position*)*: Vicki, you and your mother are very sensitive to one another and I think that you know your mother might like to be a little defiant with your father. Your mother might like not to follow his authority sometimes. (*Vicki nods in agreement*). I have the feeling that you, Vicki, in your own loyal, good-daughter way, are putting your own interests on the back burner and fighting for your mother. You are taking up her cause with your father, as this family tends to take up causes.

THERAPIST 2 [Marsha Scheinberg] (*Vicki's advocate*): I agree, but I think it's time for Vicki to act in her own self-interest and not take up mother's battle with father. Instead, she should allow her parents to work out their own problems. It is in your own best interest to go to school and get an education so you can do something interesting with your life. (*The therapist then has a brief discussion with Vicki about what she wants to do with her life. Vicki says she wants to become a doctor and the therapist says she will really need an education for that.*)

VICKI: I want to be a doctor but I also want to be my own person. I don't want to conform to society.

---

*Therapist 1 is Stanley Siegel; Therapist 2 is Marsha Scheinberg; Therapist 3 is Peggy Papp.

THERAPIST 1 (*Stability position*): You are a conformist. But you conform to the family. Above all else you will not violate family rules.

THERAPIST 3 [Peggy Papp] (*Parents' advocate*): But I don't think it's necessary for Vicki to continue to do that. I think you two parents can work out your problems without involving Vicki. Rebecca, you seem to me to be a very spirited woman, intelligent and determined. If you have issues you need to bring up with your husband I'm sure you can do it. You don't need your daughter to fight your battles for you, do you?

MOTHER: No, but I'm in the dark when you talk about Vicki fighting my battles for me.

VICKI: I think I can explain it to you. The way I see what they're saying—they're saying you have sacrificed a lot for daddy—like—for instance, your schooling. Not only for daddy but for the whole family too. You could have finished at school but you didn't. You moved here with the family and you didn't put up a fight about it. You didn't do a thing about it. You said one day I'll go back. I really doubt very much you'll go back to school, okay?

MOTHER: Yeah, I agree.

VICKI: That's just one example of a whole lot of things—living in this city—which, as you say, you didn't want to do—I didn't know you didn't want to do it until now. I'm not saying that's what I've been trying to do—fight my mother's battles for her—maybe I have and I just haven't realized it—but, you have given up a lot for daddy—sacrificed for daddy—not only for daddy but for the whole family.

THERAPIST 1 (*Stability position*): That's exactly my point and I think that you're doing that too, and that's why I disagree with you, my colleagues, here. I think mother couldn't bring her cause to her husband where it belongs because to do that would make a very strong statement that she is going to put her interests first, and the family's on the back burner. That would be very risky in this family.

THERAPIST 3 (*Parents' advocate*): I think Rebecca is the kind of woman that can do that—exactly the kind of woman that can do that. She has fortitude and courage and is perfectly capable of dealing with her husband in whatever way she has to deal with him, and if there are issues from the past—if she has issues she has buried, she is perfectly capable of bringing them out in the open and confronting him with them.

VICKI: If she is capable, she hasn't tried.

ALEX (*Oldest son*): She has tried but certain situations occurred—if she tries now—it will not be beneficial to the family. The family can't function in separation . . .

THERAPIST 3 (*Parents' advocate*): You mean if your mother brought out her issues with your father the family would fall apart? I think your father is flexible enough to listen to them.

VICKI: It's not like that. My father is very stubborn. I think I've taken after him. My mother doesn't want to destroy anything by being stubborn.

GREG (*Younger brother*): I know my mother could bring it up to him and be quite serious and do it in their bedroom alone, but I know my father would watch TV and wouldn't want necessarily to deal with the problem. It's not easy to recognize your problems.

FATHER: I don't see it that way—listen, I'm interested in the kids' perception—I don't feel that way. I don't know if my wife feels that way. Apparently there are some differences.

VICKI: But also I don't think it's only that he wouldn't listen—maybe he would—but it would take a certain amount of time and fighting to cause him to listen, and I don't think my mother would be willing to put everybody through that and to put herself through it. In a way—and I don't mean this bad at all, but in a way she is like my grandmother. My grandmother is very—like—passive. She can withstand. Like my mother would be able to withstand conforming to my father because she loves the family so much. She is willing to just forget about it for the family's sake and for my father's sake.

THERAPIST 1 (*Stability position*): It is clear Vicki has taken up your cause. And I think she will continue to do that because she believes it is the only way to hold the family together.

Bringing the Issues Out in the Open

This session brought into the open the family's fear of dissolution if mother rocked the boat. We learned that several years earlier the parents had separated for nine months after some heated arguments. Clearly, mother had made the decision to keep peace at any price. In doing so, she was assuming a typical woman's position of sacrificing her own best interests for the sake of her family. Vicki, following in mother's footsteps, was doing the same thing in a different way by offering to become symptomatic and divert the conflict between her parents so that they would not have to face a painful confrontation. The therapeutic debate was our way of making clear the price that was being paid for peace, who was paying it, and what the various alternatives were.

Mother arrived at the next session feeling vastly relieved that the issues she had difficulty raising were now out in the open. She had been given an audience in which her disagreements with her husband could be raised without being arbitrarily dismissed. She stated that she was no longer willing to sacrifice her daughter to keep peace in the family and that she had begun to fight with her husband. Father stated that he found the fights "upsetting, but enlightening," and he agreed to sessions alone with mother to deal with their disagreements. In these sessions, I focused on the relationship pattern between the parents in which mother catered to father's wishes, making them of primary importance while denying her own and then burying her resentments. Father was initially startled and defensive about mother's confrontations, but he soon began to experience the benefits of a more open and cooperative relationship. He stated, "It's actually a relief to know what's on her mind. Although I may not like to hear it, at least I can deal with it directly and don't have to keep wondering why she's upset."

As Vicki was freed from trying to resolve her parents' problem, she was able to relate to each of them in a different way. She and mother went through a stormy period for a time as mother, no longer feeling compelled to rescue her from father, began taking a firmer position with her. They fought it out together, but the fight was *between* them and not *through* father. Vicki was surprised at how strong her mother could be when she made up her mind to take a position. It was clear that she both admired and respected her mother's firmness even while fighting against it. Eventually she was convinced she could no longer manipulate either parent, and she settled into her life at school. When mother decided to go back to school and get the degree she had previously forfeited, Vicki expressed her pride by giving her a T-shirt that read, "GO FOR IT MOM!"

Summary

In this case, mother was caught in a dilemma. If she asserted herself with her husband, she ran the risk of breaking up the family. As mothers are trained to preserve family unity, she chose to bury her own wishes and comply with those of her husband. This impaired her ability to set appropriate limits for her daughter, who then acted as her surrogate in defying father and other authorities in her life. It would have been easy to see mother as an "overly protective" mother who undermined her husband's discipline. Instead, the therapists focused on the imbalance of power in the marital relationship and helped mother to express her disagreements with father. Although father initially tried to deny the conflicts between him and his wife, he was eventually relieved when they were brought out into the open. As a result he experienced a better relationship with both his wife and daughter. And when mother was able to rescue herself she stopped trying to rescue her daughter, and instead provided the strong, firm guidance that she needed.

Olga Silverstein

The Bad Mother

Feminism has forced many therapists to rethink some of their operating assumptions. The following illustrates an approach to a case in which the overriding goal might have been seen as helping a daughter separate from a mother who in fact had *not* been a "good" mother. It would be foolish to completely swing from earlier formulations of mothers as automatically "bad" medicine, engulfing, intrusive, infantalizing, and so on to the opposite pole of idealizing the idea of mother so that we lose sight of the reality. Indeed, women have been and are often cruel and uncaring toward their children, most especially toward their female children. We often hate in our children what we do not accept in ourselves.

Where a woman has been rejecting or abusing of her daughter, either physically or psychologically, the common-sense (or maybe the emotional) response is often to separate them as quickly as possible. Marianne Walters, in her introductory essay, talks about the freedom for mothers and daughters to be the same so that they can be comfortable with their differences.

The Denial of Similarity

This case demonstrates the opposite situation, that of a young woman so reactive to her mother and her mother's life-style that she has not only cut off totally from her mother but denies in herself any possibility of similarity. Only if she feels herself in opposition can she feel safe from those hateful traits she cannot accept in herself. In this case it was important for the daughter to declare her differences before she could admit any points of similarity with her mother; then she could begin the process of valuing herself as a woman, different from her mother but also the same.

The Presenting Problem

Recently, I received the following letter from a woman in Chicago.

>**Dear Mrs. S.:**
>
>I am writing to you in desperation. I have been told by friends who are in your field that you are interested in helping the relationship between mothers and daughters. We need help.
>
>My only daughter (I have three sons) lives in Denver. She has been there for the past three years. About a year ago she stopped talking to me. She won't answer my letters—she hangs up her phone when I call. She has told her brother that I am too dependent on her, and that her therapist told her that her "sanity" depended on her asserting herself. I am beside myself.
>
>If you would consent to see us, I'll try to get Susan to come. If she won't (which is probable) can I come by myself?
>
>**Mrs. G.**

Devising a Strategy

It is not unusual for a mother to call a therapist to request help in reconnecting with an estranged child. However, when an adult daughter has affected so drastic a cutoff as indicated in this letter, we can assume serious difficulty in the relationship. If a mother is then pursuing the daughter very vigorously, the daughter will more than likely tie herself to the lamp-post (read lover, therapist, career) so as not to feel carried away. In the mother's first letter we already see the extent of the problem, since the daughter quotes her therapist and speaks about the need to preserve her sanity. In this case, if a therapist were to join the mother in pursuing the daughter—in any way at all, even by gentle coaching of small moves—the daughter is apt to be driven further into flight, and perhaps even into drastic measures such as suicide. I sent back the following letter:

>**Dear Mrs. G:**
>
>If your daughter consents to come with you, you've already made progress, so by all means try.
>
>If she won't come with you—tell her that I won't see you alone because it wouldn't do any good, but I would see her alone.
>
>**Yours truly,**
>
>**O.S.**

If the daughter comes to a therapy session alone, then she is in charge of monitoring how far in or out of the relationship she wants or needs to stay at this time. The issue of separation from the mother is evident in the strong cutoff. I know that my message to mother—"I won't see you alone because it wouldn't do any good"—has been relayed to the daughter. She may find this reassuring enough to come in to see me.

Shortly after this exchange of letters, there ensued a series of phone calls from the daughter in Denver:

DAUGHTER: What does my mother want?

THERAPIST: I don't know exactly.

DAUGHTER: Why won't she leave me alone?

THERAPIST: She's your mother.

DAUGHTER: My therapist says it's a trap and I'll get sucked in again.

THERAPIST: Maybe.

DAUGHTER: You don't know how terrible she is. I'll come alone.

THERAPIST: Fine.

I knew that getting into long discussions with the daughter over the phone would be counterproductive. To pressure her to come in was to appear collusive with her mother.

I am careful to make no conciliatory statements. When she says about her mother, "You don't know how terrible she is," she's right. I don't.

The First Joint Session

Two weeks later—mother and daughter each called to give me a date when they would come in together. They both arrived promptly and met in the waiting room. Two appointments had been set up. The first was a late appointment on Friday, the second an early one on Monday. They had checked into separate hotels for the weekend.

Susan was a slight, too thin young woman. Thirty-two years old, she was dressed like a high-school girl of the fifties in a pleated plaid skirt, a cotton shirt, and beige shetland sweater. She wore no makeup. She greeted me with a formal handshake and said hello in a breathy, low voice. Mother was a woman in her early 50s dressed in a lavender pants suit. She was 30 to 40 pounds overweight. Quite elaborately made up, her flashy style was in sharp contrast to her daughter.

The Friday session began tensely. Mother described a rather chaotic household. She had married Susan's father when she was 18 and left him four years later, then married twice more and divorced twice more. She giggled girlishly as she said, "I have lousy taste in men."

Meanwhile Susan sat primly, her hands folded in her lap. She described moving away from mother to live in Denver. After her first serious relationship broke up, she went into therapy. Now her therapist was helping her to separate from her mother. Susan wept when she said that she was 32 years old and still struggling to "separate."

Interpreting the Relationship

Mother and daughter had had a close relationship until mother's second marriage. The mother then became involved with her new (very demanding) husband. She had two pregnancies and babies in three years. When that marriage ended, Susan was in her early teens. She took on much of the responsibility for her two little brothers since mother had a long bout with a debilitating depression.

Susan's difficulty in simply stepping out of her mother's life and saying she's not my kind of person or her inability (after years of therapy) in confronting her mother is partly because she doesn't fully understand the extent of her anger and sense of betrayal. In a social system that values a woman's relationship to a man as having top priority, putting a girl child on the back burner in favor of a new husband seemed appropriate to both mother and daughter.

When mother's marriage ended she again leaned on Susan, from whom she expected understanding and help. Susan, only too glad to have her mother back, moved in to take care of her and the little brothers.

When the mother married the third time, Susan, then 19, moved out of the house but continued a worried concern for her brothers. At 19, Susan was again displaced for a man. What must she have experienced of herself and of being female? We can only conjecture. That she missed whatever form of contact she had had with her mother is evident in her behavior. She seldom saw her mother, but obsessed about her constantly.

Some seven years later and after the birth of another son, mother was again divorced and moved again to re-engage her daughter.

Susan moved as far away as she could. When she found herself lost and lonely and still obsessing about her mother—sometimes in rage, sometimes with a longing she was ashamed of—Susan connected with a therapist in Denver. Her therapist was warm and empathic, and she joined Susan in her efforts to shake loose of her unreliable mother. "She only wants me now because she's alone—even the boys are growing up and they don't want to have much to do with her." As Susan moved further and further away from her mother in practice (if not emotionally) she rarely called and hadn't been home in a year. When mother escalated her pursuit of Susan, with the help of her therapist Susan cut off completely; she wouldn't answer calls, sent back presents, and refused all contact.

A Therapist's Intervention

At the end of the two-hour session, with mother and daughter each telling her story in turn and Susan frequently interrupting her mother to correct a date or a fact, I proposed the following intervention:

"It's going to be a long weekend—you will be bored and lonely—but I think it was very wise to take separate hotels. I think it's probably best that you don't spend time together, but this is what I want you to do. You are each to buy a large spiral notebook and in it you are to make a list of all the ways that you are different from each other." The instruction to fill the notebooks with the ways that they were different was the lamppost I was offering Susan against the forces that she felt were pulling her in.

> SUSAN: Did you say "different"? I don't know what you mean.
> MOTHER: Well, like—I like junk food and you don't—am I right?
> THERAPIST: That's right.
> SUSAN: I can fill two notebooks.
> THERAPIST: Good, you have all weekend.

On Monday they arrived together. Like two conspirators they confessed that by Saturday evening they had tired of doing their homework. Susan had called her mother and suggested a movie. Sunday they lunched together and went to the theater. They both seemed more relaxed.

People knowing my work might assume that my instruction that mother and daughter spend time alone, explicating their differences, was a paradoxical move calculated to bring them together. I had no such intention. I knew that Susan might need permission to remain apart and that her mother needed instructions to leave Susan alone. Giving them the same task to perform put them on the same level. Frequently in cases where there has been a reversal of roles, the therapist may attempt to put things right by requesting the younger woman to ask the older for advice or help, thus keeping in place the right hierarchical order (a notion we've inherited from a patriarchal culture). In this case, Susan was not about to let her mother "mother" her. Her enormous defense against this need was embedded mostly in her anger and determination to stay "separate." I did not wish to tamper with this determination. There is danger in infantalizing a 32-year-old woman in the service of sustaining her relationship with her mother.

Susan had filled 42 pages of her notebook, her mother, 5. I had them read alternately:

Mother read: "I'm sloppy, Susan is neat."

Susan read: "I'm neat, my mother is sloppy."

By the fifth sentence they were both laughing. I had them read on to the end. Clearly in both their perceptions Susan was the overresponsible adult and mother the irresponsible one. I then suggested that they exchange notebooks and that they pick a trait from each other's list to practice over the summer—one a week. I then asked each of them to call me at the end of the summer.

On the way out, Susan picked up her checkbook. I stopped her with, "Why are you doing your mother's job?" Her mother then said, "You pay for Friday, I'll pay for today." Again they laughed.

At the end of the summer Susan called to say that she had had a very good summer. She had to make quite a few calls home because she needed explanations from mother about some of the items on the list of traits she was practicing. Mother called to say that she had been inexplicably depressed for the first few weeks, but gradually realized what was happening. "Susan and I are really talking. I guess you meant for me to grow up. I'm really trying," she said.

Discussion of Consultation

With the help of her therapist, who called me shortly after Susan's return, Susan was able to use the consultation session to more clearly see her mother's limitations as separate from herself. Her calls to her mother concerned those items on the list of traits that puzzled her. For instance, mother had written, "I am a very dependent person, Susan is very independent." The idea that her mother (or anyone) could possibly see her as independent at first angered and then amused her.

Mother, on the other hand, came face to face with her own life. Reading Susan's list of 42 items pained her. Her previous pattern of flight into a new relationship with a man was, now that she was 51, not as available to her. She was now in danger of idealizing her daughter and fulfilling one of Susan's greatest fears, of becoming too dependent on her. I suggested to her that a therapist with a systems orientation would be helpful for her as well, and made such a referral.

Had I seen this mother and daughter ten years ago, I might have agreed to see the mother individually in order to encourage her to let her daughter go. I would have talked to her about her dependency on her daughter, and the importance of letting the young woman live her own life. Since then, I have learned that seeing such a mother individually is counterproductive when the request for help concerns a relationship with a child. The daughter can view her mother's relationship with a therapist as a "conspiracy" to hook her back into the relationship, and the effect is often to drive the daughter further away. However, I *will* agree to see a daughter in this kind of family individually because such a move respects the independence that she feels depends on her distance. I can then help her to define the difference between independence and separation.

In working with this mother and daughter, it was important to me that neither of them feel guilty or apologize for the past. I wanted to set up a context in which blame and defense were irrelevant, and in which each woman could respect her differences from the other while learning to affirm some of her similarities.

I do not mean to suggest that a single meeting or clever intervention can solve a lifelong relationship problem. I had had long telephone calls with both women before they came to see me. I could see that a shift in their behavior was already taking place. Both mother and daughter were taking responsibility for their relationship by calling me and coming all the way to see me. I saw my job as validating what was already happening, and moving it forward in a slightly dramatic way.

In my long telephone calls with Susan, I had learned that her *perception* of a relationship with her mother meant a merging, so I assigned the task of having her write down all the ways in which she was different from her mother. It was a very reassuring task for her, because she was so afraid of being viewed as *like* her mother. So she filled 42 pages with ways that she was different. Once that was done, I could help mother and daughter acknowledge similarities. After they both accepted that it was okay to be different, I instructed them to choose ways in which they could be alike.

But therapeutic techniques can only take you so far. It is the therapist's point of view that is crucial. I approach cases like this one with the very strong belief that the relationship between mother and daughter is very valuable and needs to be confirmed. When the past has been hurtful and difficult, that, too, has to be recognized and verbalized.

Issues of individuation and separation have long been confused not only in the therapeutic community but in the social climate of America in the eighties. A daughter who "fails" to make the proper gesture of leaving home by the time she's 20 is often viewed by the family, her peers, and whoever else is looking as problematic. Conversely, a young woman who leaves home at 19 is often perceived automatically as having made a move toward autonomy.

Similarly, where a mother remarries, a daughter's move out of town is too often seen as an appropriate gesture of separation. Family therapists who have been trained in a structural model may use the notion of hierarchy to elevate the spousal relationship at the expense of the relationship of a mother to her children. In a remarriage the new male-female dyad is often protected by everyone concerned. Underlying this support of the parental dyad is the assumption that (1) the protection of the mother is bound up with protecting her relationship to a man; (2) if all is well with the marriage its effects will "trickle down" to the children; and (3) the parent and not the child is the client.

Separation can be understood in its common-sense meaning as distancing. Susan had, in fact, separated totally. But in no way had she achieved that formation of an individual self that subsumes a recognition of one's own potentials as different than, but *connected* to, those of another. Individuation is the formation of an individual self, and can only be achieved in context with another.

Interpersonal relationships are unavoidably marked by ambivalence between wishes for and fears of closeness, and wishes for and fears of distance. During the process of individuation new ways of balancing closeness and distance must constantly be sought (Simon, Stierlin, and Wynne, 1985). This is especially true in relationships between mothers and daughters.

3   *Betty Carter*

Fathers and Daughters

THE RELATIONSHIP BETWEEN father and daughter is fraught with ambivalence. In middle-class families, father wants daughter to "succeed," but still sees marriage as the main goal for her; she wants to be "independent," but will spend enormous energy trying to win father's approval, and will become angry or distant if she fails to obtain it. He may spend a fortune on her education, but still not expect personal achievement of her; she may admire many of his achievements, and then push her husband and sons, instead of herself, to match them. He prides himself on his strength and competence, but then rewards compliance and dependency in his relationship with her. She values direct emotional expression, but learns that flattery and deceit work in dealing with him.

For both father and daughter, these contradictions have only increased as the role of women has changed in our lifetime. Supportive fathers have become all the more confused about what expectations and hopes to have for their daughters. Authoritarian fathers try desperately to hold on to the past so as to escape the necessity of redefining their own roles in response to changes in their daughters. On her part, the daughter wants her father's approval, even for choices or lifestyles that she knows he doesn't accept. But in seeking both approval and "independence," she may become distant, afraid to discuss these choices with him and thus incur his angry disapproval; or she may seek "autonomy" through reactive defiance and rebellion.

In the families of the poor, the roles of all family members are so determined and constricted by the effects of racism and poverty that no discussion of family dynamics can be divorced from the devastating social context. With family members almost totally blocked from access to social and economic security, the existence of problems in family functioning is hardly surprising. Thus, the absent father, or the peripheral, powerless father, are predictable problems in poor families, as is the tendency of their daughters to be pulled into complementary caretaking roles, or to remain distant and cut off from their fathers.

Interestingly, often it is the most highly successful and socially powerful men who make the greatest demands on their wives and daughters for deference and compliance. In the upper class, father's iron rule is often clothed in the benevolence of material affluence and thus fails to appear to be much of a problem outside of the family. His authoritarianism will be excused by society on the grounds that he is very important, very busy, and thus deserving of accommodation from others.

Daughters of any social class who grow up in families where fathers are physically or emotionally absent for whatever reasons often develop negative and condescending attitudes toward men and shift their energies toward more rewarding family relationships with their mothers or siblings, or they develop a fantasized "ideal man" forever yearned for and sought after.

Psychology has not helped us to understand the painful transition that is underway in our society but, on the contrary, generally adds to the confusion concerning the changing roles of women in both the family and the larger society. Both professional and popular wisdom have generally held that *father* is the key to the daughter's success in love and work, the two most important activities in life. In accordance with this thinking, women who have less than adequate relationships with their fathers will presumably have difficulty sustaining intimacy, will select inappropriate boyfriends, lovers, or husbands, will have sexual problems, will perhaps be lesbians, perhaps divorce, perhaps never marry.

With fathers supposedly responsible for all of these problems, one wonders why so many women blame their *mothers* for how they turned out. In our patriarchal culture, it sometimes seems that father gets the credit for daughter's success, and mother gets the blame for her failure.

Power

The issue of power in father-daughter relationships is difficult to identify as a problem because of its congruence with the values of the larger society.

In a world that runs on power and that values male over female, fathers and daughters are on opposite ends of the spectrum, with him in the most powerful position and her in the least. From this position, the traditional requirement of the "good father" was to protect his daughter from other men. Over most of recorded history, however, there was no one to protect the daughter from father if he abused his power. Mothers and daughters learned, therefore, to monitor his moods and needs, to try to meet them, to head off the ill humor that might be taken out on them.

Historically, daughters could consider themselves fortunate if they were protected and provided for adequately by their fathers until he "handed them over" to a husband to continue the job. Throughout most of history, father, and then husband, made all of the decisions that affected daughter's life, from childhood through old age. (Should her husband predecease her, a son would pick up the decision-making role.) The truly amazing realization is how little, not how much, these patterns have changed until this generation.

Common Triangles

Following are several "snapshots" of typical father-daughter entanglements.

Pygmalion

Consider the possibility that father, who may have had trouble dealing with his mother, and whose wife resists one way or another his efforts to control her, has, in a daughter, a final chance to be "treated like a man," whatever that means to him. If it means being able to help, always able to provide, then he will respond positively to his daughter when she elicits these characteristics in him by being correspondingly compliant, weak, dependent, and needy. She will not be "feminine" or "treating him like a man" if she imitates her brothers and appears competitive or defiant. If father succeeds in getting this message across to daughter, she will grow up to become a "perfect wife"—dependent and deferential.

Tug of War

A common problem for daughters is getting caught up on father's side in the power struggle between father and mother. Fathers help to program their daughters for this problem whenever they share with daughter comments or looks that criticize mother, or secrets that exclude her; or every time they play "Mr. Nice Guy" against mother, pleading leniency for daughter. Fathers who use the latter method of "winning" over their wives are not only contributing to mother-daughter difficulties but training their daughters to need rescue. A variation of this triangle, to which oldest daughters are particularly vulnerable, is accomplished when father "loses" to mother and his depression or complaints pull daughter in to take care of him emotionally. This triangle will also result in mother-daughter conflict, but father and daughter have switched places, with father as the "victim" needing "rescue" by daughter.

When father plays "tyrant" and mother plays "peacemaker" in the parental tug of war, daughter may be sucked into the rebellious role, opposing father in ways mother doesn't dare; or she may submit, as mother does.

My Heart Belongs to Daddy

This triangle of father, daughter, and daughter's boyfriend, lover, or husband enables father to "win" over his rivals for daughter's devotion. He may accomplish this victory, with suitable cooperation from all involved, in a number of ways.

He can form a strong alliance with his son-in-law based on business, money, or power and they can, between them, share decisions that "take care of her." Or he can criticize and antagonize his son-in-law, putting daughter into a loyalty conflict that upsets her marriage. Or he can simply ignore the "interloper," continuing to provide advice or gifts and demanding the attention that proves he's still the "number one man in her life." Everyone knows that "a son is a son till he gets him a wife, but a daughter's a daughter for all of her life"!

Get Up on That Pedestal and Stay There!

This triangle is one in which father and other men try to keep the world's work and money and power to themselves with rationalizations that it is "too hard," or "too dirty," or "too rough" for women, who are "too sensitive," "too fragile," or "too nice" for politics or business. In this triangle, daughter is apprenticed to mother, who is also "above it all" and preferably "sainted," and who trains her to be a "good wife" to one of father's protegés and a "good mother" to the next generation's sons and daughters.

Work: Entitlement or Chutzpah?

Around the issue of *work* all the questions of power, authority, entitlement, and expectations converge for fathers and daughters.

The father's crucial input is in his expectations. He may expect daughter to work, but not to engage in a demanding career. If she enters business, he may expect her to quit when she has a baby, or to switch to part-time or volunteer work that will not "interfere" with her family life. Worst of all, he may criticize her choice of work, and press advice and suggestions that lead her to experience guilt and conflict.

For the daughter, the critical questions center around entitlement. Am I entitled to pursue my dreams and ambitions even if they conflict with my father's expectations? Do I need his permission? his help? his approval? And if I *do* need it, how can I get it, or get along without it? Daughter's entitlement to pursue her goals depends on many factors. If father is the only one in the family with a "real" career, and this has always been the case, then his influence and his responsibility toward daughter in this area are, indeed, very large. He can smooth her pathway to the world of work or make work an area of eternal conflict for her. In today's world, she can probably succeed in spite of her father's disapproval, but at the expense of extra stress, and at a great cost to their relationship.

In Margaret Hennig's study of twenty-five top women executives (Hennig and Jardim, 1978), they were found to share the following characteristics:

1. All were oldest or only children.
2. All had no more than two siblings, who were *all* girls (that is, no sons in these families).
3. All had a "typical" relationship with their mothers (that is, a good one).
4. All had an "atypical" relationship with their fathers (that is, an unusually involved and supportive one).
5. Ninety-two percent of the mothers had educations equal to the fathers, and 52 percent of them had superior educations.

Since fathers have typically been given more credit than mothers for children's work success, much has been made of the relationship with father (number 4 in the list) in the literature discussing Hennig's study, while characteristics 2, 3, and 5 are generally ignored or passed over quickly (McGoldrick, 1984). It is not widely known that the work status of mothers is a more significant predictor of success of both sons and daughters than the work status of fathers (Lozoss, 1974).

In a book called *Fathers and Daughters* (1981), the author William Appleton, a psychiatrist who writes a monthly advice column for *Cosmopolitan* magazine, says that to be successful, women need their father's help and instruction in entering the world of work, learning to be judged instead of indulged, and learning that getting ahead is not the same as getting along; that being respected doesn't always feel as comfortable as being liked. Dr. Appleton's advice, although well intentioned, sounds suspiciously like a suggestion that if women are to succeed in the world of work, then we'd better act and think more like men, and learn to negotiate the work system in the same competitive style that men have established there.

This, then, is the dilemma for daughter: With or without father's support, can you enter the "rat race" without becoming one of the rats (Janeway, 1982)? Elizabeth Janeway, the feminist writer, says that as more women gain positions of power in government and business, there will be the opportunity to factor female ways of perception and behavior into the system; to humanize work, so that eventually men and women may replace the "rats." The social and political task facing today's daughters, then, is to get enough power to change the system into one that is more just and equitable, that with equal pay and equal opportunity, with flextime and child-care provisions, will support the full participation of both men and women in work *and* the family.

In order to understand these issues in a given family and to do effective clinical work, it is necessary for the clinician to keep clearly in mind the historical, social, economic and political context in which father-daughter problems arise and are maintained. If we do not keep in mind the enormous impact of the social level of the system, we will fail to address the assumptions on which fathers and daughters base their behavior, and we will be prone to pathologize the problem or to blame fathers or daughters for behaviors and attitudes that were taught to them and reinforced by our society. As we now shift attention to the clinical work at the family level, please keep in mind the social context, one level up, that organizes the family system.

Dysfunctional Father-Daughter Patterns

This discussion focuses on four major dysfunctional father-daughter patterns: cut-off, distant, enmeshed, and perverse. Each major pattern has both conflictual and nonconflictual variations; it should be conceptualized as part of a triangle rather than as a purely dyadic interaction, and as not limited merely to the nuclear family, but multigenerational in scope. We should keep in mind that even this conceptual unit (the transgenerational triangle) offers a reductive view of the relationship problem, which actually is embedded in a much more complex family system, with all its members, rules, and themes. And, of course, beyond the family level, the relationship is influenced by the complexities and mandates of the social, cultural, and political system that shapes the family. The formulations given here are meant to suggest a conceptual approach to the problem, and not to provide a complete analysis. My theoretical framework is based on Bowen family systems theory, as revised or adapted to explicitly include the factor of gender and its connections to the social values in which the family system is embedded.

The Cut-off Father-Daughter Relationship

Bowen systems theory and feminist theory are in agreement about the importance of emotional connectedness and the dysfunction that results when significant relationships are disrupted or cut off.

CUTOFF BY DEATH If a father dies when his daughter is very young, the chances are that he will continue to exert a strong influence on her life through fantasy. It is very common in this situation for father to be idealized by his daughter, who then conducts an impossibly perfect relationship with him in her head. The more father is idealized, the more negativity may be directed toward mother, who is, after all, "merely human." And, of course, if mother remarries, there is an extremely high likelihood of intense conflict between daughter and the man who tries to take her father's place. This relationship can be described by means of the following genogram:

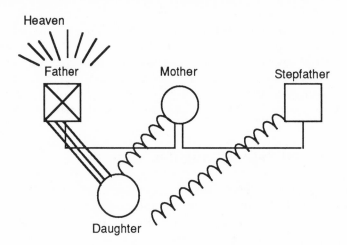

A **genogram** (family diagram) is a map that provides a graphic picture of family structure and emotional process over time. It was developed by Murray Bowen, MD, and it has become a standard form among clinicians for describing families. My version of the genogram is used in case examples throughout this book. Bowen uses other symbols to denote other details. (See M. McGoldrick and R. Gerson, *Genograms in Family Asessment*. New York: W. W. Norton, 1985.)

A complete genogram should include:

(1) Names and ages of all family members.
(2) Exact dates of birth, marriage, separation, divorce, death, and other significant life events.
(3) Notations with dates, about occupation, places of residence, illness, and changes in life course, on the genogram itself.
(4) Information on three or more generations.

Key to important symbols: Male: ☐   Female: ○   Death ⊠ or ⊗

Marriage: Husband on left, wife on right

In these interlocking triangles, father is flash-frozen in perfection, daughter's attitude toward stepfather is "you're not my father," and mother is caught in the middle. The most insidious characteristic of this situation is that since father is probably not often discussed, the adults may not be aware of daughter's fantasy relationship with him. And almost any move, positive or negative, that the stepfather makes toward the daughter will be fiercely resisted by her out of loyalty to her "real" father.

Resolution of this situation can be brought about by encouraging the family to talk to daughter about who her father actually was as a person or, if daughter is an adult, coaching her to find out about him. She needs to "resurrect" him, and then bury him again, once and for all. This means that daughter needs to replace her fantasized ideal image with an idea of her father as the real person he was, with his real strengths and weaknesses, good points and failings. She needs to grieve his loss in her life, and then to acknowledge his death in some concrete way (such as a memorial service or other ritual) so that she can let go of him and move on in her life. This may mean accepting a stepfather if she is young or, later on, being able to accept the ordinary faults of a husband rather than comparing the men in her life to an impossibly heroic ideal image of a man made up from social myths about men and fathers. Paradoxically, by reducing the dead father to human size, she connects emotionally with the person he was and rescues their mental relationship from total distortion.

CUTOFF BY DIVORCE   Some divorces result in father-daughter cut off. In this pattern, if the daughter is young when the cutoff occurs, it is more probable that daughter will grow up with a negative attitude toward her father. Unlike the daughter whose father died, she will find no excuses for his absence other than the idea that he doesn't care about her. Since the parents are cut off, there is not much likelihood of positive input about father from mother; in fact, negative input is more likely.

Children: Listed in birth order beginning on the left with the oldest:

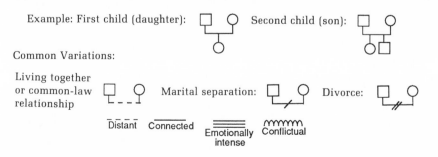

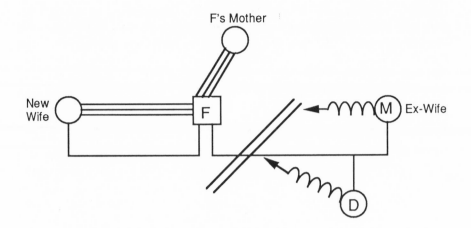

See page 96 for an extended definition of the genogram.

In their mutual anger at father, there is a collusive element in mother and daughter's relationship; and if they are isolated from extended family and social networks, daughter is a prime candidate for the emotional caretaker role. Since the intensity of other attachments on either side of a cutoff more or less matches the intensity of the cutoff, father may have an intensely dependent relationship with his mother or a new wife, which helps keep the cutoff going on his side, just as mother and daughter's mutual anger at him keeps it going on their side. Resolution of this triangle, as in the first example, can come about when daughter reconnects with father as a way of ending doubts and fantasies regarding herself and her history.

However, unlike exorcising a ghost, this daughter will find an actual person to whom to relate. And that person, although he is her biological father, will be a *stranger*. As in the case of adopted children who look up their biological parents, anyone who reconnects with a long-lost father will discover that although finding him ends one set of problems, it opens up a new set, namely, what their relationship will actually become. For while it is true that genetics has made them "significant others," only the process of "being there" for each other will make them emotionally father and daughter.

The Distant Father-Daughter Relationship

In this pattern, daughter may experience her distant father either positively or negatively.

DISTANT AND POSITIVE FATHER-DAUGHTER PATTERN   In American families, the pattern in which daughter (especially oldest or only daughter) feels warmly toward her distant father and negatively toward mother, to whom she is actually closer, is one of the most common family triangles. One of the reasons for the prevalence of this pattern is the fact that so many fathers have given most of their attention and energy to their work, leaving their wives to struggle with child rearing almost alone. Feelings of guilt or lack of familiarity with the complexities of domestic questions often lead father into the "Mr. Nice Guy" response that leaves mother holding the bag. In addition, the so-called "distant but nice" father is also suffering the emotional consequences of having established the socially mandated "polite but distant" relationship with his mother.

In this scenario, the parental relationship may be either conflictual or pseudomutual.

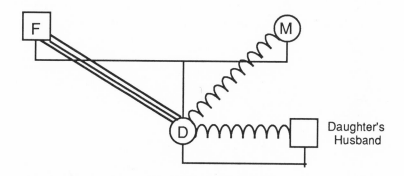

Daughter's Husband

See page 96 for an extended definition of the genogram.

The more closed the communication in the family, the more covert is the father-daughter alliance and the more vague and unclear its basis. Daughter senses without being told that she is father's favorite child, or that he prefers her to mother, or that she's like father in some ways that annoy mother. They are secret allies with an unspoken bond, and daughter stands up to mother in a way father never does. She understands that her conflict with mother doesn't really upset him; quite the contrary. Of course, if mother's upset gets intense enough to be a problem for *him*, the parental "united front" suddenly lets daughter know that she's gone too far. The more conflictual daughter's relationship with mother, the deeper her warmth and sympathy for dad for "having to put up with her." If you ask her which parent she is "closer" to, she will answer "father," mistaking the feeling of alliance for closeness. Actually, you will usually find that she knows next to nothing about father or his family. In this triangle, daughter has little understanding of the parents' *mutual* dependency, and mother's dilemma is invisible because of the triangulation. It is common for a daughter in this position in the parental triangle to choose a husband who reminds her of "dear old dad," and then to fall into a conflictual marital pattern in which she repeats, in dealing with her husband, the relationship with her closer parent—mother.

Daughter has much to gain from the resolution of this situation. Getting to know her father as an imperfect person rather than as a "saint" or a "victim" will reduce the tension with both mother and husband sufficiently for those relationships to improve almost automatically. As the daughter discovers the ways in which she is like her father, she can openly identify with him instead of blaming her mother for not appreciating dad, and blaming her husband for not appreciating the same qualities in her.

DISTANT AND NEGATIVE FATHER-DAUGHTER PATTERN   In this variation of the distant pattern, daughter has a collusive relationship with mother and feels very negative toward the distant father.

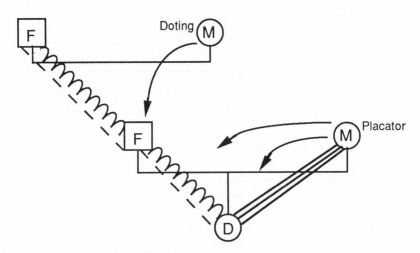

See page 96 for an extended definition of the genogram.

In a typical set of triangles illustrating this pattern, father will function overresponsibly somewhere along the spectrum from "boss" to "tyrant." He may have been close to a doting mother and so have learned early to expect compliance or catering from those close to him. His wife accepts his dominance, placating him when he's upset and generally looking "put upon" to the children. Daughter, who feels sorry for mother and is allied with her, feels anger and contempt for father. She blames him for not giving more to mother and herself. However, father is not very involved in her life, and since they are so distant, the tension between father and daughter may well remain covert during daughter's adolescence. She thinks the negative thoughts about dad that mother wouldn't dream of. She will be cold and distant, refusing to placate him and refusing his attempts, often blunt and untactful, to advise or take care of her. If they arrive at the office of a family therapist, father's distance and lack of involvement will often be seen as "normal," and mother and daughter's warm relationship will be scrutinized for "overinvolvement" and made the focus of the therapeutic work. When daughter leaves home, she'll stay as distant as duty will allow. If the stress gets high enough, however, her emotionally loaded relationship with father may explode into open conflict or cut-off.

The movie *On Golden Pond* provides an excellent illustration of this pattern of relating and how it can be resolved. Mother (Katharine Hepburn) encourages daughter (Jane Fonda) to come to terms with her father (Henry Fonda), from whom she has been angrily distant and is on the verge of cutting off. Father has never been able to relate to his daughter in a way that got through to her. Daughter's interpretation of her difficulties with her father is that he wanted a son and doesn't love her. Daughter points to him in the distance, out fishing and having a wonderful time with her young stepson. Mother reminds her that father is old and will not live long, and daughter decides to try again to relate to him.

First, she approaches him and takes the risk of being vulnerable. She tells him important personal news—that she has gotten married. Much to her surprise—in a distant relationship, people don't know each other well enough to accurately predict behavior—father's response is positive. Now daughter does something else that is different in their relationship. Instead of insisting that her father change *his* way of relating to her, perhaps through talk or through showing interest in her world, daughter accepts her father for who he is and moves toward him in his way. She reminds him that he used to try to teach her to do a backflip dive, and that she couldn't ever do it right. Now she will show him that she can.

Daughter's willingness to end the power struggle over who needs to change, and to approach her father in a way that he would understand and value, is her step into maturity. Such a step couldn't be taken as long as it was understood to be "capitulation," which is how it might appear to a rebellious adolescent or young adult. Nor could such a step be taken by a daughter overwhelmed by feelings of hurt, rejection, or anger, which is how this daughter previously reacted to her father's efforts to relate to her in his way. Now, giving up the need to "win" her battle with him, she is willing to accept his nonverbal, sports-oriented way of relating as being his best or only way of moving toward her. One would hope she is making this effort as a step in her own differentiation, and not in order to placate mother or to make Dad happy before he dies.

It is thus with a lot of unspoken but understood emotion that father gives her his old college diving medal as she leaves, and she calls him "Dad" instead of Norman. Daughter has changed her approach toward her father instead of continuing to insist that he change his approach to her. She seeks his support and a connection with him through the metaphor of the dive he had wanted to teach her, and he responds positively, using the same metaphor, by giving her the diving medal. Their closer relationship is sealed with a hug, and, by calling him "Dad," daughter signifies that she has come to terms with who he is and that she accepts him.

This is an example of the resolution on a personal and family level of a problem that relates to issues of male socialization. That is, sexist social values that might lead a man to be disappointed that his only child is a daughter, or that permit him to remain so distant and inflexible that he can't figure out appropriate ways to relate to a daughter, might have to be understood and forgiven on a personal level, although they need not be condoned socially. If we take our film example, for instance, to be a real family, one would hope that now that daughter has healed the breach with her father by demonstrating her willingness to enter and accept his world, he can be helped to find ways to enter her world and to connect to daughter in ways that *she* values.

Enmeshed Father-Daughter Relationship

In the enmeshed patterns, father and daughter are more involved with each other, in collusion or in conflict, than either of them is with mother.

NONCONFLICTUAL VARIATION: "DADDY'S LITTLE GIRL"   In the nonconflictual variation of this enmeshed pattern, father has made an ally of his daughter and is, therefore, most influential in her life. As with other dysfunctional patterns, one of the most pernicious characteristics of this variation is that it is generally experienced as benign by daughter, and is so intended by father. Its problematic aspects may thus be invisible to mother (and to therapists) because of all father-daughter patterns, it comes closest to the culture's ideal. The bargain is this: daddy will give daughter everything in his power to give and, in exchange, she will never reject or challenge his authority. In other words, she may grow old but she may never grow up.

In the parental triangle, father and mother may fight over daughter's upbringing, with mother feeling left out and angry; or mother may acquiesce in daddy's wishes, becoming more like a sibling than a mother to her daughter, with both mother and daughter equally oriented toward daddy's wishes, his rewards, and his punishments. In either case, daughter has been promised a rose garden. She has been

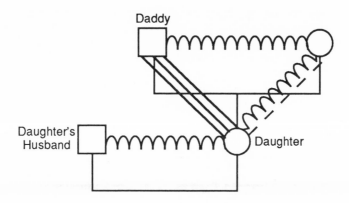

Daddy

Daughter's Husband

Daughter

See page 96 for an extended definition of the genogram.

programmed to expect a good and happy life without any effort on her part except compliance.

Push really comes to shove for daddy's girl in her marriage, where conflict or harmony will depend on a number of variables: (1) what daddy thinks of her husband; (2) whether husband lives up to daddy's treatment of her or falls short of it; (3) whether husband accepts daddy's authority or wants her to challenge his top status. Even if there is no conflict, the emptiness and loneliness of daughter's life as she ages without maturing leaves her vulnerable to psychosomatic symptoms and to overdependency on her husband and children.

If daddy's little girl responds to her midlife crisis, or to the women's movement, with the idea of trying to take charge of her life, she will dump most of the blame for her childlike status on her husband, and he may find himself divorced before he finds out what the problem is. And daughter may go home to daddy, or depend on his emotional and financial support, without the slightest realization that such behavior does not exactly constitute "taking charge of your own life." Many divorces are precipitated by women who don't know any *intermediate* way to assert themselves with their husbands since they never were permitted to argue with daddy. Therapy for daddy's girl must begin with an extended course of "assertiveness training," along with reconciliation of mother and daughter.

THE CONFLICTUAL FATHER-DAUGHTER RELATIONSHIP   In this extremely common enmeshed pattern of relating, father is once again the Boss and mother typically assumes a placating or peacemaker position regarding her own and her daughter's relationship with him. However, daughter is a lot like her mother in some way that annoys father and also a lot more outspoken in her defiance of him. She may also refuse to cater to father in the way he was trained to expect.

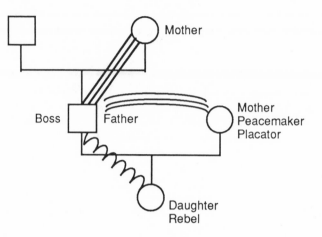

See page 96 for an extended definition of the genogram.

While she is a child, father is quite involved in directing daughter's life, on his own or through mother. During adolescence, when her growing independence threatens his role, father increases his efforts to control her, and daughter escalates her level of rebellion. She is aware that mother is often silently on her side in the battle against father, which adds fuel to the fire. Although mother's alliance with daughter may be covert, daughter knows on some level that she is fighting her mother's battles with father as well as her own. What entirely escapes her, however, is her own *collusion* with father, whereby their battles protect him from having to deal with his wife.

The major hazard for daughter is that she will devote her life to being or doing the opposite of what her father wants for her without really finding out what she wants for herself. The biggest pitfall for father is that he will let his marriage stagnate or die as he focuses on the battle with daughter, and then also lose her as she grows older and uses distance or cutoff to deal with him.

The conflictual pattern is harder for most daughters to overcome than patterns of distance. In the first place, by expressing a lot of anger directly to a man, she has broken a cardinal taboo for women; and she will feel like a bitch for doing it, no matter how justified she thinks her anger is. Secondly, during the heat of their battle, conflictual fathers and daughters will have said and done so many hurtful things that their list of grievances seems endless. Worst of all, the conflict is a power struggle, and giving it up feels like "losing." Daughter's motivation to extricate herself from this dysfunctional pattern without cutting off may depend on the ability of the therapist to reframe her moves to change the relationship as "winning" in some way. For example, the therapist might suggest: "Won't he be totally bewildered if you show up looking happy and successful instead of depressed and down-and-out?"

Perverse Intergenerational Patterns

In these father-daughter patterns there is a blurring or eradication of generational and personal boundaries to the degree that even the most basic responsibilities of parental functioning are neglected or transgressed. Examples of this include every kind of behavior in which the father functions below the minimal level necessary to promote the growth, individuation, and development of the daughter.

INCEST   Incest, the ultimate family secret, was until very recently also a social secret, with many or most cases of incest going unreported and with most people, including many mental health professionals, likely to deny its relatively widespread occurrence across economic and class lines.

A FEW FINDINGS

1. An article in the journal *Social Work* (Conte, 1984) stated that adults who sexually abuse children are strangers to the children in only 8 to 10 percent of the cases. Forty-seven percent of the offenders are members of the children's own families, and another 40 percent are known by the children although not by family members. Eighty percent of the victims are female. Eighty percent of the victims are under 12 years of age, and victims appear at all socioeconomic levels.

2. Herman and Hirschman (1977) summarized various surveys in the United States and Europe indicating that 90 percent of the reported cases of incest involved fathers and daughters. Fathers and sons accounted for another 5 percent, mothers and sons for 4 percent, with 1 percent others such as brothers or sisters, grandfathers, uncles, or the like.

3. Another study of father-daughter incest (Herman and Hirschman, 1977) reported that the majority of the daughters were oldest or only daughters; that they were between age 6 and 9 when the incest began; and that it continued for an average of three years. In general, incestuous activity with preadolescent children does not include sexual intercourse, but it is nevertheless overtly sexual and is soon understood by even the youngest child to be improper and shameful.

4. Most daughters realize the power of their secret and the risk to the family of revealing it. When they do report it, it is not usually to the mother but to some outside authority. Neither father nor mother usually reports incest to the authorities.

The most common explanation of incest in the field of mental health has been to blame mother for it, although some articles on the subject also blame daughter's "seductiveness," regardless of her age. Mother is cited as having certain negative personality traits as well as failing to protect her daughter, first by denying and then by failing to report the incest (McIntyre, 1981). Whether any of these conditions do, in fact, exist, they are in no way sufficient or even essential to the symptom of incest, for which the most significant triangle almost always involves father, daughter, and one or both of father's parents.

This triangle, connecting father to the parent who abused him in childhood, should not be understood as "past history," but is more correctly seen as an intense, smoldering, arrested, perverse relationship pattern to which father is still reacting in the present. If father has acknowledged the abuse and is available for therapy, treatment should focus on resolving the issues between him and his parents as more relevant to the current problem than nuclear family relationships. This focus on the wellspring of father's behavior in no way excuses it or eliminates the need for him to take personal responsibility for it. Quite the contrary. But on the family level, the inadequacy of the typical mental health approach has usually resulted in scapegoating the wife or the child-victim. The focus on nuclear family structure has often obscured the chaos in the extended family, its intense and *current* influence on the problem, and its possibilities as a direction for treatment.

Furthermore, the incest pattern provides a prime example of the inadequacy of the mental health profession's narrow focus on intrapsychic and interpersonal phenomena to explain and/or change it. As Conte (1984) and others have pointed out, the problem of incest cannot be separated from the broader cultural context, and the social and political ideals that set the stage for it. Socially, our patriarchal culture with its historical pattern of male dominance is linked directly to the problem of incest, which traditionally has been only one of the many abuses children were subject to as the legal property of their fathers. In our more

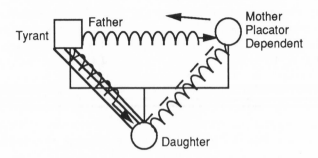

See page 96 for an extended definition of the genogram.

"enlightened" time, this tradition of subjugation by the father is maintained more subtly by society's continuing to designate as ideal a family structure in which father is in charge and mother and children defer to him, although even the economic basis of that structure no longer holds.

The incest pattern is activated in the nuclear family when two emotionally deprived, emotionally dependent, parents try to play the roles that a patriarchal society has assigned them: he blusters and she defers; she helplessly placates and he demands; he intimidates or batters and she withdraws. When this domestic tyranny has completely isolated both parents and created distance between mother and daughter, he molests his daughter, and calls it "love." *Over time, this becomes a compulsive behavior that may be triggered by any tensions in the father's life, in or outside of the family.*

On the individual level, father tries to convince himself that such molesting does no harm. Mother, when she suspects or finds out about it, is put in a double bind similar to the wife of the alcoholic: Should she plunge herself and her children into chaos and perhaps destitution, or should she try to believe that it won't happen again? As with the alcoholic's wife, she and her husband may exchange idle threats to leave and empty promises to reform for years, rather than end the marriage on which both feel so dependent. Daughter, too, knows the power of the secret, realizing that by silence she can hold the family together, or possibly destroy it by speaking out. She may thus keep the secret for years, or forever. In either case, she will struggle for life with the results of being betrayed in this way.

If the incest is current, the family's intense denial of wrongdoing must be addressed if therapy is to be successful, whether by jailing the father and/or assigning him to a sex offender's program until he can acknowledge the problem and be ready to work on it. No change will occur in any particular family until and unless the father accepts personal responsibility for his behavior, acknowledges that it is a problem, and wants to change it. Regardless of the systemic factors contributing to the problem, *the responsibility for the actual behavior is personal and changing it requires individual commitment.* As in alcoholism, drug addiction, and other compulsive behaviors, there will be no change in the symptom without its acceptance as a problem by the symptomatic individual. Individual or family therapy that proceeds with "business as usual," expecting the abuse to cease as a result of the sessions, will become part of the problem.

The restoration of a positive mother-daughter relationship is crucial to treatment in incest cases and is often the best place to begin therapeutic work. The marital relationship will require rebalancing, with father giving up and mother taking on more power. Probably the last step will be the repair of the father-daughter relationship to the extent that it is possible.

Thus, while compassion, understanding, reconciliation, and forgiveness may be personal and family options, on the social level they are not enough. Rather, institutions and social values must be changed in such a way that violence, betrayal, and exploitation of the weak female by the powerful male are no longer the values that society offers to vulnerable families.

PHYSICAL AND VERBAL ABUSE   The physical battering of a child is one of the most difficult family situations to understand or to work with because it is so deeply repugnant to us. It is almost impossible to maintain a neutral, nonjudgmental attitude toward those responsible for it. However, in spite of the widespread public view that child abuse is perpetrated by the mentally ill, it is now recognized that fewer than 10 percent of parents who abuse children are psychotic (*Social Work*, vol. 23, no. 1 [January, 1978]).

In a typical abuse triangle, father's abuse of daughter may be aimed as much at his wife as at the daughter, and he is usually abusive with his wife as well.

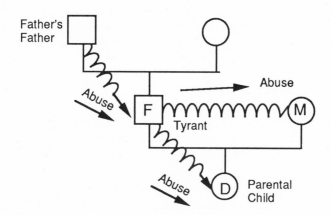

See page 96 for an extended definition of the genogram.

In this pattern, father has been abused by *his* father in childhood and has a "macho" or petty-tyrant approach to male roles. There is often open and ongoing conflict between husband and wife, in which daughter gets caught. Whatever the circumstances in which father first shoves, harangues, threatens, or strikes his daughter, the negative reaction of his wife challenges him and fuels a vicious cycle of further escalation on his part and more intensity from her until there is an explosion. Once this pattern is established through repetition, it can be triggered by any tension in the family or in the social network. And, whoever initiates it, the sequence always ends with daughter being beaten or tongue-lashed and mother thereby defeated by father. As in alcohol abuse, incest, and wife battering, this cycle is followed later by the parents' exchange of idle threats and empty promises.

Whether or not the abuser agrees to a program aimed at behavior change, it is essential in cases of physical abuse that a child-protective service be notified, as required by law. This roots the therapy firmly in open acknowledgment that a crime has been committed, and serves notice that the therapy cannot be used to bypass the social constraints created to deal with the problem.

After the abuse has stopped, if this pattern is not fueled by drugs or alcohol, and the adult participants want to change it, the cycle can be broken by helping each adult find a specific way to change behavior before the conflict becomes a runaway. Children cannot change such a pattern on their own.

Behavioral contracts and other methods of helping couples to avoid situations that lead to violence will seldom hold for long if there is an intergenerational pattern of abuse, and this triangle—the abuser and his parents—should be the focus of therapeutic exploration and work once the abuse has stopped in the nuclear family.

Women who report that their husband's abusive behavior is associated with alcohol or drug use should be told frankly that the physical abuse cannot be controlled until the alcohol or drug abuse stops. Therapeutic work should focus on helping such women do whatever is required to protect themselves and their children until the man gets substance-abuse treatment.

Daughters with abusive or aggressively intrusive fathers may marry someone who is so unlike their father that they subsequently complain of their husband's lack of initiative; or, conversely, they may duplicate the intensity of the father-daughter relationship in endless marital conflict with another tyrant. In the latter case, the relationship with father may remain the most intense one in her life, with daughter alternately placating him and fighting with him as they remain locked in intense mutual emotional dependency. Severe stress easily leads to complete cutoff, which may last for years or a lifetime.

Summary

We tend to carry in our minds a rather simple picture in which a "good father" is protective and caring. We may not notice if he is failing to teach his daughter self-reliance, independence, courage, and an ability to deal with the outside world assertively: and we may even deny or overlook the fact that he may be actively abusing her.

As family therapists, we need to examine our ideas about the role of father in the family, and particularly our views about fathers and daughters. These views have certainly been shaped by a social system that has taught, for thousands of years, that women should be raised to defer to men, to depend on them, to comply with their wishes, and to meet their needs. We have been taught that women should not openly defy men nor express anger directly to them nor compete with them. The job of raising daughters in this way has been entrusted to the family and, until very recently, good fathers and mothers did not question the value of such an upbringing for their daughters. Although family therapists, along with everyone else, are still the recipients of these centuries-old lessons, the time is now past due for us to question such ideas.

Clinical Issues

Family Therapy Theory

In my clinical work with fathers and daughters, I work with the power in the family so that it can be used to support change and not to sabotage it. This means that when the daughter is a child, or adolescent, or a financially dependent college student, I see one or both parents, but may or may not include the daughter in most of the sessions. At this stage of the family life cycle, it is my premise that the parents have the most power, so that if father changes the way he deals with his daughter, the father-daughter relationship will change dramatically whether or not daughter comes to therapy.

Somewhere between ages 18 and 21, or whenever she stops being financially dependent on her father, the emotional power shifts to daughter. Now she may not need him for survival, financial or emotional, and so she feels less obliged to put up with aspects of the relationship that she doesn't like. At this time it is unlikely that changes in father's attitudes or behavior will of themselves change the relationship unless she chooses to cooperate. In fact, between ages 20 and 30, when daughter's chief struggle is for autonomy, the most positive and well-meaning approaches by father may be perceived by daughter as critical or as threatening her autonomy (which they may well be). And, although she wishes it weren't so, father's disapproval is so hard to handle that she will become as distant, or rebellious, or as cut off as she thinks she needs to be to "feel" independent, even if she isn't. Here, the "coaching" method (Bowen, 1978; Carter and McGoldrick Orfanidis, 1976) is my clinical method of choice.

In this method, originated by Murray Bowen, it is quite possible to insert the factor of gender and to select feminist themes, thus altering the focus of the therapy through adaptation rather than basic change of the theory. At its simplest level, this means helping the client to consider the social mandates of sex-role functioning when they are thinking about the nature of their parents' lives or the characteristics and constraints of their family system. It means helping clients to recognize the sexist socialization processes that have helped to determine their lives in addition to, or through the vehicle of, their family dynamics. It means including the realities of gender in our otherwise abstract explanations of triangles, relationship patterns, and family themes. It means always talking about gender socialization when we talk with clients about autonomy, connectedness, parenting, money, career, and the like.

In my work with an adult daughter alone, I coach her to change her end of the dysfunctional transactions with her father and thus complete her passage to adulthood. If the father of an adult daughter is the client, and the daughter is unavailable or uninterested, it is usually best to encourage the father to communicate friendly but not pressuring messages to his daughter. He had best discuss his regrets, his guilt, or his anxiety about her elsewhere, and let her approach him on her own timetable.

Clinical Examples

There follow four cases highlighting the father-daughter relationship. The types of cases were freely chosen, not assigned, and it is very significant, I think, that three of us (Carter, Silverstein, and Walters) chose to present the nonconflictual enmeshed ("daddy's little girl") pattern. I think our concern with this pattern flows from its very benign appearance and the fact that it mirrors the conscious or unconscious patriarchal image that most men and women carry in their heads of the good, kindly, protecting father and the happy, protected daughter. It's not that there's anything wrong with this image either, if the daughter is young, if she has a similarly warm, involved relationship with her mother or other caretakers, and if, in addition to being "protected," the daughter is also being helped toward self-reliance.

A Feminist Direction

Interwoven in the clinical work that follows are new feminist directions based on the idea that not all problems in a family can be attributed to dysfunctional *mother*-child relationships in spite of common family therapy practice to the contrary. Furthermore, these cases show the dysfunctional relationship between mother and daughter as directly connected to supposedly "ideal" functioning on the part of the father, as all three protagonists (father, mother and daughter) live out the gender roles they've been trained for. Gender must be addressed, in thinking and in practice, by anyone claiming to help people function better, both because of its universal importance and because gender has been the unacknowledged basis of so much inequity and human suffering. Our shared belief is that feminism begins as an understanding about human behavior in a social context as well as a commitment to making the invisible visible in our clinical work.

Summary of Case Themes

The cases we present, both long-term and short-term, reflect different methodologies, various family ethnicities, and a wide range of ages in the daughters. However, they also reflect certain shared beliefs about the themes and processes of family therapy.

All four therapists avoid diagnosing the focal problems as "over-involved mother-child," family therapy's favorite diagnosis, in spite of ample evidence that the mother-daughter relationships are also problematic, and in spite of the fact that we have all been taught to focus on that issue first.

In the three cases in which the fathers were available, the therapists expected them to be fully engaged in the family and in the therapy whether they were in the emotionally "close" or the "distant" positions. We don't exclude fathers from full emotional participation because of supposed "incapacity" to relate more fully, nor do we flatter, court, or elevate men in therapy in order to involve them. We don't defer to those men who prefer to be left out of the therapeutic focus. We don't let so-called "peripheral fathers" off the hook, and we specifically reject the often quoted treatment rule: "Never chase a distancer." Expecting so little of men in therapy is actually an unflattering or contemptuous position as well as a self-fulfilling prophecy.

The three therapists who present "daddy's girl" cases (Carter, Silverstein, and Walters) show a clear understanding that a father's devotion to his daughters can readily turn into overprotection and infantilizing because of the cultural mandate to treat daughters differently than sons. Because this relationship pattern so conforms to the social ideal, fathers can easily be unaware of its elements of control and dominance, and of its negative effects on their wives and daughters. All of these therapists linked their evaluation of the father's behavior to sexist social values rather than to purely personal or family dynamics.

The Enmeshed Pattern

The tip-off that you are not in the presence of a totally "great relationship" is a certain collusive element between father and daughter that excludes significant others, most especially, the mother. If father and daughter seem to have a "great relationship," and mother is angry, distant, critical, depressed, or in conflict with either of the happy twosome, it is very hard not to think that mother is the problem, and that everything would be fine if she would just deal with daughter as father does. It is very hard to see that the "great" father-daughter relationship is actually organizing mother's behavior by excluding her. Mother plays into the pattern, of course, when she responds to her hurt and anger with conflict or withdrawal, thus looking and feeling like the one who is raining on the happy parade. And not only family members find it hard to perceive the negative aspects of this pattern; it is equally difficult for us therapists, who have been raised with the same cultural beliefs about the "proper" roles of males and females, which is implicit in every father-daughter relationship.

Father initiates such a collusive and excluding pattern as a result of many factors: he probably has an over-responsible, paternalistic approach to the male role; he may find it easier to deal with an obviously subordinate daughter than a more assertive wife; he may enjoy the complete adoration that a daughter can bestow, as well as her complete dependence; he may be in competition with his wife about good parenting; and/or he may feel he needs an ally against his wife and so, mostly unaware, he uses his daughter to fight certain of his battles with his wife.

Daughter is drawn into this pattern when she finds that she can turn to father for privileges that mothers has refused or cannot give; when father contradicts or undermines mother's rules for her; and, especially, when she feels elevated to the number one spot in father's regard as manifested by their shared secrets, winks, and looks, and by the way father openly takes her side against mother. Once programmed in this way, daughter becomes a partner in the collusion—not equally responsible, of course, but often equally active in her learned role.

Daughter is learning, along with the usual techniques of parent-management that all children learn, that men are in charge, that women can't change things on their own, and that the way to get along is through compliance, dependency, pleasing and placating, and, above all, by beating out the female competition. She is learning that other women will become angry at her if she wins the man to her side, but the rewards of her alliance with father make the struggle with her mother bearable; and the older she grows the more she can rationalize her "affinity" for men and her competitive mistrust of women.

The Distant-Negative Pattern

The father in Papp's case has a paternalistic, "daddy's little girl" *attitude* toward his daughter, but he doesn't put in the *time*. Finding direct involvement with his daughter frustrating and upsetting, father turns the job over to mother and then complains about the way she does it. He loves his daughter, but he knows how to deal with females only from the paternalistic position of the father of a young child. Father lacks the flexibility to shift gears that acknowledge and enhance daughter's growing independence, although he has no such problems with his sons, whose stages of growth and development he understands and encourages.

Mother, of course, plays her part in the problem, as women often do, by taking on complete responsibility for her daughter, although she complains about it. A crucial problem is that father is not able to listen to mother's concerns without an erratic, inappropriate response. Hampered by the social rule that prohibits a woman from saying directly what she wants from a man, mother may fail to make clear what she is asking from father when she tries to communicate with him about her daughter or herself. In fact, if she doesn't feel entitled to confront him directly with her own needs, her communications about their daughter may take on added urgency.

Aware of father's anxiety when confronted with any emotional issue involving the women in his family. and his rigid grasp on the paternalistic, one-up role in all of his relationships (giving but not receiving), one perceives vividly in this case the futility of father's attempt to substitute power politics for relatedness.

Finally, it is important to note that it is not our intention, or the outcome in any of these cases, to disrupt or block even dysfunctional father-daughter relationships or to "turn the daughters over to their mothers." The formulations and interventions were carefully designed and delivered to validate the essential caring of the fathers and the worthwhileness of the father-daughter relationship, even while seeking to remove its collusive elements and to connect the daughter *also*— not *instead*—to her mother.

cases

Betty Carter

Three Generations of Daddy's Girls

I chose this case because of the subtlety of the problematic father-daughter relationship. Because the father is a warm, intelligent, "nice" man who genuinely loves and dotes on his young daughter; and because we are always trying to get fathers more involved in their families, and this father is very involved; and because this father-daughter relationship conforms to the ideal (and sexist) stereotype—for all these reasons, it would be easy for a family therapist, male or female, to miss seeing anything problematic in the relationship between this father and daughter, and to focus instead on a more familiar problem: the cold, angry mother.

In this case, I describe a therapeutic approach that challenges our stereotyped view of a "good" father-daughter relationship and examines the process within the family, so commonplace in our society, whereby the females compete for the male's attention.

The Presenting Problem

This is a Jewish upper-middle class family in which the couple in the middle generation, Michael, age 40, and Nora, age 38, came to see me with serious marital problems. They stated that they were on the verge of divorce. Michael was a college professor struggling to get tenure at a branch of the City University. His wife, Nora, a social worker, was working part-time and planning to go back to full-time work when her children were older. Susan was age 10, and Larry, 8.

Nora was the one threatening divorce. She said that she felt trapped and isolated and could no longer tolerate her "no-win position." She spoke with coldness and anger: "Being a college professor gives him a lot of time at home," Nora said, "which he uses to supervise and criticize every move I make with the children, especially Susan. I thought of increasing my work time and letting him take care of the kids, but, of course, he's against that—and to tell you the truth, I'd really rather wait till they're older."

Michael spoke softly and earnestly, periodically reaching over to take Nora's hand, which she pulled angrily away. He appeared deeply shaken by Nora's threat, "I love her," he said, "and divorce would be crazy. I don't mean to be on her back all the time, but I truly believe that she's unaware of how coldly she treats Susan. I think it all goes back to her terrible relationship with her own mother. I know she doesn't want that to happen to her and Susan. But, listen, therapy can help her with that and I'll do anything it takes to improve our marriage."

In this case, it would be very easy for any therapist to focus first and maybe exclusively on the mother-daughter negativity, which has been the pattern for generations, and miss entirely the integral role that the "ideal" father-daughter dyad plays in mother's anger and alienation. It would be easy to find evidence in this case of "maternal fusion" and "lack of differentiation," if that's what you're looking for, and to miss the central role of the father. It would be easy for a therapist (male or female) to struggle with mother as she "resists" acting more warmly toward her daughter. It would be easy for the therapist and the "nice" husband to join forces to "help" mother to "overcome her resistance." It would be easy to urge her to try to "become a better mother" by "working things out with her own mother," while her husband offers encouragement from his superior position. Even a well-trained systems therapist, male or female, might readily decide that this must actually be an "overclose *mother*-daughter problem," with the mother "appearing" distant because she has temporarily withdrawn in anger.

Even a diagnosis that recognizes the problematic father-daughter alliance can easily lead, *in practice*, to a therapy that requires only a perfunctory "backing off" by the father and a long, long course of therapeutic work "up the maternal line" for the mother. In this event, regardless of the nonblaming intent of the theory, the metamessage of the therapy is that mother (and her mother) is responsible, if not for all of the problem, then for most of the change.

Intergenerational Patterns

The history on both sides of this family revealed that the relationship between father and daughter was and had been the central relationship for several generations. In each branch of the family, the fathers and daughters were described as loving, close, and extremely involved while the mothers and daughters experienced very tense, conflictual relationships. It was subsequently revealed that, in each case, the mother was hurt and angry, feeling that father and daughter had excluded her.

Nora, in her family of origin, was the oldest daughter with a younger brother. She had always been and still was extremely attached to her father, Murray, and had a very negative relationship with her mother, Ruth. Nora said that as long as she could remember, her father had supported her, understood her, and done everything he could to help her. She said that Michael was "ridiculously jealous" of her good relationship with her father "because he has such a bad relationship with his own father."

"That's not the reason," said Michael, "although it's true that my father is not the caring man that yours is. What bothers me is that there's some way that you put your father above *me*." Michael turned to me to explain: "I certainly have to agree that Nora has a close relationship with her father, and I think that's right, but I don't like it when she goes to him for advice that she should be getting from me. Is he still her final authority? Is that right?"

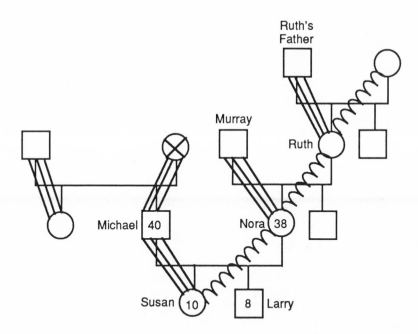

See page 96 for an extended definition of the genogram.

It was clear that Nora felt caught between her father and her husband and would need some help in making herself her own "final authority."

Nora's relationship with her mother was extremely negative and critical. Whatever relationship they *did* have rested on Nora taking care of her mother, reversing the traditional caretaking roles. For instance, Ruth complained frequently to Nora about her marriage and her life, and Nora tried, resentfully, to reassure her and to give advice. On the other hand, Nora never turned to her mother for comfort or advice, considering the very idea ludicrous. "I never get comfort from her," Nora said, "only criticism—especially about the kids. It's really a toss-up whether I get more flak from Michael or from her."

Nora said that Ruth had experienced the same kind of negative relationship with her mother, and had been much closer and felt much warmer toward her father. As Nora talked about these patterns she said sadly: "The same thing is developing in our family. Michael gets along much better with Susan than I do."

Michael reported that the same pattern of closeness between father and daughter had existed in his family. He said that his father had always had a very involved and warm relationship with his older sister, but had not supported him or spent much time with him when he was growing up. Now, Michael said, his father really disapproved of his profession, since he didn't make very much money, and he and his father had a very distant and rather negative relationship. Michael's mother, to whom he had been close, had been dead since Michael was a teenager. He frequently compared Nora unfavorably to his mother, citing mother's warmth and devotion to the "family" (meaning to his father and himself). On her side, Nora made it clear to Michael that she regarded her father as her "best friend," and expressed resentment that Michael was not able to take care of her as her father always had and in fact, still did.

Therapeutic Perspective: Family Triangles

In the (Bowen-based) theoretical framework that I use, I routinely begin some work with the family of origin as soon as the intensity of marital conflict has been reduced enough for the couple to tolerate the shift of focus away from the immediate problems in their own relationship. In this case, when Nora had given up the threat of divorce and decided to try to work it out with Michael, I was ready to move into their family tree. Typically, I move the focus of the therapy back and forth between nuclear family and family of origin, monitoring the emotional process in one subsystem while a task is given for work in the other system.

Now came the moment of choice. Ample evidence had been given of Nora's negative relationships with both her mother and her daughter. There is no doubt that both relationships needed improvement and that improving them would have a positive effect on her relationship with her husband. I think that at an earlier time I might easily have made this the focus of the therapy even though I would have technically diagnosed Michael as the "overclose" parent who, with some cajoling, might be called upon to give Nora space to "work things out with her daughter." Such a focus, of course, would have confirmed for both of them Michael's statement that most of their difficulties were a result of Nora's poor relationships with her mother and daughter.

By adding to the conceptualization of the pattern all the gender-specific aspects implied by the phrase "daddy's little girl," the power issues, thus parodied, and their connections to sexist social values, come immediately into view and loom large enough to capture the therapist's attention as priorities are set for the therapy.

Thus, keeping in mind the presenting marital complaints, and without losing my feminist perspective, Nora was pointed toward the triangle of herself, her father, and Michael; and Michael, who told me that in his family the women "adored" the men, was pointed first toward the triangle of his mother (now deceased, but idealized), Nora, and himself.

Michael, His Mother, and Nora

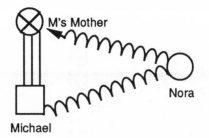

Michael

See page 96 for an extended definition of the genogram.

Through various techniques, including letter writing and conversations with family members and with me, in Nora's presence, Michael was led to consider the negative effects in his marriage of being an "adored" son. Had he expected Nora to adore him too? Did he want her to "mother" him in this way? Had he expected to hand out "adoration," or only to receive it? Did he think that comparing his wife unfavorably to his mother improved his marital relationship? Did he expect his daughter also to "adore" him, especially if his wife would not? And what impact did he think his mother's "adoration" of him had on his father and his sister? Could it have been one of the factors pushing them together? And what aspects of the relationship with his mother were lost in the "adoration"? Did it prevent them from appreciating each other as individuals? If she had lived, would it have hampered the development of an authentic personal relationship between them? When Michael realized the degree to which his relationship to his mother was mythological and idealized, he stopped trying to get Nora to be like her and embarked on a quest to discover, through family discussions, albums, and old letters, who his mother had been as a real person.

In addition to gaining "a whole new mother," Michael realized that after she died, he had replaced her in filling the distant, left-out position in his family's "daddy's little girl" triangle.

"And I hated it," Michael said, "It made me feel angry and unloved, watching my father and sister 'adore' each other. My mother must have been furious at them—so what was all that 'adoring' business about?" "Well, women tend to do that, don't they?" I said, at which point Nora said: "Not *me*. This is exactly what I've been trying to tell him—that I feel angry and unloved watching him and Susan 'adore' each other!"

Nora, Her Father, and Michael

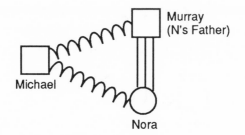

See page 96 for an extended definition of the genogram.

While Michael was engaged in the task of discovering how his family functioned, and where he fit into the pattern, Nora was being coached to change her part in the triangle that included her father and husband. The warmth and closeness of the father-daughter relationship was validated, but she was coached to eliminate the collusive elements that had excluded, first, her mother, and now Michael. For instance, Nora was not to complain to her father about Michael, or her mother, nor was she to let her father complain to her about them. She was discouraged from pursuing a long-standing pattern in which she asked her father's advice about some plan or project and then quoted it endlessly to Michael when they were discussing or arguing the plan. She thought her problem was that she was reluctant to make her husband, rather than her father, her "final authority." I explored the beliefs behind that framing of the problem.

What made her think she needed a "final authority" outside of herself? Who was her father's "final authority"? Is father mother's "final authority" or does she quote *her* father to *him*? How would father react if she stopped asking his advice and started telling him *her* ideas about things? What would happen if she told him she disagreed with him about something? What happens when he disapproves of something she wants to do? How would he react if she did it anyway? Why does she think she has to get mad at her father to do something he doesn't like? How come she is so unable to risk his anger, but doesn't really get upset when her mother gets angry at her? Does she think women have a harder time than men do in being their own "final authority"? Why does she think this is the case?

Michael and Nora

As Nora stopped acting like a child with her father, and stopped feeling responsible for pleasing him, she experienced a dramatic shift in her relationship with Michael: "I couldn't help feeling in the past that Michael was not as strong an authority as my father. Now I see I don't need that, and I'm really enjoying the idea that we're peers, Michael and I, and we can discuss and negotiate things as equals, with no 'outside authority.'" "It's kind of a paradox," Michael said, "she's much more independent than before, but much nicer. I guess I'd still like to be an 'authority' to her, but I'll settle for retiring her father from that job."

In the next phase of their work, Michael reconnected with his father, and Nora tried to become a daughter to her mother.

Michael and His Father

Michael began a correspondence with his father, who lived in a distant city, and opened up to him some of the issues in their relationship, particularly his father's disapproval of Michael's choice of profession. He had learned from watching Nora with her father how to phrase things so that he could stand up to his father without attacking or placating him. He also told his father how childish it had been for him to withdraw in the face of the special relationship father had with his older sister. "Now," Michael told his father, "I've learned from experience that a father is able to relate perfectly well to two children, and I'm returning to claim my patrimony."

Nora and Her Mother

Meanwhile, Nora was having a very hard time trying to become her mother's daughter.

"I've been her mother, her competitor, her enemy, and a thorn in her side," Nora said, "But I've never been her daughter—only my father's." She was instructed not to defend her father when mother complained about him to her, but to get mother off that subject by asking her advice on some matter, asking her for help with the kids, or in other ways reversing the usual flow of advice giving in their relationship. Although thunderstruck at the very idea of such a new way of relating, Nora committed herself to it with alternating gritted teeth and a sense of humor. After much work on the "climate" of their relationship, she was able to broach deeper subjects with her mother, such as their competition for father's attention. Although their relationship didn't become easy, it became considerably warmer and more respectful. After several months they embarked on a regular schedule of mother-daughter activities that ranged from ice skating to museum going. Although she did not articulate it in this way, I saw Nora's withdrawal from the collusive intimacy of Michael and Susan not only as the natural left-out feeling of any person who feels excluded, but also as a reflection of her profound lack of trust in her own capacity to mother adequately. Her own mother had felt invalidated in her mothering of Nora and so did not pass along the sense of womanly competence needed for the job. Nora found that as she developed empathy and respect for her mother and actually began to enjoy her company at times, she felt a strong enhancement of her own sense of herself as a woman, and of the importance of the emotional connection between mother and daughter, which she had tried to deny and to live without. This had a profound effect on her motivation to strengthen the bond with her own daughter, which, she now realized, was as important for her daughter as for herself.

Michael, Nora, and Susan

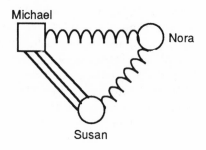

See page 96 for an extended definition of the genogram.

During the course of all the work outlined above (which proceeded on and off over a period of three years), I always monitored its effects in the nuclear family, with particular attention to the "daddy's girl" relationship that replicated those in the extended family and fulfilled the patriarchal ideal of the social system.

In this triangle of Michael, Nora, and Susan, I believe many therapists would have seen Nora as the problem, deploring her strict and angry manner with Susan and admiring Michael's warm doting on his daughter. Many a therapist would have prescribed more father and less mother for this child, and/or would have tried to get Nora to be more like Michael in dealing with Susan. It took careful scrutiny to see the warm father-daughter relationship as a problem.

I thought that the collusive father-daughter alliance had several problematic consequences: (1) Michael put his daughter in the number one spot, thus disenfranchising his wife; (2) Nora withdrew in hurt and anger, thus intensifying the pattern and making herself look like the bad guy; (3); mother and daughter now had to vie for father's attention, with the result that (4) daughter is now in a high-anxiety spot, vulnerable to a variety of symptoms.

Throughout the therapy, tasks were prescribed that changed the nature of Michael's relationship with Susan and moved Nora closer to her daughter. Michael and Nora were now working cooperatively to change the very intense triangle with Susan. In keeping with their style (and with mine), there was extensive use of humor and absurdity, as reflected in the following excerpts from therapy transcripts.

THERAPIST: So how would it be for you if Nora took over the job of supervising her homework?

MICHAEL: (*Laughing*) Are you kidding? Why not throw lighted matches on gasoline?

THERAPIST: That bad? I thought . . .

NORA: He's right, actually. I could never sit there laughing along with her goddamned homework for two hours a night!

THERAPIST: Well, how would *you* do it?

NORA: (*Laughing*) Well, we all know I'm a short-tempered bitch, right? I'd probably tell her to just do it herself.

THERAPIST: And could she?

NORA: Well, I don't know. I think so.

MICHAEL: But she might have questions . . .

THERAPIST: Well, okay, whatever. Why don't you just take charge of it, Nora, however you want to do it. Could you let her do that, Michael?

MICHAEL: Well, if she can do it successfully.

THERAPIST: (*Laughing*) You mean *your* way?

MICHAEL: Yeah, I guess so.

THERAPIST: Could you let her do it *her* way?

MICHAEL: Even if . . .?

THERAPIST: Even if. I mean we're only talking two weeks.

MICHAEL: Yeah. Okay. I can do *anything* for two weeks.

NORA: Thanks a lot.

During the first week of this task, Michael experienced Susan's increased involvement with Nora as a loss. He said he was sort of shocked to realize that the exclusivity of his relationship with Susan, which he intellectually rejected, meant so much to him. But he kept to his new position because he realized he had inadvertently been doing a disservice to Susan and Nora. Several weeks later, when Susan started seeking him out for advice or companionship, he reported with great happiness what a new and wonderful experience it was for him. "I used to be always seeking her out," he said, "and I never gave her a chance to need me or miss me. It's wonderful!"

Michael agreed not to interfere when Nora was disciplining Susan, whether or not he thought she was being "too strict." Needless to say, I would not have taken such a cavalier stance if this were an abusive situation. Nora's frustrated displays of anger at her daughter, while not pleasant, nevertheless occurred within the context of a stable, caring relationship.

THERAPIST: Well, how come you always butt in, Michael?

MICHAEL: Listen. You'd butt in if you were there. Do you think it's right to scream at a 10-year-old?

THERAPIST: Why do you think she screams, Michael? Is she just a natural-born bitch?

MICHAEL: (*Smiling*) Well, I guess she gets frustrated.

THERAPIST: And what does our dimpled darling do to frustrate her?

MICHAEL: Well, she has a pretty smart mouth, I guess.

THERAPIST: And does she expect the Red Cross to arrive in time to save her from this beast—her mother?

MICHAEL: You're saying I encourage her.

THERAPIST: Do you?

MICHAEL: I don't mean to.

THERAPIST: But she could take it . . .

MICHAEL: Yeah, I see what you mean. So how far do I let them go?

THERAPIST: Well, I think if Nora's about to throw her out a window, you should intervene. (*General laughter.*)

And Nora, instead of withdrawing in hurt and resentment, learned to bounce Michael out when he got in the middle:

NORA: Boy, did I let him have it.

THERAPIST: What do you mean?

NORA: Well, I was talking to Susan about how to make lasagna, and Michael yells in from the other room—"Lasagna, I thought we were going out for pizza tonight." So I said, "Yes, we are." And he said, "Then what's this about lasagna?" So I said, "None of your goddamned business, Michael, I'm talking to my daughter." (*General laughter.*)

Finally, after about six months of concentration on the breakup of this rigid triangle in the nuclear family, the work was deemed a success when Michael gave Nora a Valentine card that said, "You're number one." "In the past," Nora said, "he would have given this card to Susan and then would have been all bewildered and amazed that I was angry. But now that I know that I am really number one with Michael, and I have a much better relationship with Susan, I am perfectly happy for them to have a good relationship too."

> MICHAEL: Long live fathers and daughters!
> NORA: And mothers and daughters!
> THERAPIST: And husbands and wives!

Summary

The question that needs to be addressed is whether the same or similar results could have been achieved in this case with the use of conventional Bowen theory, without a feminist perspective, and without explicit use of gender themes in conceptualization and in therapy.

I think the answer is "yes, but": *Yes*, the symptoms could have been resolved, and the relationships could have been improved, and the individuals could have emerged more mature and "differentiated" than they were; *but*, it is not possible to separate "differentiation" or sense of self from gender, since the two are braided together in an integral way. The goal of therapy, after all, is not to produce genderless persons. Becoming a "person," when requisite attributes such as being independent, objective, and competitive are called for, seems to mean to most people, including therapists, the same thing as becoming an *adult male*, as the well-known Broverman study showed (Broverman et al., 1970). Therefore, it is especially important that gender issues and differences be addressed in therapy, to clarify for therapist and client alike that in helping women to "differentiate," the therapy isn't inadvertently urging them to become more like men in ways that are dysfunctional for both men and women, that is, becoming emotionally disconnected or inexpressive. Nor is it helpful if therapists define "differentiation" differently for women, that is, by assuming that women require less "autonomy" in the decisions affecting their lives or less economic control than men do.

The emotional development of males in therapy is also enhanced by addressing the issue of gender, since the male sense of self includes, in all cultures, ideas and attributes that are harmful to men themselves as well as destructive of their relationships with women and children. But at least male self-esteem has been traditionally supported and enhanced in the family, in society, and in therapy, whereas women often have problems in both *sense of autonomous self* and *self-esteem*.

Femaleness has always been equated with inferiority, and the female sense of self as a mature adult has been attacked and disparaged from time immemorial—in the family, in society, and in therapy. Thus, for therapy to become helpful to women, both a woman's sense of herself as worthwhile and her sense of herself as a competent mature adult need explicit attention, with reference to the influence of her gender socialization. If a woman's problems with "lack of autonomy" are not connected in some way during therapy to the social mandate that produced them, she and her family (especially her mother) are left to assume that this problem is a matter of personal or family pathology.

Thus, female selfhood—once a contradiction of terms—needs to be specifically redefined to include "self-reliance" along with the already existing "connectedness to others," which the therapy should validate, not disparage. For instance, the widespread use of the term "close" or "overclose" to mean fused, enmeshed, or entangled in a dysfunctional way lends itself to abuse by many therapists who destroy the positive meaning of the word "close" by using the term pejoratively to discredit the genuine involvement and concern of women, especially mothers.

Addressing gender issues openly will also enhance male differentiation, so that Michael, in this case, could learn that he can be a good husband and father without having to be overresponsible toward his wife and overprotective toward his daughter.

For women, as with Nora, it is always essential to address the influence of gender socialization, since so much of women's problematic or misunderstood behavior, in the family and in therapy, is gender-based, as are the obstacles to her more complete differentiation, which, let us remember, means *autonomy with emotional connectedness*. While it is true that men have featured one of these attributes and women the other, the world has certainly favored those who emphasized autonomy over those socialized in emotional connectedness. Redistribution of power in such a way that women have as much choice in the world and as much control over their lives as do men would radically change our society in ways we can only guess at. I think this is frightening to all of us and is the reason "gender" is such a hot issue whenever it is raised.

Peggy Papp

The Godfather

Introduction

This case involves a father/mother/daughter triangle in which the
father has not only incorporated, but exaggerated, certain stereotypical attributes of male functioning. His professed ideal image of himself
as *The Godfather* is an extreme version of the macho cultural hero—
powerful, paternal, independent, self-possessed, emotionally detached—a world unto himself. He is comfortable only when he is in
control of relationships, which to him means having others beholden to
him and never needing their help. The way he keeps others beholden to
him is through a common male source of power, money, showering
family, friends and business associates with gifts and favors.

When his daughter becomes a teenager and he can no longer
function as provider, protector, and playmate to his "little girl," he
distances himself, turns her over to mother, and leaves all the daily
worrying and caretaking up to her. Mother, following the dictates of
what she considers to be her maternal responsibility, automatically
accepts this job. Father then blames the daughter's problems on mother's "overinvolvement," unaware of the connection between her "overinvolvement" and his distant relationship to both mother and daughter.

In the following case, I avoid accepting father's definition of the
problem as mother's "overinvolvement." Instead, I concentrate on helping father to let go of his ideal image of himself as "The Godfather."
This change requires him to become involved in a give-and-take relationship in which he learns also to receive from his daughter rather
than trying to control her through giving.

The Presenting Problem

Seventeen-year-old Penny was brought to our clinic by her parents
because she had dropped out of school, refused to work, and spent
most of her time shut in her room behind closed doors.

Penny was the youngest of five children and the only one currently living at home. She reluctantly accompanied her parents to
therapy, where she participated minimally, responding to questions
with shrugs or monosyllables. Mother spoke in quiet desperation,

imploring us to help her daughter. She gave a detailed description of her daughter's gradual withdrawal from family and friends, her dropping out of school, her erratic moods and hibernating in her room. Father, a huge, impressive-looking man with a hearty personality, expressed his concern about both Penny and mother. He was concerned about mother because "her whole being is consumed with worry about Penny." He spoke of her as being "obsessed with Penny. She watches her every move and talks about nothing else day and night." He had suggested that mother enter individual therapy, but mother insisted they come as a family.

Although father complained about mother worrying too much, he also conceded it was reassuring to him. "Worry is also taking care of. If I know she is worried about Penny I know Penny is going to be taken care of." The therapist commented that this attitude let him off the hook, and he replied laughingly, "You're damned right. I planned it that way too. If I didn't have my wife I would go crazy."

Mother states, "It's not fair. It makes me angry. Why should I have to do all the worrying? It's 'our' daughter, not 'my' daughter." Father then categorized mother's worrying as a character trait, saying that if she didn't have something to worry about she would manufacture it because she was a born "worrier." She had been that way with all the children, but especially with Penny. He believed she had inherited this trait from her own mother, who was also a worrier.

Mother denied she needed to worry, saying it would be a big relief to her if she could give it up; but she complained that whenever she tried to discuss her worries about Penny with father, rather than his listening and understanding, he either cut her off with "I don't want to hear anymore," or he felt compelled to take action and "fix" the situation. His idea of "fixing" the situation was to charge into Penny's room and lay down the law to her. When she refused to respond to his commands, he would fly into a rage and threaten violence. Mother would then interfere to protect both of them.

Father conceded, "There is no real communication between Penny and me and there hasn't been for a long time." All messages between Penny and father went through mother, who acted as the mediator and tried to keep peace between them. Mother remarked, "I go back and forth between Penny and my husband. I don't think that's good. They should have their own communication, but I'm afraid someone will get hurt."

Therapeutic Perspectives

Knowing what we do about this family, one common way of diagnosing their situation (which this therapist herself might have done in the past) would result in the following evaluation: mother is overly involved with her daughter, probably because she is the last one to leave home. Father is hooked into mother's anxiety, and acts as her "policeman" or "strong arm." He moves in to control Penny because mother is unable to do it herself. Mother then interferes with father's efforts to discipline Penny because they are too violent. Father's anger toward Penny is actually misplaced anger toward mother for having to do her "dirty work." By placing herself in the middle as the mediator, mother prevents father and Penny from developing their own relationship.

Treatment based on this evaluation would be focused on defining mother as the focal problem, exploring her excessive worrying and "overinvolvement" with her daughter, perhaps relating it to a tradition in her family of origin or to the impending empty nest. Mother would be instructed not to tell father about her anxieties so as not to provoke his excitement. She would then be coached to "pull back," get involved in outside activities, stop mediating between father and daughter, and trust father not to become violent. Father might be advised to take charge of Penny in order to relieve mother and "dilute" the mother-daughter relationship. Or the problem might be handled as a marital problem, and Penny excused from the sessions in order to focus on the issues between the couple. Or it might be turned into a management case in which the parents were instructed in how to join together to form a united front.

The issue to examine here is the way in which the particular perspective of the therapist influences the course of therapy. It determines which areas are explored, the kinds of questions asked, the therapist's responses, and, finally, the hypothesis on which further treatment is based. All of the hypotheses discussed here contain elements of truth and any one of them or a combination of them could lead to symptom removal. But all of these hypotheses would focus primarily either on mother's "overinvolvement" or on problems in the marriage rather than on father's avoidance of emotional engagement. I chose to focus on the latter issue since I believed it was central to the presenting problem. I, therefore, explored further father's lack of communication with Penny. In the course of our discussion it became clear that the relationship between Penny and her father changed when Penny reached her teens. Father was conflicted about her growing up, and didn't know how to treat her as an adult woman. He stated in his abrupt and forthright manner, "I know I'm part of Penny's problem. I tried to hold back the clock. I know she's 17 and a woman and I respect her but I tell you straight out, she's still a little girl to me. My sons are my sons and the age they are, but my girls are little girls to me."

PEGGY: How young do you want Penny to stay?

FATHER: About eight. No, really, I'm just kidding. But that's what I miss. I want to give others everything and make them happy, buy them things, and take care of them. She doesn't respond to that anymore and I don't know what else to do.

MOTHER: He's a giver, but he can't receive. There's nothing he will let me do for him. He likes to become completely independent—which in a way is wonderful. I never have to pick up his socks, take things to the cleaners—and it's always "Let's go out to dinner so you won't have to cook."

FATHER: I can't stand anyone doing anything for me. If it's my birthday I want to give you a present.

MOTHER: It makes other feel not appreciated, not needed.

PEGGY: (*To mother*) So you feel deprived when your husband doesn't let you give him anything?

MOTHER: Yes, when he has a cold he won't let me take care of him. On Father's Day he won't even open his presents.

PEGGY: (*To father*) Do you deprive everyone in the family in this way?

MOTHER: Yes, deprive—that's the word.

PEGGY: (*To Penny*) Penny, does your father let you do anything for him?

PENNY: (*Shrugging her shoulders*) I don't care.

MOTHER: The way I see it is you're doing others a favor by allowing them to do things for you. Independence is a great thing but there is another word—interdependence. That I think is better. I see this as his being one up. He's like this with friends and in business.

FATHER: Very true. Every time I take one I want to give you three.

MOTHER: I see it as one-upmanship.

PEGGY: (*To father*) You feel it's better to have others obligated to you rather than you being obligated to them?

FATHER: Yes, I can't stand to feel obligated. If I do a favor for someone I don't ever want them to pay me back. I was watching *The Godfather* the other night and I said, "I'd like to be the Godfather."

MOTHER: And I said, "You are. You don't know it."

FATHER: And she's right. I can't call in my favors. That's my problem. I have to pick up the check all the time.

MOTHER: (*To father*) I feel sorry for you that you can't get more pleasure out of things being done for you. It keeps people from getting close to you.

FATHER: If I get too close I have to worry about you—you become a responsibility. When someone gets close to me I start backing off.

PEGGY: And how does that work between you and your wife?

FATHER: I don't know if there's a relation with that. I know when I'm sick I don't want her to take care of me. I don't want to feel weak. If she takes care of me too much I am weak. I don't want others to take care of me. I'll take care of them.

After having gathered this additional information my hypothesis was as follows: father's extreme paternalistic attitude, his avoidance of the obligations of intimacy, and his insistence on being in a one-up position in personal relationships keep mother and Penny infantilized. Mother asks for cooperation and understanding in coping with the daughter's behavior, and father responds by either withdrawing or using physical force. Mother, accepting her stereotypical role of peacemaker, mediates the fighting between father and daughter and thus protects father from having to come to terms with his daughter as an adult woman. Penny responds by remaining a little girl, dropping out of the adult world, and staying cloistered at home.

Therapeutic Aims

My first therapeutic goal, based on this hypothesis, was to help father experience a personal relationship that involved receiving as well as giving, and to help mother and Penny out of their infantilized positions. I began with father's relationship with Penny, since she was the presenting problem. I instructed them as follows: at least twice a week, father was to ask Penny to do something for him and allow her to do it. It could be anything but a task that involved her welfare such as going back to school, getting a job, or leaving her room, for example. It had to be something that involved the father's well-being. Penny was asked to comply with his request and in that way to teach him how to receive.

By reversing their positions of giver and receiver, the therapeutic task removed Penny from her little-girl position and instead placed her in the position of a competent adult who had something valuable to teach her father. By having to ask and receive, father was compelled to relinquish his "Godfather" position and become involved in the give-and-take of a more equal relationship with his daughter.

I have found that prescribing a task around a central issue is one of the simplest and quickest ways to change the rules of a relationship. It immediately provides the participants with a new experience in interacting, upsetting their old familiar relationship patterns and opening up new possibilities.

For the first time since we had been meeting, Penny came alive in the session. She raised her head and joined her parents in laughter at the thought of father receiving anything. She doubted he would be able to do the assignment, saying, "I can't imagine anyone teaching him anything. He knows it all." Father was surprised by the turning of the tables and agreed it would be difficult. But true to form, he declared, "It will kill me, but I'll die trying." Mother looked relieved.

Father made two requests of Penny, with great difficulty: one was that she go to the corner drug store and buy him the Sunday newspaper, and the other, that she get him a book he needed from the library. Both of these activities got Penny out of her room and put the father-daughter relationship on a different footing. As father began to move out of his "Godfather" position, the distance between him and his daughter was reduced, permitting a more open and honest exchange. Mother became less worried as Penny showed signs of becoming more communicative and began to leave her room.

The Process of Change

Within a few weeks Penny had a job and no longer wanted to attend therapy sessions because she was too busy. Father's first reaction was to get furious and yell at mother because she was the one who set up the therapy; why should he be willing to go and expose his head if Penny wasn't willing to expose hers. Penny became very upset over her parents' argument and retired to her room. This time, however, father broke the old cycle by doing something different. He went to Penny's room without mother's prompting and said, "Penny, I'm wrong. I'm learning too and that's why I'm coming to talk to you. I took it out on your mom and I didn't mean to. I'm really angry at you. So that's why I'm coming here with what I've got to complain about." They had a long discussion during which they argued with each other, became angry, cried, and finally reconciled. During the course of this intense exchange, Penny convinced father she was old enough to make up her own mind about whether or not she wanted to continue coming to therapy.

The parents continued for several more sessions without their daughter since they decided they themselves were reaping benefits. They wanted to better understand their own relationship, and during this process I helped father to receive from mother.

When we terminated therapy the parents reported that Penny seemed much happier and was enthusiastically making plans to go back to school the next fall. Father said he thought they didn't need any more therapy because "I couldn't take it much better. This is fine."

Summary

This case demonstrates a way of dealing with a mother/father/ daughter triangle other than by focusing on the problems of the "over-involved" mother. Instead, the family problem was conceptualized as an imbalance of power in the family as a result of father maintaining his one-up distant position through giving. A simple task changed the relationship between the father and daughter by reversing their positions of giver and receiver. This shift in the father-daughter relationship relieved mother of her position as the mediator and sole worrier in the family. Following this realignment, the power imbalance between mother and father was addressed and modified.

Olga Silverstein

The "Independent" Daughter

Introduction

Following is an example of a systemic therapy with an individual. In working with a single person in the room I frequently use a genogram. A genogram is a family diagram, commonly of three generations, linking the two sides of a family and tracing the emotional patterns through the generations.

Such a device identifies the family process as intergenerational and contextual. Then, it effectively brings the absent family members visually into the room. The genogram enables the therapist (and therefore the client) to identify relationship patterns through the generations in order to place the presenting problem into context.

This case exemplifies the common problem of a young woman torn between attending to her own needs and the often conflicting pulls of the people she cares about. A common error in treatment is to conceptualize this problem as difficulty in separation, which then can lead the therapist into helping the young person to cut off, "do her own thing"—reactively. The opportunity to relate differently is then lost.

The Presenting Problem

A 27-year-old student here from Italy for the two years of an externship at the Ackerman Institute came to see me in tears. "I just got an anguished letter from my father asking me to come right home. My training is over in two weeks and I was planning to travel around the country for the summer and then go home, but he says, 'Please—right now.'"

THERAPIST: Do you understand what the urgency is?

MARIA: Oh, yes, both my sisters are in trouble and he needs my help. (*She starts to cry.*)

THERAPIST: Okay, lets start from the top—you have two sisters?

MARIA: Yes, and two brothers—I'm the oldest. The boys are both away at school. I think they're all right. I came to America to study two years ago, and then a year ago Angelique went to London, to study acting, and then Laura went to the university—she's the youngest, 18. But now they're both home. Angelique had some kind of breakdown—I don't know just what—but the school called and my father went and brought her home.

THERAPIST: How did he feel about her going to England in the first place?

MARIA: Oh, he was against it. He was against it. Acting—pooh. He comes from a very respectable family, clean, clean, clean—no, he cut her off—he wouldn't talk to her. She's not my daughter, he told everyone.

THERAPIST: And your mother. What did your mother do?

MARIA: Oh, she protected her. She never confronted my father, but she sent her a little money and she secretly called her.

THERAPIST: And Laura, what's with her?

MARIA: I don't know because no one tells me much, just that she dropped out of the university and she cries all the time.

THERAPIST: Now what are you supposed to do about all this?

MARIA: Well, I always took care of all of them. When I was still in Milan—I had finished school, I had my own apartment—they always came to me when something went wrong at home. My father always sent them to me. My mother would get very angry. She'd call and tell them to come right home.

THERAPIST: So you were a little mother—

MARIA: Oh, yes. Now since I'm here I try to stay out of it. They call me and I say, I'm sorry I can't help you—but it's hard. I don't know what's going to happen if I'm right there. I want to be able to stay out. My friends all tell me, stay out of it, and I try.

Systems Therapy with an Individual

Because I know this is a one-session consultation, I move directly into the genogram. Since Maria has been a student of family therapy for the past two years, the introductory process of getting connected to each other and the induction into systems thinking is not necessary. She has also, in her training, been encouraged to accumulate information about her own family and knows much.

I do not mean to suggest that every single-session consultation can have dramatic results. A more naive client would obviously need more time for both preparation and execution.

Her mother, Rosa, is still a young woman. Maria describes her as very beautiful, gay and lively. Rosa is ten years younger than her brother Emilio. When Rosa was 3 years old and Emilio 13, their father, Dominick, deserted the family and went to live with a younger, more attractive woman. Although there was no divorce, Rosa never saw him again.

MARIA: (*Continuing the story*) My uncle Emilio was 13 when his father left, and he became very sad. My grandmother was also very sad. They were very poor. By the time my mother was 12 or 13 she was the family's main wage earner, the independent one. My mother cleaned for the rich, she took care of babies, sold things in the market, and there were some hints that she maybe did some other things as well. I don't know. I know all the men were after her and she had no protection. Her brother never left the house, and Anna stayed home and took care of him. Oh, she tried, my grandmother tried, but my mother was very independent. And they were very poor. You know in those days in the villages in Italy, if your husband leaves it's a disgrace. Every one assumes that if a man leaves, a woman did wrong.

THERAPIST: What do you know about your father's background?

MARIA: My father is twenty years older than my mother. He is different. Very serious. He comes from a very respectable family. Very respectable. His name is also Emilio. (*Therapist continues to map out genograms.*)

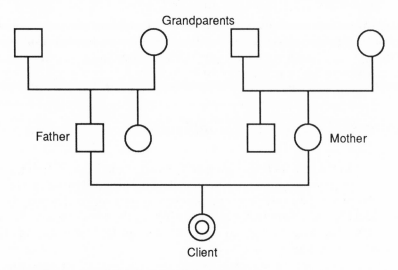

See page 96 for an extended definition of the genogram.

Emilio, my father, is the oldest of two children by six years. He has a sister, Maria. I have her name.

His father died when he was 10 years old. The opposite to my Uncle Emilio, my father became the man in the family. They were not poor. Oh no—very respectable. So he was educated. But he always took care of his mother. And always protected his sister Maria.

THERAPIST: What's his sister like?

MARIA: My aunt is very nice. A very good woman. She never married and she stays with her mother. Very nice. A very good woman. Serious.

We could, with this information, begin to formulate some hypotheses about Maria's fear of going home.

THERAPIST: So when did these two people meet? (*Writing on genogram*)

MARIA: At a dance. The story is that she was in love with another man, but he was poor and my father was a very good match for a poor girl. He says he liked her because she was beautiful and gay. He rescued her from the gutter. My mother was without prospects and my father rescued her.

THERAPIST: Whose story is that?

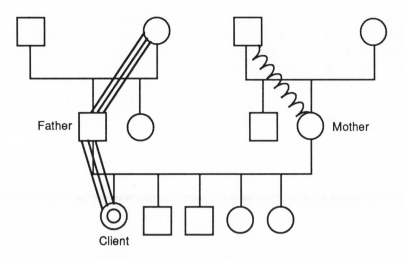

See page 96 for an extended definition of the genogram.

MARIA: My grandmother Theresa's.

THERAPIST: Tell me a little about your parents now—what's their relationship like?

MARIA: Oh, they are very polite, but the relationship is not good. Years ago, maybe ten, twelve years ago, I heard them arguing—threatening separation.

THERAPIST: Who was doing the threatening?

MARIA: Both of them. He says she's too pushy—too frivolous, too disorganized. She says he's too biased—too tired—he works all the time. He doesn't allow her any independence.

THERAPIST: Whose daughter are you, whose side are you on?

MARIA: Oh, his, his! He's a very hard worker—very generous with his children. He never denies us anything. Then I look just like his mother. People always said, you're your father's daughter!

THERAPIST: You like that?

MARIA: Well, sure—since I was a very little girl he talked to me about things he wouldn't discuss with my mother.

THERAPIST: Did your mother ever confront him about that?

MARIA: Oh, no, she never confronts him—only about money.

THERAPIST: I thought you said he was very generous.

MARIA: With the children—not with my mother—he says she's very frivolous. He acts like her father and she acts like a rebellious kid. But he's marvelous—he's a hard, hard worker and he'll do anything for his children.

THERAPIST: Okay, now let me see if I understand. You say your father is a good man who seems to be at the mercy of a foolish woman—your mother, who is still young and wanting to have a good time. About two years ago you left home, followed by your two sisters—the brothers were already away at school—is that right?

MARIA: Yes, a few months ago we were all moving along and then, poof—I feel terrible—(*Crying again*).

We now know a number of things about Maria's family:

1. Maria's mother, Rosa, is a young and beautiful woman married to a serious man twenty years her senior.
2. She grew up independent, unprotected (in the family's language). Maria's father, Emilio, grew up as a protector.
3. Rosa's father abandoned the family for another woman. Her brother and mother grieved inconsolably. The family lived in disgrace. Emilio's father left the family in a more acceptable way—by death. Emilio, the father, was elevated rather than shamed. He became, too early, the too serious man of the house. His family lived in respectability.
4. Rosa and Emilio shared a common experience of early loss and abandonment.
5. They most probably shared an uneasy feeling about the reliability or vulnerability of men. Emilio handled it by overfunctioning and Rosa by never confronting Emilio's controlling caretaking of her and the children.
6. Emilio married down, thus incurring the disapproval of his mother and sister.
7. Maria was handed over to Grandma Theresa—as a consolation prize, an effort to win back her favor.
8. Maria now had a collusive bond with her grandmother as well as her father, a bond that excluded and criticized Rosa. Maria's physical appearance helped in the handover, but this alliance was preordained as soon as she was given the aunt's name.
9. Maria's position in the family as father's ally and grandmother's confidante left her alienated from her mother.
10. What's more, she was secretly contemptuous of her mother.
11. And therefore she took on the job of "little mother" with her father's and grandmother's approval.
12. Maria's "moral superiority" to her mother—handed down directly from Grandma to father to daughter—limited her ability to function as an independent adult who was still caring and connected to her family.

Having gathered the information on which to base this systems hypothesis, I now can confront the current problem directly.

THERAPIST: Now your father wants you to come home and take care of the younger daughters who are, like their mother, dependent and needing care. Is that right?

MARIA: Yes. Right now, he demands that I come home.

THERAPIST: Do you think you could do something very different when you go home?

MARIA: I've been trying that—not to get involved. (*As stated earlier, "I won't get involved" is the first line of defense when you feel the old tide pulling you off shore.*)

THERAPIST: No, you've tried that and it doesn't work. Could you go home as your mother's friend? (*The first attempt at an intervention is put in the right frame, a shift in positioning from daddy's girl to mother's friend, but in an unacceptable context—"Could you go home?"—which I know she is reluctant to do.*)

MARIA: I don't know. Because she complains to me and I don't like that.

THERAPIST: What does she complain about?

MARIA: My father—how he doesn't give her any independence. He doesn't let her have any money. And then she tells me how many men look at her.

THERAPIST: And you—how do you respond?

MARIA: I tell her she uses that as an excuse. (*Another example of Maria's confusion about her place in the family.*)

THERAPIST: So you lecture her.

MARIA: I guess so.

THERAPIST: I'm going to explain what I'm thinking to you, Maria, and then I'll tell you what I think you should do—the problem is that you might not be so willing to give up being your daddy's number one girl. Well, we'll see. It seems that your mother has been unhappy for a long time under your father's tight rein. Would you agree?

MARIA: Oh, yes!

THERAPIST: But as long as they had children at home—she took care of them and stayed home. Then for a little while it looked like the children were growing up—then I don't know what happened—something, maybe she pushed for more independence—I don't know—but we do know that now she has babies again. And things are back to where they were. Your father has very good daughters—they look out for his interests.

MARIA: I feel very sad for them both. And for my parents, too.

As Maria expresses feelings for her sister, and then for both parents, I separate the notion of doing something different from the need to go home. Perhaps she can "help" her family and still follow her own plans.

THERAPIST: Good, now that's some progress. You can start your change even before you go home. Perhaps you can continue with your plans for the summer and still do your family work.

I then tell her, "I would like you to write your mother the following letter":

Dear Mother,
    When I was home and you used to talk to me about wanting your independence, I used to get impatient. Forgive me, for I didn't understand how important that was.
    Now that I've grown up and had two wonderful independent years, I keep wondering how you were able to convince Daddy to let me achieve my independence even though you felt so helpless about achieving your own. I will always be grateful to you.
    As for Angelique and Laura, I'm sure that even though they are back in the nest now, you will be there to help them get on their way again.
                              Your grateful and loving daughter

THERAPIST: Can you do that?
MARIA: (*Doubtfully*) I think I can.

A Feminist Intervention

At one time my assessment of this case would have led me to feel that as a therapist I needed to help her separate from her controlling, demanding, albeit benevolent father. However, Maria needs to be helpful to her family and to stay connected in a meaningful way. Helping women to be uncaring of others and narcissistic in the name of autonomy seems a poor exchange.

    The first step in the process of change for Maria was to connect her to her mother—not to disconnect her from her father. My task in this one-session consultation was to use the information on the genogram in such a way that Maria's perception of the family, and her place in it, would shift so that she could see her options, and act, differently.

Maria's notions about her mother as a frivolous and foolish woman had its payoffs in her warm and cozy collusion with her daddy, and her identification with the "good," respectable side of the family. Wherever there is this kind of perceived difference in a couple in which one is seen as respectable, the other as disreputable—one good, one bad, one serious, one frivolous—the children can get caught in a loyalty bind that can be paralyzing; that is, they can't be good and they can't be bad. Or they may shift back and forth between the two sides trying desperately to be both. Or, like Maria, they can be induced to take one side. We could conjecture that the sisters may be balancing that position by joining mother.

It is obviously more difficult to give up membership in the respectable, high-functioning side of the family, to join what she sees as "the other." The task is to elevate the position of the mother enough to help Maria overcome her natural resistance. Why would anyone give up a good position in exchange for a dubious gain?

So knowing Maria's conflict about being a good daughter to her father and going home, or acting on her own wish to join friends on a trip, I now unhook the notion of going home from the notion of being a friend to her mother. So maybe she can stay here and still help the family. But I know that her reluctance to change her position in the family is based on several things, which, as we sit there winding up our hour, can hardly be in her awareness.

1. What will my father say? He'll be disappointed or angry or both.
2. I would be "abandoning" my father if I join my mother.
3. I don't like my mother—she's weak.
4. I have to rescue my sisters.
5. If I join the distaff side I will be weak and disreputable.
6. I like things the way they are—I just don't want to go home yet.

These are just a small sample of the possible points of resistance to change. So I begin: "Perhaps you can continue your plans for the summer and still do your family work." This statement addresses both sides of the conflict, and it offers immediate reassurance. That's what she came in asking for. I think it's possible. "Write your mother a letter—what's more, I'm going to tell you what to say."

Dear Mother, (*Maria's letters are generally addressed to father with postscripts to mother, or to "Dear Parents."*)

When I was home and you used to talk to me about wanting your independence, I used to get impatient. (*That sentence immediately elevates mother and joins her with Maria as*

*women wanting independence. "I used to get impatient" signi-
fies a change.)*

Forgive me, for I didn't understand how important that was. *("I
couldn't hear you then, but I do now.")*

**Now that I've grown up and had two wonderful independent
years, I keep wondering how you were able to convince daddy
to let me achieve my independence even though you felt so
helpless about achieving your own**. *(By acknowledging herself
as a grown-up woman who has enjoyed her independence,
Maria is reassured that she is not being asked to join her
mother as a child, but as an adult daughter.)*

By giving her mother recognition for, at the very least, not interfering with her growth, it becomes possible for her to honestly say, **"I
will always be grateful to you."** It also makes it easier for Rosa to
respond positively.

**As for Angelique and Laura, I'm sure that even though
they are back in the nest now, you will be there to help them
get on their way again.** *(This sentence implies that you are a
good and enabling mother. You have been a good mother to me,
and I trust that you are to my sisters. We both know the value
of independence as women.)*

MARIA: *(Doubtfully)* I think I can. *(This was not an easy letter for
Maria to write. It disrupted every image and perception she held about
her family and her place in it.)*

I added one more "strategic" statement before she left:

THERAPIST: I don't know if you will be able to send that letter.
But I want to tell you one more thing before you leave. I don't think
that men, and most particularly your father, are weak and need
to be placated and mollified, but I understand why you might
think so.

Maria's fear of her father's "anger" might be the rationale she
gives herself for not making a change. She might then say the letter is
"foolish" or "dishonest" and go home, thus perpetuating the old system
and actually helping no one, least of all herself. Reframing her behavior
toward her father as not respectful of his strength but protective of his
weakness may help her, since it throws her whole sense of herself in
relationship to him out of balance.

During the summer I received a few postcards from various parts of the country, and in September a long letter from Maria:

Dear Olga:
     So much has happened. I don't know where to start. After I wrote the first letter, I got an answer from my mother. She wrote, "My darling daughter, please do not disturb yourself about home. We will manage here. Angelique is already a little better—she goes to work every day with your father, and Laura, too, looks better. So finish your INDEPENDENCE. Your loving mother."

The word INDEPENDENCE had become the connecting link between Maria and her mother.

Can you imagine that? When I called my father to say I would come home in September as planned—he was first angry and said my sisters needed me, and I followed your lead, took a deep breath, and said that Mama was there to look after them.

Maria's response to her father was appropriate but not uncaring, and she responded to his story about the younger girls as she gently suggested that Rosa and not she, Maria, was their mother. And that Rosa was competent to care for them.

Then I got letters from my grandmother and aunt, both telling me that my father did not look well. I answered that I was sorry to hear that, but I was sure my mother would look after him. This went on all summer. Each time I got a letter I wrote to my mother and told her how I had replied. She always wrote me—encouraging me to enjoy myself.

The letters from grandma and aunt were to be expected as moves to bring things back to "normal." Again Maria was able to reply not by writing, "I don't care—I have my own life" but by saying, "If that's so—his wife is there. She will care for him." In fact, Maria went way beyond my expectations by writing to her mother and sharing her contacts with her father and grandmother. In effect, she told her, "I will not be a party to keeping secrets from you any more." Mother always responded by reassuring Maria that Maria was free to enjoy herself.

Now I have been home two weeks. I can't believe how my mother has changed. She confronted my father about Angelique and told him that he made her sick by sending her to London in such bad spirit. And, wonder of all, he has agreed that if it's

acting she wants—well, why not. So she's leaving for London this time with his blessing. Laura will re-enter school in a few weeks.

I don't know how all this came about, but I guess if we have patience things work themselves out.

Now I am trying to find a place for myself in this family. I always thought I knew exactly where I belonged. It feels strange but not bad. I guess I understand for the first time in a real way what you always said. Change is hard even if it's for the better. Maybe it will make me a better family therapist, knowing that.

                                        Affectionately, Maria

Summary

Maria needed to be helpful to her family. She needed to stay connected in a meaningful way. By the same token she needed to be free to live her own life. Women, through the generations, have known how to do the first. This generation of young women struggles to do the second. As therapists, it's our job to help them achieve both connectedness and autonomy.

Helping women toward autonomy by supporting narcissistic cut-offs and confrontations is not merely the flip side of the coin, but also invalidates what women have learned from their mothers and so silences "the woman's voice" in all of us.

Marianne Walters

The Different Faces of Close

Fathers of teenage daughters are particularly susceptible to the generalized male mystification of woman that is best illustrated in that plaintive query, "What *do* women want?" At best, teenagers confuse and confound their parents. For fathers and their adolescent daughters this is exaggerated by that general "state of confusion" men have about women's needs, emotions, style, and even biological processes—a state that is not only expected of men but about which there is considerable social acceptance, for instance, in the form of media images, male camaraderie, humor, and the like.

This confusion or mystification is "reason enough" for fathers to defer to their wives when it comes to direct dealings with their adolescent daughters. For daughters, the inherent danger in this paternal attitude is that they will experience themselves, during those crucial formative adolescent years, as not being taken seriously. If their moods, conflicts, aspirations, and ideas are somehow seen as simply the unfathomable workings of the female psyche—charming, but not quite understandable to their fathers—daughters will learn how to charm rather than how to take charge. Fathers of adolescent girls will protect them or avoid them; they will indulge them or be strict with them; but they will seldom deal with them directly concerning their own emotional and intellectual issues. Of course there are exceptions to this attitude. But so often in our work with adolescent girls we see them in conflict with their mothers and detached or worshipful with their fathers; they tend to engage their mothers and circumvent their fathers. So again, the system will look like another "overinvolved" mother and "peripheral" father. And family therapy will frequently mirror this system with moves directed toward hierarchy, boundary, or function. A father may be called in to restore order or to keep the peace; he may be advised to turn his attention to his wife; but seldom will the father be encouraged to "enter the fray" and engage directly with his daughter around the developmental issues with which she is struggling.

The following case illustrates how the mystification of the female experience can, on the one hand, obscure and trivialize the behaviors of an adolescent daughter and, on the other hand, make her father feel unqualified to deal directly with them. In this family the father is functioning as a single parent. Having enjoyed a warm and loving relationship with his young daughter, but unable to "turn her over" to his wife as she enters adolescence, he is rendered inept as a parent when his daughter begins to have problems, act out, become moody. Having tried to deal with her as he would a son—with rules, sanctions, discipline—and failing, he feels lost and unsure. At the same time, his confusion about her developmental processes as an emerging woman makes his daughter feel diminished. So they both fall back on earlier behaviors: he cajoles, she becomes petulant.

The therapist for this family was one of my trainees (a clinical psychologist) in a practicum training program at the Family Therapy Practice Center. Supervision in this program includes both direct (live) supervision and video review of sessions, on an ongoing weekly basis. The supervision group is made up of trainees who work and learn together, observe each other's sessions, discuss clinical issues and debate techniques, but do not enter directly into the supervisory process during the conduct of a session, for instance, by making suggestions to the therapist/trainee or by providing a clinical counterpoint. Any peer supervision that occurs is informal.

In describing this case I have included some of the supervisory discussion that framed the therapy. It seems to me that supervision and training is a crucial place for developing a consciousness among therapists not only about what to do and what will work, but about how our social, cultural, and methodological contexts shape our choices and behaviors, our attitudes and values, in conducting therapy. This, I believe, helps to create the dialectic between the personal and the technological, between imagination, intuition and professional calculation that is the key to the heart of therapy.

The Family

Sam, a man of about 44, brought his 15-year-old daughter, Barbie, to the center requesting therapy for the two of them. An epidemiologist at a local medical research center, Sam was very concerned about the "sudden" changes he was experiencing in his daughter's attitudes and behavior toward him, and most especially in her attitude and deteriorating performance at school. At home, with him, Barbie had become surly, sullen, and disobedient. She disagreed with almost everything he said, and resisted most of what he asked of her. At school her grades had taken a nose dive, from mostly A's, to C's and D's. For the first time, teachers at the school Barbie attended were calling him about their concerns instead of their praise. They complained that Barbie had become negativistic and seemed to have lost interest in academic achievement as well as in other activities at school. Sam had tried "reasoning" with her, getting "tough," imposing sanctions. But each thing just seemed to make matters worse. He was running out of options and was very disappointed. Now, he said, they seemed to be locked into two opposing positions, facing each other down across a deep chasm.

Barbie, a very bright, sophisticated high-school sophomore, vehemently disagreed with her dad. She believed the problem was that *he* had locked himself into an extreme position and that *he* could get out of it if *he* really wanted to. He was just stubborn, insisting on treating her as if she were a two-year-old. School was her business. She knew what she had to do to manage it, and he should just get off her back. Did she tell him how to do his work?

Interestingly, their interactions in the first therapy session belied both the alienation from his daughter that Sam was describing, and the anger toward her dad that Barbie was expressing. They were obviously affectionate and even relaxed with each other, smiling over private jokes and making constant eye contact as they responded to questions. The therapist, a psychologist I was supervising in an advanced training program at the center, later described feeling almost like an intruder in their private world. Although their language was often harsh as each described mounting disagreements and conflict, their manner with each other was playful and gentle.

Barbie and her dad have enjoyed an almost exclusive relationship since Sam and his wife, Rose, were divorced when Barbie was 3. At the time of the divorce Rose was seriously depressed and returned to her parents' home in another city. She and Sam agreed to his retaining custody of Barbie until she was on her feet again. After something over a year of treatment Rose returned to college, which she had dropped out of after marriage. Upon graduation Rose came back to the city, set up her own household, started work, and began seeing Barbie regularly—weekends, vacations, overnight. She and Sam had another go-round on custody and sought mediation. The result was the continuation of Sam's custody of Barbie, then 7, with Rose having flexible, unlimited visitation rights. There was another period of negotiation over custody when Rose remarried, the results of which pretty much maintained the status quo. Barbie sees her mom regularly. She describes their relationship as "up and down," and says that lately they've been talking a lot about their feelings toward each other, and about the past.

Clearly Sam and Barbie have made a winsome duo over the years. Both are wiry, dark, energetic, attractive, with a kind of pixie charm and wry humor. They obviously adore each other despite their current conflicts and differences. Sam reminisced about how they used to "hang out" together, and how they enjoyed so many of the same things, with shared tastes in movies, books, music. He worried that their present differences would destroy their closeness.

In recent months Sam had been dating a woman with whom he has become quite serious. In fact, they are planning for her to move in with him in two months. It was actually Elly, Sam's woman friend, who had precipitated his seeking therapy, although he has for some time been concerned about the problems with his daughter. Sam, Elly, and Barbie had taken a trip together over the Easter holidays, and Barbie had behaved "horribly," making it miserable for all of them. Elly and Sam had fought about Barbie's behavior, with Elly demanding to know why he "put up with such crap." Finally, she suggested that he and Barbie get some help, to which Sam agreed, when Barbie did not object.

The First Session

In the first session the therapist relabeled Barbie's sullen rebelliousness as a normal developmental transition of adolescence. While admiring their close relationship and appreciating Sam's concern about maintaining it, the therapist cautioned against Sam's tendency to "peer" with Barbie, pointing out that an adolescent, even one as precocious as Barbie, needs a parent who has clear expectations and is in charge. Dad could not expect to seek Barbie's opinion on every family rule and household decision, and then be upset when she differed with him. The therapist worked with Sam to establish some small but precise expectations with Barbie regarding school performance in the coming week, while at the same time helping him to agree not to actually monitor Barbie's schoolwork at home. With some reluctance, Sam delineated the consequences for Barbie if she failed to uphold her part of the bargain. While Sam felt that the first priority for change concerned schoolwork, since it had taken on crisis proportions, he cautioned that they would have to deal, in the very near future, with Barbie's attitude toward him. Barbie insisted that her dad would have to stop treating her like a baby if that attitude were going to change. The therapist helped both of them to call a truce concerning who and what was to blame for their current conflicts, and to agree to focus— this one week—on managing school more successfully.

Supervision: Feminist Perspectives

The issue for family therapists seeking a feminist perspective is to challenge our own assumptions and therapy traditions in order to probe the ways that sex roles and gendered power systems structure family relationships and influence our own thinking about what is happening in the families we see. Within this framework, my supervision between therapy sessions is focused on analyzing and critiquing the concepts and assumptions underlying alternative interventions.

The supervisory group was concerned that Sam treated Barbie "like an equal" and that they functioned "very like a married couple." The therapist saw Barbie as participating in a triangled relationship with Elly and suspected that it had roots in unresolved issues with her own mother. Her current symptoms were thus probably precipitated by the increased commitment between Sam and Elly. He suggested that the therapy be directed toward helping Sam establish more appropriate boundaries with his daughter, and restructuring the hierarchy of the family system by setting clear-cut expectations and firm monitoring of her school performance. The group suggested that it would be useful to have Elly in for some sessions, and wondered about working with Barbie and her mother, who could well be undermining Sam's authority at this crucial time in their daughter's life.

We rightly assume that hierarchy, boundaries, authority, limits, and rules are necessary systemic regulators of healthy family functioning. Yet, seen in a larger social context, these properties, or areas of functioning, will be understood to have very different meaning and significance for men and women. They are manifested or expressed in different ways for mothers and fathers, sons and daughters. For instance, fathers will tend to use their authority with their daughters in indirect ways to avoid conflict and maintain the posture of "benign paternalism." (With their sons they will tend to be more direct, risking conflict along with the expectation of achievement.) Similarly, a hierarchical relationship with daughters will often be manifested by fathers around entitlement, protection, and permission; with sons it will be centered more on management, control, and responsibility.

I thus cautioned the group to use these systemic concepts with reference to their differing meanings for each sex. For instance, while supporting Sam's authority, we would challenge its "paternalistic" features; while working with boundaries and rules, we would pay careful attention to appropriate ways of empowering Barbie.

Certainly, the chronology of events in this case suggests that Barbie's negativistic behavior is connected to Sam's serious interest in Elly and their intention to live together. And, surely, unresolved issues between Barbie and her mother, her anger and fear of being left, are part of the current scenario. Yet if we were to work with either Elly or Barbie's mother at this juncture, there is the danger of reproducing a transaction that would both conform to and confirm (to this family) the widely held assumption that if the women in families would work out their conflicts and contradictions, the men would be free to behave in their less complicated, more straightforward ways.

This belief—that the more direct, less emotionally laden dealings of men are often impeded by the indirect, emotional, even mysterious dealings of the womenfolk—is so generalized in our culture that we hardly notice it, and are frequently moved to sort things out between the women while the men await a "higher" ground on which to enter the fray. Though clearly Sam is deeply engaged with his daughter, he just as surely experiences the relationship between Elly and Barbie as emotionally volatile; and they could all (including the therapist) easily slip into the "comfortable" culture of woman-focused change (and problem) if either Elly or Rose were brought into treatment at this juncture!

The nature of the relationship between this father and daughter is forged as much in the crucible of cultural images as in the particulars of their personalities and family system: the "besotted" doting father of the teen daughter, not understanding "what girls want," but adoring them for being so complex and emotional even while berating them for not being more logical and direct (straight out of a dozen renditions of *Pygmalion*). The loving lament, "Why can't she be more like me?" is accompanied by the clear message that she would lose her special place in his heart if indeed this miracle could be performed. The daughter knows the way to her father's heart is through charm and guile; that to get her own way she needs only to have him wrapped in loving embrace around her little finger. If this doesn't work she can always "go off the deep end" and so completely mystify him. Straight out of a million TV soaps and paperback novels!

With these cultural stereotypes in mind, I suggested that the therapy remain centered on Sam and Barbie for the present, and that the therapist focus on the theme of their closeness, using it as the basis for a range of personal skills that each has, and can use, in exploring new styles of connectedness more appropriate to the current developmental changes in their lives.

Since I work *within* the therapy session to challenge habitual interactional processes and to create new perceptions and experiences among family members, I counseled the therapist to pay attention to the gender constructs in the behaviors and interactions of this father and daughter *as they occurred*: Barbie's lowered eyes, secret smiles, ready tears, coyness, and coquetry as she struggles to win acceptance of her growing up and her search for self-definition; Sam's pleading, cajoling, but half-amused efforts to articulate his concerns. The therapist needs to validate their closeness, as both a value and a competence, while persuading both of them that in its present manifestation it is getting in the way of new directions that each is independently seeking. Father's wisdom could be affirmed by helping him to articulate his expectations and parental values without benefit of the pleading glance and cajoling stance; daughter's intelligence could be highlighted by helping her to discuss her needs without benefit of the lowered eyes and secret smiles.

Finally, Barbie needs to experience the power of her own resources and skills before she can begin to relinquish the derivative power she has found in being "daddy's little girl." Her resistance and ambivalence about change can be understood not only as developmental, or as a system's homeostatic impulse, but also in terms of the real conflict for a young woman (even in these enlightened times) in seeking a self-definition that is not male-identified. Similarly, for Sam— with few male models on which to base his role as primary parent—he employs the acculturated relational skills he knows best, vacillating between "buddy" and instrumental agent. Without social supports that value his parental function, he will need help in affirming his own "knowing" as a parent before he can begin to reach for new areas of connectedness that encourage autonomy.

Ongoing Therapy

Sam began the second session by reporting that Barbie had not followed through on the school expectations on which they had agreed in the initial interview. He said he had been leaning on her pretty hard. Barbie was furious. Sam was frustrated and sad. The therapist defined Barbie's negativistic behaviors as inexpert ways of seeking to establish her own "identity," her separateness, rather than as simply oppositional. Her efforts to "be my own person" scared them both because it threatened their special closeness and sharing.

The therapy sessions with Sam and Barbie were used to redefine and reorganize their relationship, working with such issues as Barbie's school performance, household rules, behavioral expectations, parental values, and the "crisis of growing up." The direction of therapy was based on the belief that a more functional relationship between Sam and Barbie would not only free each to deal more successfully with significant others in their lives—for example, Sam with Elly, Barbie with her mother—but also would serve to reduce the anxiety and ambivalence exacerbating Barbie's rebellious behavior. In working to expand their range of skills in dealing with their differences, change was framed with reference to personal style, "old" assumptions that underlie current behaviors, and the flexibility to experiment with alternatives. Guided by the conceptual framework we had evolved in supervisory sessions, the therapist could provide Sam and Barbie with a new perspective on their interpersonal process, one that challenged their usual transactions in terms of the gendered messages they implicitly conveyed. For instance, in the second session we chose to highlight the way Sam's protective behaviors reinforced Barbie's anxiety about using her own resources, and at the same time we held Barbie accountable for her own ideas as a measure of respect for them.

BARBIE: (*To her dad*) If you'd just get off my back, leave me alone! I'm okay the way I am. I like it this way.

SAM: No you don't, no you don't, honey. It can't just go on this way. You'll get into trouble that I won't be able to get you out of, no matter how much I want to. Than you'll be up the creek, and it'll be too late.

THERAPIST: Hold it a minute, Sam, I think I know what you mean, and how much you want to help. But the idea that's coming across, Sam, is that Barbie should behave herself in school because she won't be able to handle the troubles not behaving will get her into. My guess, Sam, is that you're afraid she might just fall into that hole she's digging and your safety net won't be strong enough to save her. (*Smiling*) You want she should shape up so she'll fit into your safety net?

SAM: (*Chuckling*) No, no—that's not what I mean. (*Seriously*) It's just that she needs to know that there is just so much I can do to set things right for her; that there are limits to what I can do.

THERAPIST: For sure. And if she understands that then you believe she'll begin to think for herself and do what she needs to do to get along in school?

SAM: Yeah, yeah. You see—she really counts on me even when she's always saying—no, screaming—leave me alone!

THERAPIST: You bet she does. Sam, you sure do know her. Yet I think it's something you both do, in different ways. Well, what I mean, Sam, is—you want Barbie to take care of things herself and at the same time you want her to continue to depend on you. That part—the depending on you part—is the stuff you think keeps you two close, I'll bet. Lots of fathers have learned to think this way about their daughters—especially about their daughters. With their sons it's more like, "Get out there and learn to depend on yourself." With daughters it's more like "I'll take care of you" (*Sam and Barbie grinning at each other*).

BARBIE: That's right—you got it! Daddy just won't let me do anything for myself.

THERAPIST: There's an old song—Sam, you may remember it, (*Singing*) "It seems to me I've heard that song before, it's from an old familiar score, I know it well, that melody. . . ." Oh, Barbie—you're soooo quick to sing that old refrain! (*More seriously*) I wonder—if just maybe—you're kept so busy working the angles, playing both sides of Dad against his middle—so to speak—that you don't have any time left to think for yourself. Do you think, Barbie, that other girls learn to do this when they feel like they aren't being taken seriously, hummm? (*Barbie, sitting up, very attentive*). Well, anyway, Sam, how about trying to find out if Barbie has some ideas about how she's going to manage school differently—other then beseeching you to get off her back and proclaiming her independence.

SAM: Well, Barbie—what do you say? What do you have—sooo, is there something . . . (*Barbie looks sad and wipes away some tears*). Now honey—it's nothing to cry about. We're all here trying to help you, to make things better.

THERAPIST: Oh, oh—Barbie really knows that, Sam. But she's learned that crying is one way to get to you—or maybe get around you! Or maybe it's her way of protecting you—maybe she doesn't believe you can stick with getting at *her* ideas—and she doesn't want you to fail.

BARBIE: That's all bullshit!

THERAPIST: How so, Barbie?

BARBIE: I can damn well take care of myself.

THERAPIST: No—I mean, how is what we've been talking about bullshit?

BARBIE: Well, it's just crap, plain crap! All this is just about *his* wanting to get *his* way.

SAM: Barbie, I want to hear why you think it's crap.

BARBIE: It just is.

SAM: That won't do.

BARBIE: Tough . . .

SAM: Look, honey—the thing is, I'm trying to sort things out, make things better between us and . . .

THERAPIST: Hold it a minute, Sam; has Barbie said why our discussion is bullshit? You see, if she has trouble saying what she means, and you get out your safety net, she's going to get the idea that you don't believe she can use her own very good head when she's in trouble—or otherwise.

SAM: You have a point, a point. (*Reflectively*) Barbie, honey, I think we have got to get past this; we're stuck. And you can do better than just calling everything bullshit—you've got to do better. It's the damnedest thing how we go back and forth. So what do you think about my safety net, or your tears, or what is going down in school? Begin . . . wherever . . .

BARBIE: You're gonna be sorry you ever asked!

SAM: I suspect I will . . .

The therapist has constructed a sequence that moves Sam from engaging Barbie as a petulant child to beginning to encourage her to feel safe in expressing her differences and her viewpoint in less reactive, more self-defined ways. Using different content, such interventions are repeated throughout the next several sessions as the therapist works with Barbie and Sam to redefine and reshape their relationship. For instance, a sequence in the fourth session exemplifies the therapist's persistence in pursuing this frame of reference.

BARBIE: The problem, Daddy, is—you treat me like a baby and then you expect me to be all grown up.

SAM: That's because one minute you act like a baby, and the next minute you act like you think you're a grown-up.

BARBIE: So, what are you going to do about it?

SAM: Not much, young lady. I think you're going to have to decide which act . . .

THERAPIST: Well, now, it looks like you all are moving toward another brilliant no-win contest! Figuring out "who's on first" and who started what isn't going to change it. Sam, do you think Barbie's made a point worth pursuing?

SAM: Well, maybe . . . you mean . . . I'm not sure . . . well, anyway, so continue your thought, Barbie.

BARBIE: Soooo, all right. Like . . . see . . . so I guess . . . ummm . . . well, I think . . . sooo, you see, it's like sometimes I feel really, really on top of things; sooo, okay . . . and then I get, well . . . maybe scared, or pissed about something and like it's going to be too much . . . and then, then I don't even want to be on top of my own shit . . . so then, then maybe I act dumb—like a baby—but I'm not . . .

SAM: (*Tenderly*) I know you're not, honey. And when you feel like that you can always come to me and we'll talk it over.

THERAPIST: Sam, Barbie really, really knows she can do that. Have you any other suggestions for her when she's feeling low? What do you know about her that would help?

SAM: Well . . . that everyone feels that way sometimes and that it's OK. And that a person doesn't always have to be on top of things.

BARBIE: (*Muttering, with lowered eyes*) . . . except you.

THERAPIST: What do you know about Barbie, in particular?

SAM: Ummm, well, that she's resilient—and she has a great sense of humor, and that, yes . . . that she's inventive.

BARBIE: What do you mean?

THERAPIST: What do you think Dad means?

BARBIE: (*Smiling*) That I make things up . . . no, only kidding folks . . . inventive . . . get it? Ha, ha! (*Getting serious*) Oh, I know what he means . . . he means that I can figure some ways out of my own shit pile. Use my imagination.

THERAPIST: So why did you ask?

BARBIE: Like you're always saying—habit—bad habit!

This sequence illustrates interventions in the ongoing therapy that affirm Sam's parental competence—here, his knowledge about his daughter—as the foundation for his beginning to risk giving up some of the perks of paternalism. At the same time, Barbie is encouraged to trust her own competencies—here, her ability to explain her thinking—without fear of losing Dad's protection in the process. They are exploring new ways of being close.

The following excerpt from the fifth session illustrates a similar process with different content.

SAM: Look, Barbie—you're just not getting any new clothes if you can't take care of the ones you already have.

BARBIE: I don't give a shit . . . when Elly comes I can borrow some of her stuff—she already said I could.

SAM: That isn't the point. That's nice of Elly but I still want you to learn to take care of your things, and for that matter, Elly's too, if you borrow something of hers.

BARBIE: That's really up to Elly, Dad. That's none of your business.

SAM: Yes it is, and Elly completely agrees with me on this issue.

BARBIE: Elly's not nearly such a fiend about junk like that as you are.

THERAPIST: Whoa—it's interesting, Sam, that you started out talking about what you expect from Barbie, and now you're talking about Elly. Smart move, there, Barbie—when in trouble bring in new troops!

BARBIE: (*Lowering her eyes*) Welll . . . maybe. Anyway, my clothes aren't any of his business and I'm tired of being threatened.

THERAPIST: OK, that's better. What do you propose instead?

BARBIE: Instead of what?

THERAPIST: Instead of the threats.

BARBIE: That's not the point.

THERAPIST: What is the point?

BARBIE: That he should leave me alone.

THERAPIST: OK. What do you propose instead? How do you think things should go between you?

SAM: Barbie—let's say I back off . . .

THERAPIST: Wait, Sam. Your safety net is out.

BARBIE: (*Relaxing a bit*) Well, we could . . . like, maybe . . . well, maybe your standards are too high. Don't get me wrong . . . I'm not suggesting they should be as low as mine! (*Everybody smiling now*) But, Dad . . . well, why don't we talk about what in hell "neat" means . . . you know, let's define our terms!

THERAPIST: Reasonable approach. Would you agree, Sam? (*Nodding*) So . . . who's going to begin?

In the sixth session, Barbie and Sam arrive furious with one another, avoiding eye contact and hardly able to speak to each other. It seems Sam had refused to let Barbie go to a party on Friday night because she was late with several school assignments. Despite the anger, they had already begun to self-correct.

BARBIE: (*Slumping in her seat; "sotto voce"*) It's no use, he just throws his weight around and doesn't trust me no matter what I do. It's no use. I'm a prisoner in my own house.

SAM: Barbie will just have to learn the hard way that there are consequences if she doesn't do what is expected of her.

THERAPIST: Do you think, Sam, that Barbie fully understands what you mean?

SAM: (*Struggling to explain*) Barbie, I can't let you off the hook . . . I can't let you mess up and get away with it. If I did, in the end you'll suffer more.

BARBIE: Oh, I see . . . so now I can't even do my own suffering in my own time!

SAM: (*Startled, then laughing*) Right, right . . . you're right! (*Seriously*) It's not about your suffering more or less. It's about my own decision in the matter. There will be consequences when you . . . with no real reason . . . abrogate your responsibilities at school.

BARBIE: Abro . . . who?

SAM: Give up on . . .

BARBIE: Oh, yeah—well, I don't think the consequences should jeopardize my peer relationships! How's that for big words—I guess I can sling 'em around with the best of them!

There were eight sessions with Sam and Barbie. These were followed by three sessions with Sam and Elly, with Barbie being seen separately. With Sam and Elly, the focus was on sorting out their own arrangements and intentions as a couple and in relation to living together with Barbie. With Barbie, the sessions were devoted to dealing with her issues at school and some concerns she had about friendships, especially with boys. In a situation like this one it is important to see the teenage daughter alone a few times so as to demonstrate in deed as well as word her capacity to sort out some things on her own. The last two sessions, after Elly moved in, involved all three of them. The therapist continued to relate to Sam as the primary parent and to support him in not relying on Barbie and Elly to organize the newly formed household. Barbie was encouraged to resist the natural temptation to form a right flank (with either Elly or Sam) when the left flank wasn't working well, since she was a born strategist. And Elly was welcomed into the family.

Outcome

Barbie's schoolwork improved, but she did fail one subject, having fallen behind too much to recover. This meant summer school, which she hated; but since she was "suffering" anyway, she took a job for the first time—and loved it. Camp was forever foresworn in favor of "gainful employment"! Sam called six weeks after therapy ended for a consultation session—to help in figuring out some of the dynamics of their new family constellation. Ten weeks later he, Barbie, and Elly came in for a "checkup." Needless to say, there was plenty going on, this being a rather lively crew! But they felt they were coping and even enjoying being a family. At the checkup session Barbie asked permission to come in with her mother a couple of times. Sam agreed, and Barbie and her mother were seen together for three sessions to talk about their own relationship.

As within most families, this father and daughter needed to restructure their relationship as Barbie traveled from childhood to adolescence. What is often missed in understanding this interpersonal realignment is the profound influence of our cultural mores and social expectations on the process of change. Certainly Barbie's symptomatic behaviors could have been improved and change brought about between father and daughter in a number of ways. Yet, if in the process Sam had continued relating to Barbie in the manner to which they had both become accustomed—as daddy's little girl—the danger is that she might have grown up to be one.

Adolescence is a volatile time; feelings are intensified and behaviors are exaggerated. Defining oneself, seeking autonomy, and struggling with dependence are all mixed up, for both girls and boys, during these years. But for fathers and their daughters the expectation is that the struggle will be played out between mother and daughter.

In this case, the therapy was intended to create a context in which father and daughter would feel safe engaging directly with each other—in common cause as well as in struggle around their differences—without needing to resort to role stereotypes. It was a therapy intended to demystify the daughter, empower her by encouraging self-defined behaviors for which she would be accountable, and to offer her father alternatives to the paternalism of one who protects and entitles a dependent.

4   *Olga Silverstein*

Mothers and Sons

ALTHOUGH POPULAR IMAGES of the ideal woman have been challenged in recent years by feminist analysts, the mythology of the mother-son relationship seems to remain inviolate. Few women have the courage to deflate those myths. Mothers have helped to perpetuate it with a view toward building the armor that they think their sons will need to face the outside world. The fear of alienating a male child from his culture and thereby subjecting him to ridicule and shame goes deep, even for women who reject that culture for themselves and their daughters.

Woman's covert role in the maintenance of the status quo in the family and, consequently, in society at large has until recently been shrouded by a conspiracy of silence. Despite the increasing volume of feminist scholarship in the last twenty years, there is precious little writing by women on the subject of mothers and sons. Such a conspicuous silence results largely from the fact that the dynamics of the mother-son relationship still lies at the very foundation of our contemporary social structure, yet paradoxically is seen as the source of all dysfunction in the sons.

Myths of Gender

Verbal conceptualizations of motherhood have come traditionally from the sons. In *Every Mother's Son*, the feminist writer Judith Arcana (1983) points to the Orestes myth as one of the typical cultural models of our expectations of motherhood. In this myth, matricide is committed and male heroism is defined as a son's ability to destroy his mother's hold upon him. Arcana discusses Erich Neumann's interpretation of the Orestes myth. In his analysis, Neumann praised Orestes' "identification with the father" because, in his view, it enabled Orestes to defy the maternal principle and thereby avoid emasculation.

Ever since the middle of the nineteenth century, when industrial capitalism severed the bond between the nuclear family and the public world, women have been charged with most of the responsibility for raising children of both sexes. As work, education, childbirth, and religion moved out of the household and into larger public institutions, women became imprisoned in a narrow interpersonal structure (Goldner, 1984) that was to serve as a refuge for men from the pressures of the workaday world. In this rarefied atmosphere, women were charged with preparing male children for their roles outside the home and female children for their future homemaking functions within the family.

In her book *Reproduction of Mothering* (1978), Nancy Chodorow traces the sociohistorical context of the institution of motherhood and defines its relationship to the economic structure. She asserts that the modern division of roles in the family and the personality characteristics needed to perform each of them were historically determined by specific functional relationships among caretaker, wage earner, and consumer.

This division of social and psychological roles is currently reflected in many institutions, products, and media creations intended for the molding of children (Hare-Mustin, 1983). Criticisms of mothers by family theorists in the 1950s and analyses of the historical determinants of motherhood by feminist theorists in the last fifteen years have to a certain extent shaken the confidence that society has placed in the institution of motherhood, yet without any discernable change in our expectations.

Although some of the tenets of the women's movement have trickled into the media in the form of watered-down clichés, the practice of child rearing, which inculcates many of the values a person will hold for life, still largely maintains gender-role distinctions. Motherhood itself today remains tacitly defined much as it was in the isolated milieu of the nineteenth-century "sanctified home." The fact still remains that the traditional postwar triad composed of an involved and nurturing parent (the mother) and a detached primary wage earner (the father) is still fundamental to the economically and socially functional family; but this fact has not prevented the mental health profession from ascribing many disturbances in children to "too much mother and not enough father."

In today's loosening family structure, women who become mothers and thereby take on the primary responsibility for building their children's system of values have lately been faced with some complex and contradictory choices in a world that is still largely dominated by men. These contradictions are especially aggravated when it comes to the mothering of sons.

The Paradoxical Role of Women
in Mothering Sons

To perform her tasks as defined by a patriarchal society, a woman must be warm, responsive, caring, nurturing, and self-sacrificing. This stands in complementary opposition to masculine objectivity, detachment, autonomy, aggression, and sexual freedom—in short, all those characteristics that make men function successfully in the world of enterprise outside the family. The mother of sons, then, stands in the position of having to create her complementary opposite, someone destined to behave in a way that works to keep both mothers and sons locked into the established social structure, and perhaps also locked in opposition to each other. A mother does not necessarily act to her personal advantage when she acts as the agent and nurturer of male authority.

As a mother raises her son, she must be careful to be loving and nurturing without being seductive. She must be available and attentive but never appear to be smothering. And she must always be aware of the right moment for her to pull out and turn her son over to his father and the world of men.

The mother who feels that she has been competent during the early years of her son's life will often draw back when she feels it is time for him to assume male roles, or if she feels there is some failure or lag in his development. The son's failure carries the stigma for the mother of having created a "momma's boy." If her child is to be seen as functioning successfully as an adult, he must learn to abandon the intimacy of the mother-son dyad and join ranks with his peers. And the mother—no matter what her deepest instincts may be telling her—is expected to facilitate the son's move into the male domain. Thus, the "good mother" is expected to facilitate a pattern of emotional development in her son that stands in direct opposition to her own.

In shaping her son's manhood with a view toward his successful functioning in the outside world, a mother acts as the agent of power in a hierarchy that rests on her obedience. Such obedience may conflict with feelings of resentment about her own sense of disenfranchisement and her ideas about the nature of ethical or reasonable behavior. Or she may never develop such ideas because of a blind identification with the sources of power that control her.

In a much publicized study of obedience to authority, Stanley Milgram (1974) demonstrated that most individuals will obey authority even when its demands seem to conflict with personal ethical values. Milgram defines obedience to authority as the loss of autonomy when such loss is prescribed by a specific hierarchical structure. As soon as an individual enters a specific hierarchy, some degree of personal responsibility is abdicated to make the hierarchical system function smoothly. In those individuals whose scruples conflict with obedience to an authority that appears to them as malevolent, Milgram identifies *conflictual strain* and enumerates the various mental and behavioral mechanisms that are employed to alleviate it. These include avoidance, denial, subterfuge, the search for social reassurances, irrationally blaming the victim against whom one has acted aggressively, and paying lip service to dissent without actually rebelling. Anyone who has had some experience working in one of the mental health professions will recognize that the majority of these mechanisms have been widely applied to analyses of female pathology.

In clinical practice it is not unusual to find any or all of the above behaviors when a woman is acting on the instructions or orders of an authority figure she cannot openly defy. The mother in the following case—unsure of her ground in the face of the apparent certainty of the father and the therapist's support of the father's position—first tries pseudocompliance, then avoidance ("I can't, I don't know how"), finally anger at her son for not performing.

A Clinical Example

A family is referred to therapy because their only son, a 12-year-old boy, has been diagnosed as learning disabled. The problem, as defined by the father, is not the learning disability, but what he perceives as a lack of structure in the home. The school authorities as well as the examining psychologist had both stressed the fact that the boy needed structured help at home to enable him to concentrate on tasks in a focused way. Father told the therapist that he expected his wife to spend time daily with the boy and his homework. "I work long hours and by the time I get home it's too late. She has to be the one to help him." Mother complained that she was not able to help. She didn't remember her arithmetic, the boy didn't listen to her, and so forth. This argument was waged between the parents session after session while the boy sat sullenly and silently.

The therapist attempted two maneuvers. First he tried negotiation. Mother could help the boy on weekdays, father on the weekends. When that failed, as the mother reported her inability to keep her end of the bargain, the therapist, trying not to lose patience with her seeming noncompliance, interpreted it as the mother's unwillingness to "let the boy go." Feeling bullied by the therapist's interpretation, the mother agreed she would try again. Two weeks later they returned and reported that the mother had indeed tried. She sat with the boy day after day, insisting that he attend to his work. She reported that it seemed he was trying, but he was very upset. She wept. The therapist indicated that (having complied) she was "overinvolved."

Father was pleased and was encouraged to compliment and reward both mother and son, thus maintaining his hierarchical alliance with the therapist as well as the school and the psychologist. The more mother complied, the more miserable she appeared and the unhappier the boy seemed.

The therapist then asked the mother what she felt was her son's problem and what she thought were possible solutions. He apologized for not asking her sooner and merely assuming that the authorities were right. After all, as a mother, she knew her son better than anyone else.

The mother, with tears in her eyes, looking nervously at her husband, said, "Bobby is a very creative and sensitive child. It's true he doesn't learn in the conventional way but he is intelligent. The pressure to conform to those rules makes him very unhappy. I think we make him feel inadequate. I think he should be in a different school which values what he has to offer. I told my husband that, but he says I'm pampering him." By the end of that session, with encouragement from the supervisor and then the therapist, attention was respectfully paid to the mother's point of view as well as to the boy who spoke for the first time, attesting to his intelligence. Then the therapist was instructed to ask the father to express his concerns. "I don't want him to be a mama's boy—sensitive and creative. He needs to grow up."

The three members in this family were then helped, first, to listen to each other, and then to agree that *both* parents had something important to contribute. A month later they had located a school with a much less structured learning program that still paid attention to what the father saw as the need for discipline.

At times a mother who finds herself relegated to the isolation of family life when she had ambitions in the outside world may express a distorted version of her own needs for competence and validation in covert or devious ways. She is aware that she must ensure her husband's freedom to pursue economic and status goals while she herself remains responsible for the climate of emotional commitment in the family. And she has often learned to displace her own aspirations for power and autonomy.

In an attempt to cope with the frustrations inherent in this situation, some mothers project their squelched dreams for influence onto their sons by encouraging them to be overly ambitious or aggressive. Sometimes these mothers are very successful.

Other mothers may distort more petty disagreements involving male children into psychodramas that covertly express marital conflicts. The overdramatized emotionalism of "Pick up your clothes, I'm not your slave," cannot be ascribed solely to a mother's response to an intractable four-year-old son. In statements such as these, a woman is also expressing half-conscious feelings about her husband, her marriage, and her own feelings about her place in the social structure.

Feelings of powerlessness may result in the forming of alliances between mother and son against a distant or domineering husband that both have learned to resent. But underlying this temporary alliance is the mother's fear that her own skills and talents provide no viable role model for her son. If her son is to survive in the male world, he should not turn out to be too much like mother nor should he be overly disturbed when their bond is disrupted. And if she flounders when he leaves her, her loss should not be taken too seriously lest he feel guilty. There are no established traditions for guiding a woman through this difficult period of loss, nor are there any specific therapeutic models for treating its effects, despite the fact that mental health professionals are well aware that the majority of high-stress events in an individual's life have to do with losing or gaining a family member.

Role Conflicts Facing Women Family Therapists

A silence paralleling the silence that conceals the meaning of woman's contemporary role as a mother of sons also shrouds the conflicts faced by women in their role as family therapists. Such conflicts can be understood in the context of the history of the mental health establishment, which itself stands in complex relationship to changes that took place in the family and in society at large in the latter part of the nineteenth century.

Historically, the American mental health movement has always fluctuated indecisively between the need to help individuals achieve autonomy and self-direction and the need to influence them to adjust, or conform, to the functional demands of specific social conditions. These conflicting aims are often confused. The therapeutic conflict is no more clearly revealed than in the case of the family unit, where autonomy and self-direction—especially on the part of women—are often in direct opposition to a smoothly functioning family.

Some female family therapists were initially attracted to the structural/strategic family systems model because they felt it would provide a means of reorganizing the balance of power in the family. Others merely learned the systems model and used it without any consciousness of its relationship to larger social issues. However, it was not long before many female therapists realized that imbalances in the family power structure were one of the very factors that sustained it and made it functional in the larger social order. When a family therapist comes to this realization, she may begin to regard certain traditional therapeutic interventions as thinly disguised alibis for protecting or concealing power inequities.

The family's gradual retreat from the outside world has been paralleled by its conceptualization in family therapy as a nearly autonomous organism in which individuals play equal parts. Because this approach amputates the family from the larger social context that the family actually models and sustains, the responsibility for pathology has been placed on family members without acknowledgment of the inequitable balance of power in the family, as in society at large.

A dysfunctional mother/son dyad is most often thought of as one in which a mother's "overinvolvement" with her son has been interfering with his psychic and social development as a "normal" male. In conventional family therapy, the mother's central conflict—the fact that she is being asked to show total dedication to another without overinvolvement—is usually deemphasized in favor of a focus on the therapeutic needs of the son. The therapist strives to move the son out of the "smothering" mother-son bond into a new relationship with his father, with whom he is expected to achieve identification, and from whom he will learn coping skills that will help him in the outside world. The father is encouraged to return to the family circle in order to foster this new involvement, and the mother is encouraged to develop her own life and asked to accept the loss of her son as inevitable.

When a therapist acts as one of the agents that sets this shift in motion, she is acting to curtail mother-son intimacy in an attempt to prevent the mother's feminine personality characteristics from influencing the son as a result of his growing identification with her. As a result, the mother's most socially valued characteristics—sensitivity, empathy, the ability to communicate—are suddenly portrayed during therapy as negative, because they now threaten to "contaminate" the male child.

A female family therapist in the process of shifting a male child from the influence of his mother to that of his father must necessarily experience some conflictual strain herself. She must face the fact that such derailment of mother-son intimacy cannot be effected without encouraging feelings of severe self-doubt and guilt in the mother, and that both parties, mother and son, will somehow have to recover from the trauma of the loss of intimacy. She would have to convince herself that empathy, sensitivity, and communicativeness are so limited in their value that a son would be irretrievably scarred were he to develop these traits instead of more aggressive, independent, and competitive characteristics. And she must face up to the fact that taking such a position as a therapist covertly devalues some of her own abilities as a therapist in influencing and shaping others.

A female family therapist often finds herself in the conflictual position of having to endorse and protect the male values. In this role, she is like the woman in Milgram's experiment who is being asked to obey an authority that she implicitly feels is acting neither in the best interests of herself nor in the interests of those on whose behalf she is being asked to act. Thus, in the role of therapist many women face the same conflicts that are faced by mothers within the family setting.

Clinical Models: Reestablishing the Mother-Son Bond

Male children in adolescence are assumed to be well functioning when they are athletic, do reasonably well in school, show signs of leadership qualities and bravado at the same time that they are basically attentive to authority. That they may also be detached, uncommunicative, and emotionally sealed off is seldom perceived as a problem. The mother may silently suffer her own sense of loss and her knowledge of what the boy may be losing emotionally. Often she sees in her own marriage the possible deficits of male functioning as her "successful" husband in middle years struggles with his loneliness, emptiness, and sense of alienation, often paying a heavy price in physical symptoms or depression.

The double bind for the mother is obvious. If she worries openly about this paragon of a son she is in danger of being labeled "an overinvolved mother." If she tries to share her concerns with her husband, he may intuitively hear her concerns as critical of his own behavior, and thus respond with anger and denial: "Can't you leave the boy alone?"

The clinical cases seen as dysfunction in male children center on issues of passivity, dependency, lack of athletic initiative, and defiance of male authority manifested in school failure and antisocial behavior.

In response to these and other issues facing the contemporary family therapist, new clinical models are emerging. A strong feminist component is being felt in family therapy. It remains to be seen whether this new component will merge successfully with other therapeutic models or engage in conflict with them. The clinical cases we present are feminist-informed to the best of our understanding.

All four of the following cases center around the mother–son relationship as central to the organization of the family. Carter's case emphasizes the negative aspects of a relationship where a mother shields her son from his father's disapproval, with the underlying belief that right or wrong, a father's leadership is more important than a mother's. Papp's case deals more directly with a mother's fear of "squelching" her young son if she exerts some parental authority. Walters presents a case where a mother's sense of responsibility for family functioning is counterproductive. Silverstein's case dramatically demonstrates the cultural indictment of "mama's boys" and the reactive fear and withdrawal of a woman who has been made to feel she was destructively close.

All four cases avoid the pitfalls of pathologizing the mother-son relationship either implicitly or explicitly. No relationship is sacrificed for another; fathers are respectfully validated without denigrating the value and importance of a warm, empathic mother-son bond.

cases

Olga Silverstein

It's All Right to Love Your Son

The Presenting Problem

The original call was made by the father in this family. The intake sheet indicated that the 17-year-old son had made a suicide attempt. He was hospitalized and had been subsequently treated as an outpatient for the past six months. Now it seemed that he was getting more depressed again.

When I called to set up an appointment with the family, I again spoke to the father. I requested that all members of the family come to the session including the two other children in the family, a 19-year-old son and a 14-year-old daughter.

Only mother (Anna), father (José), and Harold, the 17-year-old patient, arrived. Father, appearing very much in charge, informed me that the other two children were not coming. The older son was working and the daughter was too young to have to listen to "all this." I decided that challenging this Puerto Rican father at this time would serve only to antagonize the family, so I consented to see the three without further comment.

The First Session

Anna, a serious-looking woman, sat with her coat on, her hands in her lap, and her eyes on the floor. The two men positioned themselves on either side of her. José perched on the edge of his chair, feet planted firmly on the floor in a ready-to-start position. Harold was a neatly dressed, delicately built 17-year-old with smooth skin and shiny long-ish hair. He sat meekly by his mother, with a vacant air, looking at no one.

JOSÉ (*Father*): Did Mrs. K. from the hospital call you?

THERAPIST: No, I'm afraid not. Perhaps you can tell me the story.

JOSÉ: (*With the air of a man who has told this story too many times*) On Thanksgiving, the family was invited to friends for dinner. Harold refused to go. He had been moping about the house for a few months and his mother wanted to stay with him. But I was angry. I told her there—"Leave him alone. He wants to sulk, let him sulk." So we went. But Anna, she was worried. So we came home early and found him on the floor. That's it. That's the story.

Both Harold and Anna declined comment, so José continued.

JOSÉ: Harold spent three weeks in the hospital where he was seen by a psychiatrist. The family (all of us) was seen by a social worker. The treatment continued for the next six months on an outpatient basis. And now the social worker, Mrs. K., is leaving and we had to start all over again (*This in an aggrieved voice*).

He then assured me that things had changed. The therapy had worked, but now Mrs. K. was leaving.

THERAPIST: (*To Harold*) Are you less depressed?

HAROLD: (*Shaking his head, whispering*) No.

ANNA: (*Eyes still on the floor, also whispering*) I'm afraid he's going to do it again.

JOSÉ: (*Angrily turning to Anna*) I told you and told you to stop worrying. (*He shook his head wearily.*)

THERAPIST: (*To father*) Why do you think Harold is so unhappy? What's your idea about why he would try to kill himself? Why is Anna so worried about him?

JOSÉ: Well, getting back to your question, then. He—how can I tell you? He has an identity problem. Like—on one occasion he told me that he wanted to be a girl. My answer was that God made him a man, but he's not happy being a man, he—he wants—he wants to be something else—and at one time it was hard for me to—to accept that, but like I told him on many occasions, the problem is getting to be critical to the stage that he tried to commit suicide and I want him alive because whatever he is, he's still my son and I love him, see? So even though I didn't agree with it, I told him that I would accept him. Accept the fact that he's that way. See? So, that is his—the problem. You know.

THERAPIST: Is that one of the things that changed in therapy—you learned to accept him as he is?

JOSÉ: Yes.

THERAPIST: Who in the family do you think might not accept him the way he is? How about you? (*To mother*).

ANNA: I love him very much because he is my son and I have said to him because he's my son, but I know—I can't accept the fact that he wants to change.

THERAPIST: Anna, in Puerto Rico, when a boy like Harold is homosexual, is it a mother's fault? Is the mother considered to be at fault?

ANNA: I don't know.

THERAPIST: (*To the father*) Hmm? No? What do you think?

JOSÉ: That's—I think the father is to blame everywhere.

THERAPIST: You think so?

JOSÉ: Yes.

THERAPIST: Yeah? You think it's your fault?

JOSÉ: No, I don't.

THERAPIST: Aha. Oh, good. Anna, is it your fault?

Anna does not answer at this point, but her husband's words seem to indicate that she has not been alone in placing the blame for her son's homosexuality on herself. Her husband, by his very emphasis, demonstrates his bias.

FATHER: I have told her many times, many times, and she can attest to that, that we cannot blame ourselves for this because I don't think there is anybody to be blamed. (*Angrily pointing finger at mother*) Am I right or wrong? Right? Hmmm? Did I tell you many times that it's not your fault? Hmmm? (*Anna keeps her eyes down and doesn't respond.*)

HAROLD: (*For the first time*) But she takes it out on me.

THERAPIST: She takes it out on you? In what way?

HAROLD: A lot of different ways. I can't go anywhere. If I tell her I'm going, she gets mad, she doesn't want me to go. Sometimes she doesn't let me breathe. I don't bring friends over because she doesn't trust me.

THERAPIST: Trust you to do what?

HAROLD: Anything! She doesn't want me out of the house. She wants my kid sister to watch me.

THERAPIST: Does she think you're going to try to kill yourself?

HAROLD: (*In a whisper again*) No. The other thing. She doesn't like my friends.

Harold had been a very good child. All three of the children were good and hard-working. Harold was an excellent student. He had a partial scholarship to college and expected to graduate with his class— this in spite of his many absences. In the light of his high functioning, the depth of his sadness was puzzling.

HAROLD: (*Continuing*) Now she hardly talks to me except to give me an order. Do this, do that. Don't wear that. Come right home. (*His eyes filled with tears.*)

THERAPIST: Anna, you still think you can change him? You think if you try harder you can still change him? (*To father*) Why do you think she blames herself so much?

JOSÉ: I—I never thought that she blamed herself until lately. I always told her there's nothing—see, I have asked a lot of questions to different people. You know? And like for instance going back to the past—like maybe your relatives—grandfathers and things, and try to find out whether this is something that could be carried on by the—

THERAPIST: In the family?

JOSÉ: Yeah. In the family. And according to what I have heard, this is nothing that is passed on from one to the other. It is something that somebody wants to be that way and his inclinations are that and that's it. I know that there is a saying, especially in this country, that they call a kid that is attached to his mother a "mama's boy," where the mother wants to protect the kid so much that it will harm him in a way that is—he will sort of become dependent so much on his mother that he will become the feminine type. Since we—we never had that problem in the house or maybe in my family or I don't know about her family, but I don't agree with that.

The father's good will and ambivalence are clear in this exchange. The family had received two contradictory messages in their previous therapy: It's nobody's fault if a boy is homosexual, no one is to blame; the son has been too close to his mother, but can still be rescued if only the father would move in to loosen that bond. The latter message is covert, of course, but implicit in the direction of the therapy.

José was trying valiantly to hold on to both messages. He readily admitted that he left the children pretty much to their mother; as he remarked very defensively, he worked two jobs to support them. And although both mother and father denied blaming anyone, or that anyone was to blame, they each felt blamed. He felt guilty for not being there more, she for being there too much.

THERAPIST: Anna—Anna, were you close? Were you two good friends at one time?

ANNA: That's why it—it—it hurt me so much. He was special.

THERAPIST: Because he was special. What made him so special for you?

ANNA: Because when he was born he was sick. Since he was a little boy he was always with me and he was the one who helps me a lot in the house.

THERAPIST: Right. Um-hmm. And the older boy was more with your husband?

ANNA: No—just maybe more alone. My husband worked—he always worked hard.

THERAPIST: All right. So that's why you think that maybe it's your fault. Hmmm?

ANNA: He used to help me a lot around the house and sometimes I think he—ummm—because I would—you know—I didn't know what was going to happen so maybe if I don't—(inaudible)—to make those kinds of things, I don't know. Somehow I feel so . . .

THERAPIST: (Checking for early signs of depression) What was he sick with? What was the trouble when he was little?

FATHER: He had a heart murmur. He still does, I think.

Some family therapy models might regard Harold as having failed to develop proper masculine qualities and might attribute that to an inadequate male model. Even if the homosexuality were not perceived as problematic, many practitioners would still stress the need to pry the son away from his childhood involvement with his mother, if not for his gender identification then in the name of autonomy. Structural models would certainly stress the need to draw the uninvolved father back into the family, if not to model masculine behavior then to help loosen the mother-son bond.

It would appear that the earlier family therapy had served to bring the question of homosexuality into open discussion. It had effectively put a stop to any overt blaming. It had made acceptance of the son's homosexuality a key issue, and had in fact successfully achieved a high level of overt acceptance. Although that issue was still a difficult one (and might always be), the father, if not the mother, gave more than lip service to accepting his son "as he is."

More striking was the degree to which the father was now "in charge" (although resentfully) and the mother and son locked in an unhappy, uneasy distance by which mother was trying desperately to undo her past errors.

If, when a mother discovers the nature of her homosexual son's sexual life, she is flooded with sorrow and shame, she communicates a devastating message to her son. The implication is clear that what she has just learned about him is so bad that it has erased all the pride she ever had in him. Without doubt, this will be a mortal blow to the son's self-esteem (Klein, 1984), as we find in the case of Harold.

THERAPIST: (*To Harold*) When did this start, this trouble between you and your mother?

HAROLD: About a year ago, when I told my father that I planned to be a nurse, and he said that was a girl's job. I told him I wanted to be a girl. He slapped me. After that she (*pointing to his mother*) wouldn't talk to me—never again. Just like that.

José's explanation for Harold's suicide attempt had been reinforced by both Harold's individual therapist and the family therapist. They had indicated that Harold was despondent because his father had not accepted him. Given that understanding, it might follow that the suicide attempt was a gesture calculated to bring the father around. Given that hypothesis, the therapy had proceeded logically and successfully—except that Harold was still depressed and possibly not out of danger.

I explored more carefully the relationship that had been primary in Harold's life. The change in that relationship had occurred when Harold declared that he wanted to be a girl. Anna's withdrawal was her reaction to her sense of having wronged her beloved child.

But the previous therapy's prescription to put father in charge had not only *not* relieved Anna's guilt and sense of failure, it had exacerbated it. Although the father was now ostensibly "in charge," it was clear that the bond between Harold and his mother was strong and that the currently tense and distant relationship between mother and son was extremely painful for both. On this premise the following intervention was made.

THERAPIST: (*To Anna*) I think part of the problem right now is that you blame yourself so much that you're afraid to love your boy. You're afraid that somehow your love hurts him, so you don't show him how much you care about him, and that seems to hurt him very much.

ANNA: He thinks I don't love him?

THERAPIST: That's what he thinks.

ANNA: It's not true.

HAROLD: You don't show it (*Not looking at her, and starting to cry*).

THERAPIST: Um-hum. But you've been afraid to love him ever since he said he wanted to be a girl because you think your love harmed him. Right? I want you to think about that.

Therapeutic Strategy

The strategy in therapy was to strengthen again the bond between Harold and his mother on the assumption that Harold had not tried to commit suicide because he was homosexual, nor because his father didn't accept him, but because he felt he had lost the primary relationship in his life. In attempting to reestablish the bond between Anna and Harold, I felt that I was improving the chances for both of them to regain their sense of self-esteem. Anna needed to realize that the intimate relationship that she had enjoyed with her son did not have to be viewed in a negative light.

I was aware of the fact that I was implicitly devaluing the need to turn male children over to the male power structure. I knew that Harold would have to face that power structure in the near future outside the home and would have to cope with it to the best of his ability, but I did not think that Anna's feminine characteristics had no value for him. If Harold's continued closeness to her would instill him with a sense of empathy, sensitivity, or the ability to behave in a nurturing manner, that would serve him well.

The fact that Anna's feelings about her son and about discipline in the family were often expressed through her husband showed her implicit endorsement of the conventional belief that the husband is the decision maker of the ideal family. When her son was younger, they had enjoyed an easy, loving, open relationship. He would help her with the chores, and the two of them shared many feelings. It was only when he announced his homosexuality that she reinterpreted their fulfilling, warm relationship as harmful to her son and, therefore, wrong.

If I had worked more conventionally to shift Harold into his father's sphere, I would also have risked reducing Anna's already diminishing self-esteem and would have increased her feelings of powerlessness. Such a blow to self-esteem curtails a mother's clear-headedness and diminishes her potential for positive, influential behavior. As soon as a mother becomes convinced that the love she feels for her son is detrimental, her sense of herself as poisonous will infiltrate *all* areas of her life, and of the son's as well.

At the end of that first session, Anna touched my hand on the way out, Harold gave me a wan smile, and José thanked me rather profusely. I interpreted that as possibly indicating some relief on his part because he sensed that maybe I would help them restore the old order in the household.

I saw the family four more times. In the next session with just the three members present, Anna's competence as a mother was connected with Harold's high achievement in school, his independence in making life choices, his good manners, and his obvious devotion to his family. José was also credited for the example he set for his children—of hard work and devotion to the family.

Without urging from me, all five family members attended the next three sessions. The themes were the same, although they now involved the roles of all three children in the family. As in the previous sessions, the contributions of both parents to the family were validated.

THERAPIST: Did you decide together that it would be best for Anna to be home with the children and for José to work two jobs to make that possible?

JOSÉ: Well, I told her, in this neighborhood when the mother works the kids run wild in the streets. I told her, "You stay and be with the kids. I'll worry about paying the bills."

ANNA: (*Nodding*) I worry that he works too hard. When she (*pointing to the daughter*) gets married, I'll go to work. (*The whole family laughed.*)

The last session was late in May—a week before high-school graduation. Harold was graduating with honors and was preparing to leave for college on partial scholarships. He had a summer job as an orderly on a hospital psychiatric ward. The family was teasing him with "Watch out, they won't let you out."

Anna joined in the teasing by saying to Harold, "Well, you got something from me anyway. You can go away from home because you can do your own laundry. That's more than I can say for your brother." Everyone laughed.

Of course, all of this means nothing if we persist in defining the imbalance of power that currently exists in our society as functional. Awareness of the outmoded assumptions and cultural imperatives upon which our discipline's theories of human behavior were built is the first step in changing them. In our willingness to reexamine the premises of our parenting lies the hope for all future generations of mothers and sons.

Peggy Papp

"Too Much Mothering"

This case of a single mother and her son highlights the confusion and contradictions that surround the use of maternal authority in raising a son. Since women are socialized to be passive and submissive in relation to men, they are understandably uneasy about exercising parental control over a male child. They seldom experience this kind of hesitation in relation to their daughters. Cultural expectations lead them to believe that male children, more than female children, should be raised to be aggressive, self-assertive, independent, and competent. They are not nearly as concerned that their parental discipline will harm a daughter as they are that it will emasculate a son. Restraining the aggressive impulses of a daughter is likely to be viewed as teaching her to be a lady and thus enhancing her femininity. To curtail the same impulses in a son creates the fear of robbing him of his masculinity. Most mothers are phobic about homosexuality and have been led to believe that "too much mothering" causes it, even though the most recent studies disprove this notion. For example, according to the latest research findings from the Kinsey Institute for Sex Research, there is little or no support for the traditional theory that a dominant or seductive mother causes homosexuality in men. However, there is little wonder that mothers still worry about this since words such as "castration" and "emasculation" have for so long been connected with "domineering" and "overly protective" mothers.

   In the following case, the single mother was unsure of her right to discipline her son because she was afraid of robbing him of his masculinity. Rather than viewing her inability to assert her parental authority as pathologically based, I saw it as a mistaken notion, culturally induced. This mistaken notion was challenged through a task that released her from her fear of "too much mothering." At the same time, it relieved her son of his burden of inappropriate power and paved the way for him to enter the world of his peers. As a result of becoming more assertive with her son, mother was able to consider her own emotional needs in a new way.

The Presenting Problem

Mother, a 34-year-old working woman, divorced eight years, requested counseling for herself and her 10-year-old son, Jimmy, because they argued a great deal and became involved in frequent power struggles. She said she knew she was inconsistent and couldn't follow through on discipline. "I don't think I'm definite enough, not persistent enough, and as a result nothing seems very definite in terms of rules. I think I should have started earlier or perhaps believed what I said. I keep backing down. I don't know why because intellectually I know what I'm doing is wrong."

She made it clear from the beginning that she felt this was primarily her problem and did not involve Jimmy's father. Jimmy saw his father on a regular basis and the parents had remained on friendly terms. There were no arguments over visiting rights and neither parent interfered in the other's relationship with Jimmy.

Jimmy, a precocious child with an innocent cherubic face, sat close to his mother throughout the session and frequently stroked her arm affectionately or gave her hand a paternal pat. Mother responded with an amused smile. In a soft gentle voice, she described the following cycle of interaction: she would ask Jimmy to do something and he would say, "Why should I do it if you don't have to do it?" to which she would reply, "Because I'm the mother and you're the child, and the rules aren't the same for each of us." Jimmy would then say, "That's not a good enough reason. Adults have rights and children should have them also." Mother would then become confused and back down.

Exploring the Issues

In the following exchange, the mother expresses those fears that prevent her from asserting her authority with her son:

MOTHER: Doubt comes into my mind about whether I'm being arbitrary or just asserting myself to be assertive.

THERAPIST: What's wrong with being assertive?

MOTHER: Probably a fear of not being fair.

THERAPIST: And what if you were unfair?

MOTHER: I would be afraid that I would squelch him—that he would lose confidence in himself. If he sees me as too much of an authority figure I'm afraid he will feel overpowered.

THERAPIST: And what if he feels overpowered?

MOTHER: Well, you see, I'm the only parent in the home—there's no father there. If he sees me as too much of an authority figure—it will be too much mother.

This is an example of the kind of anxiety that is generated in single-mother families. Therapists also have a tendency to become anxious about the lack of male influence, and may call in a male therapist to assist them, try to get the father more involved, or refer the child to a Big Brother agency. While male influence is important in any child's life, it is not the solution to a problem between a mother and child. These are two separate issues. To bring in a male to assert authority in dealing with the son would imply that mother was incapable of resolving the problem herself.

MOTHER: I know this sounds silly—but . . . it would be different because his father is a man and his father would make a man of him.

THERAPIST: Ah, I see. And what will you make of him?

MOTHER: I guess I do feel that if I use my authority as a mother I will destroy his masculinity.

THERAPIST: So in order for him to grow up to become a man he must be disciplined only by his father? And what will his mother do? Allow her son to discipline her?

MOTHER: It's clear I've given him a lot of power. I get very angry about it though. I don't feel good about myself when I back down.

The degree of power mother had given Jimmy not only disadvantaged him with an inappropriate burden but it caused mother to feel badly about herself. Turning to Jimmy, I asked, "What percentage of the time do you win the fights with your mom?"

JIMMY: Oh, I'd say about two-thirds. If I think I'm right and she says something else, like "I'm the mother and you're the son," I'll know that but it doesn't change anything because if I'm right it doesn't matter if she's the mother and I'm the son because what's right is right. Children should have rights too.

THERAPIST: (*To mother*) And you're worried about his self-confidence?

MOTHER: (*Laughing*) It does seem foolish.

There was a comic incongruity between Jimmy's appearance and the way he talked. He had not yet lost all his baby fat and yet he spoke with the authority of a young man. He went on to tell me about a tape he made of a fight he provoked with his mother just before they came to the session. He taped the fight so he could bring it for the therapist to hear.

JIMMY: I didn't think when we got here—sometimes you know my mom is a little shy (*He strokes her arm reassuringly.*) and I didn't think she would be totally open so I started a fight and I taped it. But when my mom found out I was making the tape she stopped me.

THERAPIST: It seems it's very important to you that you solve these difficulties between you and your mother.

JIMMY: (*Speaking like a little husband*) Well, yes, because we're always yelling at each other. I go to work—I mean school—hurt, and she goes to work hurt and then you know we even go to sleep in the evening hurt. It's terrible. It's really bad. I want to find out what's wrong and solve it. I expect we'll have some fights but—you know—we already have so many fights.

THERAPIST: What are some of the things you do to keep from having fights.

JIMMY: I guess most of the time—we yell at each other for awhile and then we separate and come back later and she'll say I'm sorry and I'll say okay, I'm sorry too.

THERAPIST: How do you have a good time together?

JIMMY: We see movies and we play games and sometimes, you know, we just have a nice quiet evening at home, and I'll say, "Let's not fight tonight, it's a good night (*Playfully slaps his mother's thigh*). Let's just enjoy each other's company . . . We'll just eat and watch some TV and then just go to sleep and we won't fight tonight.

Jimmy gave a perfect imitation of the conventional husband. He took complete charge of the situation by setting the rules about right and wrong, and then was alternately possessive, protective, and seductive with his mother. Mother passively allowed him to take charge, observing him with a combination of amusement, admiration, and irritation. She was clearly proud of his precociousness, was afraid of crushing it, but at the same time resented being controlled by it.

Mother then expressed concern over the fact that Jimmy had no friends his own age. As she described his problem, it was clear that he behaved with his peers as he behaved with mother. He was bossy and uncooperative with children who did not defer to him, and soon alienated them. This was another area in which mother did not intervene in a firm way to correct his behavior for fear of being too hard on him. Jimmy stated, "Most of my life I've been hanging around with adults. As long as I can remember, most of the people I hang around with are adults. I don't get along with other children very well."

In exploring mother's social life, I discovered that she broke off a relationship with a man named Sidney just two weeks before she came to our clinic. She had been going out with him for a year and was seriously considering marrying him. Jimmy was extremely jealous of Sidney, and constantly tried to interrupt their relationship. Mother allowed Jimmy to get away with such behavior out of her fear of neglecting him. However, Sidney resented mother's constant giving in to Jimmy and finally broke off the relationship. The final incident occurred just two weeks before, when mother and Sidney had planned to go away for the weekend; Jimmy was to spend the weekend with his father. However, his father had become ill and wasn't able to take him. Rather than making other plans for Jimmy, mother decided to stay home with him. This was the last straw for Sidney, and he walked out of the relationship. Mother was unhappy about it but she blamed Sidney, explaining that he had a problem in dealing with children that stemmed from his own childhood.

Defining the Problem

There are several ways in which the information we have gathered about this mother and son might be used in conventional family therapy. One approach would be to interpret mother's choosing to be with Jimmy rather than with Sidney as her way of avoiding a closer relationship with Sidney. The therapist would then focus on exploring mother's problem with intimacy and concentrate on her fear of getting involved with a man. Or the problem might be posed as an "overcloseness" between mother and son, with the "oedipal problem" becoming the central issue in therapy. Either of these premises would have made it mother's psychological problem.

Instead, I saw the problem as stemming from mother's having been handicapped by the belief that "too much mothering" would emasculate her son. She was afraid of stifling the son's aggressive take-charge personality since she knew it would stand him in good stead in the outside world. She so admired his standing up for his rights that she allowed his argumentativeness to impair her common sense. Although it was true that she was allowing Jimmy to interfere with her relationship with Sidney, this did not necessarily indicate a desire to avoid a romantic involvement with a man. Rather I saw the problem arising from her being torn between her own needs and her distorted perception of Jimmy's needs; like a good mother she had decided to sacrifice her own needs for those of her son.

Prescribing a Task

I excused Jimmy from the session and told mother it was important for her to take back her power as the mother. I reassured her that her assertiveness was not likely to rob Jimmy of his masculinity: "It is better for him to learn to deal with an effective mother rather than an ineffective mother."

I then suggested a task that was designed to give her permission to exercise her authority on the basis of being a mother rather than on the basis of being "fair." I told her that once every day she was to deliberately ask Jimmy to do something that she considered to be arbitrary. This must not be something that he was ordinarily expected to do, such as his homework or taking a shower, but something completely arbitrary. She was not to back down and if Jimmy objected or asked her why, she was simply to say, "Because I said so." Mother responded with a knowing smile and said, "Yes, I understand—something unfair."

My task challenged her notion that good mothering always meant being fair, and that she would damage her son's manhood if she was unfair. It gave her the right to make rules arbitrarily solely on the basis of her rights as the mother. Since she already showed an intellectual understanding of her problem, a logical discussion of discipline and the importance of being consistent would serve little purpose. The task bypassed discussion and interpretation, aiming directly at changing her behavior. My authority as a therapist was used to support her in what she otherwise would never have considered doing.

Outcome of the Task

During the first part of the following session in which mother was seen alone, she reported that she had followed through on the assignment and it had worked well. There was much less fighting between her and Jimmy. "I realized I had felt abused by Jimmy. I wouldn't let others speak to me that way. Why should I let him? I had allowed it. But I've stopped it now. I had your authority behind me. It felt very supportive. I even began thinking it would be nice if we could do things for each other. Up until now I've done everything for him but I've been reluctant to ask him to do anything for me—like helping me to shop and carry the groceries upstairs or do some of the housework. I felt I never had the right to." Then, with a beaming face, she reported, "And another thing, that man I told you about is back in my life and we're considering getting married."

She had taken the initiative to call Sidney, and he was delighted to hear from her again. She had asked him to participate in a therapy session in order to try to work out a better relationship between the three of them, and he had agreed. In giving herself permission to make demands on Jimmy, she had become more aware of her own needs and had begun to take the initiative to try and satisfy them.

Jimmy was invited to the session, where he discussed the changed relationship between him and his mother with a slightly wistful expression, "Lately she's been telling me to do these things—you know— that I've never done before—like vacuum the rug, bring her a glass of water, put the dishes away. At first I thought she was kidding and I told her, 'You must be kidding. Get out of here.' But then I found out she wasn't kidding." He heaved a sign of resignation and continued, "So I did the things. Finally I caught on and I told my mom, 'You're just doing these things to prove you have authority, okay, so you have authority, I'll do it.'" Mother and I laughed at Jimmy's way of giving his mother permission to have authority over him. He was still young enough to feel relief at being released from his adult position.

Recognizing that Jimmy would have a difficult adjustment to make as Sidney became a part of their family, I discussed what the changes would mean to him. He said he liked Sidney and was glad his mother was going to marry him, but admitted he was afraid of feeling jealous and left out sometimes. I suggested it would be helpful if he could make some friends; he said he would like to but didn't know how. I then made a suggestion that gave him a way of using his precocious skills in making the transition between the adult world and his peer world.

> You know, Jimmy, I'm sure there will be times when you will feel that you are being treated unfairly and left out by your mother and Sidney. Whenever you feel that way I think it would be helpful if you went to your room and wrote it all down in a notebook or diary. You are a very sensitive and intelligent boy and you see things in a very interesting way. I think it might be helpful for other children to read about your feelings because probably a lot of them feel the same way as you do. Maybe you'll put it in a book some day for other children to read. But if you ever decide to let someone read it, it should only be another child because only another child could really understand it.

He smiled and seemed pleased with the idea.

Conclusion

This case has demonstrated a way of avoiding the following common pitfalls in dealing with mothers who fear exercising authority with their sons: accepting the myth of too much mother; viewing the problem as mother's fear of a close relationship with a man; imposing male influence in the form of a male therapist, the father, or a Big Brother; pathologizing mother's inability to be assertive and consistent. It offers an alternative feminist perspective that connects mother's difficulty in disciplining her son with the cultural myth that too much mothering can destroy a son's masculinity.

Betty Carter

The Good Son

This case is an example of the way in which my work has changed since I started to think seriously about sexist assumptions, including and especially my own. I think that if I had met this young man earlier, I would have believed (as his mother did) that he would be better off to overcome his ambivalence about following in his father's footsteps in a law career than to pursue the low-paid, low-status, uncertain field of music. Of course, I would not have told him what to do, but we all know the power of therapists to lead, point, explore, ignore, question, and respond in a way that indicates what our own beliefs and values are.

Presenting Problems

John, age 30, came from a New York Irish family. He had moved to Washington, D.C., several years ago, after completing law school. After several years at a Washington law firm, he had been asked to resign because he didn't fit in with the firm's "pace." He told me this meant that he had expressed reluctance to work nights and weekends on a regular basis, and that he didn't usually arrive at his desk before the official starting time unless he actually had urgent work to do. He expressed a lot of contempt for his colleagues' total involvement in the "rat race."

Depressed, anxious, and unable to mobilize for a new job search, he had been referred to me by his girlfriend, Anna. He was polite, soft-spoken, but strained in manner. He announced with shame that he was the first member of his family to "enter therapy" and that his parents would be shocked and devastated if they knew about it.

It became clear during the evaluation that most of John's current life would "shock and devastate" his parents if they knew about it: (1) he was living with his Italian girlfriend, Anna, although they maintained two addresses for his parents' edification; (2) he hated being a lawyer and couldn't seem to succeed at it; (3) he didn't care very much about money, or life in the fast track, and he wasn't planning on voting for Reagan. He thought his mother might suspect some of these secrets, but they could never be discussed openly for fear of his father's wrath, which dominated the family's life.

Family Background

His older brother, Don, had rebelled in high school, refusing to take prelaw courses and concentrating instead on rock music and drinking, both of which he was still involved with. The whole family was musical; everyone sang and played several instruments with a high level of proficiency. John's maternal grandfather had been a Big Band musician, his mother had been a musical prodigy, and the children had inherited their talent.

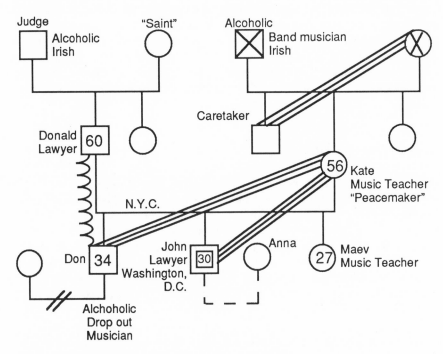

See page 96 for an extended definition of the genogram.

John felt that the most crucial turning point—and disappointment—in his life had occurred when his mother, Kate, to whom he was very close, sat him down when he was leaving for college and explained gently and sadly, knowing his disappointment, that "music is not a fit occupation for a man." It was too uncertain financially; made you keep "abnormal hours"; led to too much free time, drinking, and drugs ("look at my own father and your older brother"). "It's all right for your sister and me to be music teachers, but your father will never support or respect you if you do this to him. You'll be a fine lawyer."

John said he had felt betrayed by his mother, and, although he had never confronted her about it, had been angry with her ever since. "She gave up her own career because of Dad, and then she blocked mine. She's just a wimp and a chicken and she always will be."

John had not felt able to defy his parents, and so had embarked on a career in law. Things had gone well for him through college and law school, and when he moved to Washington for a job with a prestigious law firm, he felt that his life was "clicking along perfectly."

The first dilemma occurred when his father took a dim view of his choice of a girlfriend ("Italian *and* a bleeding heart liberal"), and his mother, acting as spokesman for father, phoned him at work to suggest that it would be better *not* to bring her home for Thanksgiving as planned. During the past two years, John's involvement with Anna, along with the number of secrets to be kept from his parents, had grown enormously. Some day soon, he said, he would "have it out" with them about his wish to marry her, and he'd have to let them know that he wasn't really doing that well in law because he found so much of the work "boring" and the pace "killing." When asked which parent would be harder to "have it out" with, he responded immediately: "My mother. Definitely. I used to be very close to her. I'm her favorite and I suppose she thinks she's advising me about my life for my own good. I know she can't stand up to dad. He'll explode and probably cut me off, and then she'll be all upset."

When I am coaching an adult to change his or her relationships with parents and other family members, I frequently suggest that difficult or taboo issues be raised by letter, instead of in face-to-face contact. This technique has many advantages: the communication can be precise, and it can be edited, with the help of the therapist, to delete hostility or defensiveness. The client does not have to experience the first intense emotional reaction of the parent, but can plan calm, appropriate responses for the future. Further, the client's own intense reactivity to toxic issues with parents can be more easily controlled in a letter than in a verbal encounter. The idea, central to the work of differentiating from the family, is that the client take an *I-Position*, which is to reveal one's own thoughts, feelings, or position without attacking the other's position, or asking for the other's approval for one's own position.

Letters to the Family

Following are excerpts from a series of letters John wrote to his parents over the following year, with help from the therapist, with whom he met monthly. I think many therapists would have tried to get John to resolve his ambivalence about being a lawyer by focusing on his relationship with his father. I encouraged him to work out his problems with both parents, and I saw that he really yearned to try working at music and song writing, even though it meant following in his mother's footsteps.

His first task was to start being honest with his parents about the facts of his life.

> **Dear Dad,**
>   . . . I have some bad news for you. In spite of everything that you and mom have done to help me get launched properly in life, I can't seem to put my heart into law. I'm thinking seriously of trying something different, although I'm continuing to support myself with a legal job. It is very hard for me to disappoint you. I know that both you and grandpa were born lawyers and I have tried to follow in your footsteps. I am afraid that this will make you very angry, and I keep trying to prepare myself for your reaction. . . . I will certainly understand if I don't hear from you again. . . . Mom has warned me that you would never tolerate my doing this. . . .
>
>   Love, John

> **Dear Mom,**
>   Your letter made me very sad. I was afraid that you would get all worked up over this, and you have. I do realize that everything you have advised me to do was for my own good— and it was good advice; I just seem to be marching to a different drummer. . . . You were certainly right about dad's reaction. He phoned and blasted me for half an hour. . . . Anna and I had been hoping to come up for Christmas to announce our engagement, but I think it would be best for everyone if we didn't come right now. . . . I know that you're feeling upset about all of this, but when things calm down, you'll love Anna. She's a lot like you— musical talent and all. . . . I don't expect to hear from you soon because I know how you hate upsetting dad. I do too.
>
>   Love, John

In the following letter, John reacts to his father's threat of cutoff by reminiscing about tender moments in their past relationship. In order to affirm the affection between them, John had to control his anger and the impulse to counterattack. After much discussion in therapy, he had acknowledged that his father probably cared for him even though he was unable to express it verbally. This letter served as a reminder of that to both of them.

> **Dear Dad,**
>   . . . I know you told me that I'm "no son of yours" and I keep trying to integrate that thought, but I'm having trouble

with it. I keep remembering times when I *was* your son. . . . Do you remember when you told me to tell Kevin Cavanaugh that if he didn't stop bullying me, you'd knock his block off? . . . Do you remember the big game with the Indians—and how you gave up a business trip to be there? . . . Do you remember how much time you spent teaching me to drive? Do you remember the *really big* check you gave me when I graduated from Georgetown? . . . I know I should get all of these pictures out of my head, but it's hard to do. . . .

Love, John

John had a harder time understanding and forgiving his mother because he felt she "should have understood." After much discussion with the therapist and several talks with his sister and, especially, his aunt, he began to understand his mother's position. She wanted him to "succeed," to be a financially secure and respected man, as his father was. Being a lawyer would assure that. If he took after her side of the family, she thought, there loomed chaos, insecurity, alcoholism, and failure, or the poorly paid, low-status career of music teacher. In keeping with the view of society, mother found the latter satisfactory for herself and her daughter, but not for her son.

Once he understood her position, he was able to address some of her fears while still letting her know that he did not plan to back down in order to placate her. In the following letter, John assures his mother that he understands her worry about his choice of a music career, that it *is* a difficult path, but not necessarily disastrous in the ways she fears. Anticipating her negative reactions, he also decides to be open about his relationship with Anna.

Dear Mom,

I really appreciated the letter you wrote warning me about what's ahead. . . . You know, mom, just because I "take after" your father doesn't mean I have to become an alcoholic. I don't know whether I'll go into music as a profession or not, I'm just exploring possibilities . . . you know, I used to think you were afraid to stand up to dad about a career in music for me, but now I realize you were just trying to protect me from the hard knocks on that path. Now I guess I'll just have to choose my own path, hard knocks and all. . . . I was glad to hear that you think we'll all get over this someday. I'm not so sure of that, and I'm trying to prepare myself for the worst. . . . Yes, you were right—the next thing I'll be telling you is that Anna and I are living together. I suppose mothers always guess these things. I'll try to understand if you and dad can't come to the wedding.

Love, John

Opening up more of his life to his mother, he sends her some of his musical work, especially songs about the family.

Dear Mom,
   I'm glad you liked the song I wrote about your father, Big John. . . .
                                                                Love, John

As his mother began to accept John's intention to live his life in his own way, John's attitude toward her softened further. The more clear he felt about himself and his own decisions, the closer he could afford to move toward his mother. In the following letter he thanks his mother for giving him the gift of music and enabling him to try to follow in *her* footsteps.

Dear Mom,
   . . . Did I ever tell you how grateful I am to you for all those hours you spent on me? Whenever I sit at the piano, I remember the afternoons we spent over the keyboard. I wasn't always such a great pupil and I am so glad that you persisted and helped me stick with it. I used to dream of getting to be as good a piano player as you are, and I still do! . . . I remember how I loved to hear of grandpa's adventures on the road. They sounded so exciting to a kid, though, of course, now I realize how lonely he must have been so much of the time. . . . I've been doing some more songwriting lately, and it's not bad, if I do say so myself. I'm enclosing one I wrote about all of us.
                                                                Love, John

The change in the family's reaction to John can be seen in the above letters. When he resisted the urge to fight or flee from his parents' disapproval, and instead stayed friendly while raising personal issues, his parents finally accepted the fact that he was making his own decisions, and gave up their opposition to his choices and his life-style.

Although John had initially been most angry at his mother for not supporting him, he came to understand that her problem was not that she didn't dare stand up to her husband, but rather her own belief that a young man would be happy and "successful" only if he entered a high-status profession. She found her own field appropriate "only for women," thus denigrating herself and her daughter and trying to elevate her son, as society requires. In the process of trying to follow this prescription, she had risked her close relationship with her son. When John freed himself from the social and family programming that was driving him into a life he didn't enjoy, mother and son were restored to harmony and father accepted the inevitable.

After months of persisting with warm, personal communications to both parents—always addressed separately—John finally reports a call from his father:

Dear Mom,
. . . Yes, it's true. Anna and I are going to be married in October. I was so surprised to get a call from dad that I told him about it without thinking. I was even more surprised at his invitation to bring her up for a weekend soon. He sounded different. Did you play "Lovesong" for him or something? Anyway, we'll see you soon.

Love, John

Marianne Walters

"Oedipal, Shmedipal— As Long As You Love Your Mother"

Benji was sort of like the "incredible hulk" as he stormed through the door with his parents and little brother. He towered over the other members of the family, who seemed to diminish in his presence. One arm was swathed in a huge cast reaching almost to his elbow; the other hand was stuffing an "Egg McMuffin" into his mouth. He took no notice of the one-way mirror, being totally involved with himself. His younger brother slipped into a far corner of the room, while their parents used the mirror to adjust hair and clothes. There was a general flurry, father slapping his folded newspaper against his legs, mother folding jackets, gloves, and hats. When they sat down, Benji's presence still seemed to dominate the room. Mom sat between Benji and her husband, with shoulders slumped and feet turned inward. Father fidgeted and slapped his newspaper. Little brother, with downcast eyes, slouched in his chair. Benji sat bolt upright, devouring his breakfast. Hyman and Adele W. had come to see me with their two sons, Benji, age 17, and Noah, age 12, following an episode in which Hyman had had to call the police to restrain Benji, who had assaulted him.

MW: (*To Benji*) What happened to your hand, dear?

BENJI: I broke my wrist.

MW: Ohhhh—how awful. How'd you do that?

BENJI: I hit a wall.

MW: Owww—you hit a wall! What did you hit a wall for?

BENJI: 'Cause my Dad wants to aggravate me enough so I'll hit him and then he can call the police—so I hit a wall.

MW: 'Cause your Dad wants you to—and you—I don't understand. Mr. W., could you . . .

BENJI: (*Interrupting*) 'Cause he was provoking me.

MW: He was provoking you . . . ?

BENJI: Or . . . in my opinion he was provoking me.

MW: To . . . to hit him?

BENJI: Sometimes he, well he just eggs me on. (*Imitating his Dad most disrespectfully*) "I'm gonna call the cops . . . you won't be here anymore . . . I don't need this . . ." Stuff like that.

MW: And so what did you do? You just went and hit the wall?

BENJI: Yeah, yeah.

MW: Well, that seems pretty sensible. Did you hurt the wall or just your hand?

BENJI: The kitchen wall.

MW: Oh, the kitchen wall. You broke the wall, or you made a dent in it? Was it plaster . . . dry wall . . . or . . . ?

BENJI: Naw, naw, it's like that . . . what do you call that stuff?

MR. W: Plaster board.

MW: Oh. Is that sort of like fiber board?

MR. W: Yeah, yeah.

MW: It's pretty easy to go through that stuff . . . make a hole . . . (*Dad nods agreement*). So, Benji, how did you fix it?

BENJI: I didn't.

MW: (*Incredulous*) You didn't! For heaven's sake, why not? Don't you know how to fix plaster board?

BENJI: Well, it messed up the wallpaper—you'd have to redo the whole wall, you know . . . the wallpaper too, and all.

MW: So, when will you be doing that?

BENJI: I won't be doing it.

MW: So who will?

BENJI: No one—he hung something over it.

MW: Huh . . . I don't understand.

BENJI: He hung something over it . . .

MW: Who did? Dad?

BENJI: Yeah.

MW: Well, that was most helpful. So, Mrs. W, do you like the way it looks now? Is it okay? Does it look funny?

MRS. W: The whole world there looks funny.

MW: The whole world at home looks funny? How do you mean?

MRS. W: It's just one more dent, one more dent . . .

MW: This is just one more dent in your world? Oh, my—that seems so sad. Obviously you both [Mr. and Mrs. W] are feeling really up against the wall, a wall full of dents. Yet it's clear to me in your coming here today, and in the way you've sought other help, and explored different possibilities, how much you're concerned and that you're all trying to get these family dents straightened out—or you wouldn't all have come. So, let's see . . . in some way, Benji looms bigger than life in your family?

MRS. W: A good way to put it.

MW: How so?

MRS. W: He's very much a presence in our home, I guess. He seems to have a lot of needs and wants and . . . he needs them. I mean, somehow he can't seem to get any part of his life in order and . . . well, he's very vociferous and he's abrasive; and I guess he's angry inside over something that hurts him . . . and that maybe he's not aware of where his rights begin and where his rights end . . . or how to get there.

MW: Why would he be angry? You look like lovely people.

MRS. W: We're not . . . (Looking at her husband) . . . We're a lousy couple.

MW: You're a lousy couple? And that makes him angry?

MRS. W: I don't know—I don't know what came first—the chicken or the egg.

MW: So you're angry, Benji, because your folks are a lousy couple?

BENJI: You can't just say what am I angry about . . . there are a lot of little things. It's not just the way they are—the way he [dad] is to her [mom], to me . . .

MW: So, a lot of little things make you angry—and when you're angry you go punch walls?

BENJI: Mostly . . . when my father . . .

MW: You mean your father is there when you punch the walls? Or you're going past him into the wall? I don't understand.

BENJI: Ummm—how can I explain it? . . . He starts trying to provoke me . . . pushing me to my limit so he can be pushed to his.

MW: Mr. W., what do you make of what your son is saying?

BENJI: He won't tell the whole story—he won't say what he does to me . . . he knows how to turn things around his way.

MW: Oh, I see. So you have a smart father. I'm pleased to know that. (*Benji, mumbling in the background, protests that his Dad is "sly" rather than smart.*) Tell me, Mr. W, so you've needed to call the police a few times? Tell me why.

MR. W: (*With Benji still mumbling in the background*) Yes, yes—because he gets physical, out of hand. He hits, threatens, pushes, shouts obscenities . . .

MW: (*Incredulous*) He hits you?

BENJI: (*Interrupting*) Maybe once . . .

MW: Now I'm talking to Dad, Benji—this is a time for you to listen. That's important.

MR. W: Yes, he has—a few times. And he makes threats . . . so I think it's important to . . . you know . . . his violence . . . damage to person, property. He pushes and hits and spits. It's been going on for some time.

MW: And so when it seems to be getting out of hand, what you've done a couple of times is call the police? That seems prudent.

MR. W: Exactly.

MW: Have they been helpful?

MR. W: Yes, yes. Somewhat. They are an authority he respects. He doesn't want to be put away.

BENJI: (*Protesting*) Oh, sure . . . yeah . . . they just bully . . . like him, and . . .

MW: So, Mr. W, one of your son's problems is that he can't contain himself? He just spills over into what goes on between you and your wife, into every conversation. Like he's doing now?

MR. W: That's right. He doesn't know when to stop. He'll go on talking, arguing, shouting—even if we've left the room.

MW: So this is something that you and your wife agree on—that Benji sometimes gets out of hand, and that you need to bring in the police when all else fails?

MRS. W: (*Who has been sitting with downcast eyes and lowered head throughout this conversation*) We-elll, no, not exactly.

MW: How not exactly?

MRS. W: I don't know . . . oh, it's just all too much. I don't want him put away . . . (*She starts to sob. I go to her, put my arm around her, hand her a tissue.*)

MW: What is it? What's too much?

MRS. W: I don't know. It's so bad, so bad ... (*Gaining her composure*) I'm so worried. I don't want to talk against Hymie—God knows he's had a rough time; it's been real hard on him. But he does ... he does provoke Benji. He engages him constantly. All the time he's pushing, pushing. He provokes ... he can't leave him alone ... he's always got something to complain about. He eggs him on—never, never satisfied no matter what Benji does. I try, I try ... oh, how I try. But they are at each other all the time. It's so ugly, so ugly—not like a family should be—not like a family should be at all ...

Impressions

This is how the first session began with the W family. Surely here was enough data to evoke impressions about this family in any one of the many old familiar ways: the indulgent mother and beleaguered father; the mother-son alliance that excludes father; the overinvolved, overprotective mother and the ineffectual, reactive father; the symptom that diverts the couple from their own issues, or that keeps the marriage together; the faltering hierarchy accompanied by poor generational boundaries. And just as surely such ideas will lead to thoughts like putting father in charge of his son while asking mother to back off; or exploring unresolved alliances in their families of origin; or reinforcing the hierarchy by urging parental agreement on how to deal with the problem; or going to work on marital-couple issues.

But I was filtering my impressions about this family through the prism of gender, which sheds light on another set of configurations. Was there a different experience and meaning for the same and opposite-sex parent in having a son—a teenage son, verging on manhood and yet so angry and troubled about the prospect of growing up? And if there was, as of course I believed, how were these different experiences and meanings valued, and understood, and manifested within the family? Outside of the family? And how had these different experiences, values, and understandings shaped and organized the relationships and interactions that were being presented to me? And what of the son? Was he so angry and being so difficult because he hadn't gotten it together with his dad, or because he is "too close" to his mom? And had these two rather polarized relationships evolved out of a particular skewed family system, a set of skewed social and cultural contexts, or both?

For the mother of a teenage son who is angry, rebellious, and out of control, the overwhelming response is one of having personally failed. His behavior is a constant reminder to her that she's done something wrong. Even if she blames others, she knows that her job—

to raise her son right—has gone wrong. With a son she is almost always in an ambivalent and compromised position: "If I'm too close, he won't become a man; if I'm not close enough he won't learn how to be caring." In this family it translates: "If I protect him in his battles with his father, he won't learn how to take care of himself; if I don't protect him, he will be damaged by the anger and conflict between them." If women learn that the best way to help their menfolk feel "big" is for the women to play "little" (to be the power *behind* the throne, never *on* the throne), then they must, even as the primary parent, look elsewhere for the exercise of authority with their sons—obviously, to their husbands. What a dilemma, then, if it is not forthcoming. And if it is forthcoming, how must mother feel to know that for her son she is never enough—although she is always in danger of being too much.

For fathers, the presence of a teenage, acting-out son in the family arouses a somewhat different set of feelings and reactions. While father will also feel failed, particularly in the area of authority, his responses to his son will be tinged more with feelings of alienation and disappointment. The dream of the son who takes the reins of manhood in his eager, confident hands is threatened, and confusion sets in about who or what is to blame. For fathers, I think, there is less ambivalence about what is to be done. They are clear that more authority, control, and discipline are needed, and are less given to searching for causality in the interplays of familial and marital relationships. Their sense of failure is less rooted in the interpersonal than that of mothers. It is felt more as a breakdown in management.

Therapy that is responsive to these different meanings and experiences is difficult to achieve. When we get involved with interpersonal issues and child-rearing concerns, mother will "hear" evidence of her failures. If we go for authority and control, she will feel blamed for not having provided it, or for counting on her husband to do so and then not trusting his efforts. If we explore the triangle in which the mother-son alliance is grounded, mother's worst fears may be confirmed: that their closeness is harmful to her son. And if we suggest that her son's problems "serve" the family, we are in danger of compromising the mother's function as family caretaker. So, at the very least, before entering into any of the systemic interventions and techniques that our particular model of therapy dictates, we will need to counter the prevailing family model that assumes mother's primary responsibility for family well-being; that presumes that mothers damage their sons by their tenacious attachments; and that vests authority in fathers as an essential feature of the male role model boys need in order to become successful men. It will be necessary to find, and to highlight, clinical material that will validate the power and confirm the significance of the attachment between mother and son, and that will encourage role models in the family that offer a range of relational and instrumental behaviors from both parents.

The Family

Returning to the first session with the W. family: Adele and Hyman look older than their years. Now in their early forties, they have worked long, hard hours in what has become a very successful family delicatessen. Hyman is heavy; Adele, painfully thin. Their younger son, Noah, age 12 and soon to celebrate his bar mitzvah, is a small, pale replica of his older brother. Benji is 17; large, glowering, and verbose, he is not reticent about giving his opinion on anything. When not playing the angry young man, his face is open and very expressive. In his dark good looks, he takes after his mother. His favorite sport is telling his parents, especially his father, what's wrong with the rest of the —— up world! And they listen, and they argue, and they defend themselves.

Clearly, both parents are deeply involved with Benji. Though he and dad endlessly do battle, they "read" each other constantly. They are forever checking each other out. When one lets up, the other begins. According to mom, even when Benji isn't being intrusive and angry, dad will find something wrong in his room, or with his clothes, or about school, and the battle will commence. Mom listens to Benji's complaints and tries to reason with him. She listens to her husband's complaints and tries to placate him.

Benji is abusive verbally and sometimes physically. He is angry much of the time, uses "foul" language, is argumentative and extremely intrusive. He does well in school academically without half trying, but has few friends. He doesn't do much sports, except wrestling, at which he excels. He gets into trouble at school for minor infractions of rules and classroom expectations. Hyman is viewed by his wife and son as an ineffectual bully. Adele is viewed by her husband and her son as soft and conciliatory. Adele thinks Hyman is too hard on Benji. Hyman thinks that Adele undercuts his efforts to discipline Benji and enforce consequences when he disobeys. Adele agrees that Benji can, and often does, come to her to get around punishments that she and Hyman have agreed on (especially involving allowance and lunch money—after all, you can't let a growing boy go hungry). Anyway, she is sure that Benji is "hurting inside," upset by the general unhappiness and discord in the family, and especially in their marriage. Hyman thinks his son is just plain disrespectful and out of control.

Framing Family Relationships

Early on in the session I challenged the parents about the way they both listen to Benji criticize them and their relationship, and allow him to "read" their motivations and behaviors. I suggested that mom allows it because she believes that Benji has a lot of pain locked up inside that he needs to express, and that dad allows it because he feels unable to control Benji. I told them that what worried me about all this was that they are blaming each other, and that they mistrust, disqualify, and pick at each other. They feel powerless in coping with Benji, so they direct their frustrations at each other. I expressed concern for their well-being and the continued viability of their relationship. Did they plan to stay together? Both parents assured me they did—after cautiously checking it out with the other; they did so with little sense of either pleasure or conviction, but rather because of the lack of any alternatives. Yet both also assured me that they were very keen on improving things for themselves and the family. I suggested that their alienation from each other had prompted each of them to turn their attention to Benji, but in different ways: mom to experience closeness and affiliation; dad to exercise his management skills and feel more in charge of his family. On the other hand, it was clear that their relationship had sustained them through some really hard times together—with their business, illnesses, Benji, extended family crises, and the like—and was important to them. Despite the severity of Benji's current behaviors, I suggested his problems were less serious than either parent believed, and assured them that we could help. But in the meantime I was concerned about their own well-being, physically and emotionally. At some point in this back-and-forth, Adele began to cry and Hyman put his arm around her comfortingly:

MW: Oh, that's so very nice, Hy—comforting Adele like that—reaching out for her. She really needs that. I imagine that sometimes it's easier for you to reach out to her when she's really down like this—perhaps then you feel more able to give to her, and she's, maybe, more available?

HYMAN: Absolutely. When we're not fighting . . . when she's not criticizing. I want to help . . . I know she needs . . .

BENJI: (*Interrupting, forcefully*) I've never, never, never seen him do that before—he never comforts her!

Turning to Benji, I commented on how observant he is and how he feels she needs to describe what goes on in his family, and especially between his parents. I assured him that I thought his viewpoint was interesting and informative. In fact, I found him quite an unusually perceptive young man. However, when he interrupts the way he does, his thoughts tend to get lost and the result is confusion and arguments rather than discussion. And this I wouldn't allow. So I offered him the alternative of writing down his ideas and comments on a yellow pad so that he wouldn't forget them, and assured him that before the session was over we would discuss the thoughts he'd written down. Benji accepted the pad and pencil and started writing vigorously.

MW: (*Returning to Benji's parents*) So this is one way that Benji gets to be bigger than life in your family—he grabs the stage, announces his views—he comments and criticizes, and you both listen! It's as if you believe he always has something important to announce—something new—something you haven't heard before—but I'll bet you've heard most of it a zillion times.

BENJI: (*Mumbling while frantically writing*) I just don't want anything to be misrepresented—he never did it before . . .

HYMAN: (*Mildly, with a little smile*) Benji, I want you to quiet down, right now. You can talk when Mrs. Walters asks you to. Otherwise, write it down.

MW: Thanks, Hy. Do you ever wonder how Benji got to believe he is the owner of the truth in your family? We-ell, anyway—I wonder if Benji knows you're serious—I mean, do you think he knows you really mean it when you ask him to cool it? I wonder because—well, it's hard to be sure because you're sort of smiling—and you keep looking over at Benji—checking him out—even when you're talking to me. I think maybe being serious with Benji makes you uncomfortable and . . .

HYMAN: Marianne, he doesn't listen to me either way. It doesn't work if I take it seriously, or if I'm light-hearted. It's like talking to a wall either way. But I am sure that he knows what's expected of him here. . . . he knows not to interrupt.

ADELE: (*Sadly, with downcast eyes*) But Benji's right—we don't comfort each other much—what happened—it's not typical . . .

BENJI: (*Mumbling*) Like I said—it was weird—the first time he ever comforted my mom . . .

HYMAN: You should be writing, Benji.

MW: Adele, you know what? I think you're protecting Hy now—kind of getting us away from looking at what goes on between him and his son—maybe you thought I was getting on his case a bit much, so you turn it back—back to what you're all more used to. How did you put it earlier? Oh yes, that you're a lousy couple. But I tell you, what concerns me right now is that Benji thinks you need him to tell me that Hy doesn't comfort you often. Or maybe he thinks that's the way to be on your side. Is it?

ADELE: Well, I guess he does think that he's being nice to me, Marianne.

MW: Oh, it's clear he means it to be caring. But, Adele, if Benji has to tell me what's going down between you and Hy—well, is it that he doesn't think you can say what is happening for yourself? It's strange—he protects you, you protect Hy . . . hmmm . . .

ADELE: Yes, uh huh . . . he does, but actually he knows I can say . . . that I really don't need him to speak for me. It's just that . . . well, I think Benji needs to get something out . . . there's something bothering him . . . something inside that he can't get out.

MW: So you think he has accumulated a lot of hurt, a lot of pain? That he's full of *tsuris* [Yiddish for suffering]. Well, that's our heritage—we're supposed to suffer, right? Seriously, Adele, I'm just not convinced that's the case. I think it's more a case of Benji being real smart—that's our heritage too, don't forget! I mean he's really clever, intuitive—the kid has good genes—and he knows just where to get to you, to you both. He knows what will touch you, both of you. He knows he can grab you when he talks about what happens—or doesn't happen—between the two of you.

ADELE: Yes, yeah—I can see that. And we're his buffer on the world—so he concentrates on everything we do. And I guess I give him more—physically and emotionally—so he is nice to me; he's concerned for me. I help him to control his environment. (*Leaning towards me, almost whispering*) Marianne, I believe he has a kind of oedipal . . . (*Tears well up*) . . . I think we have an oedipal problem in our family.

MW: (*Taking Adele's hand in mine, and smiling broadly*) Adele, my dear—like I'm fond of saying—oedipal, shmedipal, as long as he loves his mother!

ADELE: (*Laughing through the tears*) I knew my psych courses at Ohio State would come to no good!

MW: Psych courses do tend to get in the way! But you know what, Adele, I think you are just so scared that this young man is too attached to you—too close. You want closeness, you like it, but you're afraid it's wrong—that it's not good for him, that Benji will—God forbid—be a momma's boy! Well, that's not the problem. The problem is that you think his attachment to you has something to do with his anger generally, and particularly with the conflict he has with his dad. That's not so . . . not so. These are two different things, two different issues. And the sooner you start enjoying your son's attachment without fear . . . what is it that Roosevelt said, Hy?

HYMAN: Ummm . . . uh, yes . . . you have nothing to fear but fear itself . . .

MW: Right, right—a good thought. Adele, your closeness to Benji—enjoy it, stop being afraid of it. I want to be clear with you. Your closeness with Benji doesn't cause the conflict between him and Hyman. And their conflict is not the reason you and Benji are close. You each have your own relationship with your son, and it comes from a lot more than just what goes on between you all. Sure, you all live together and so how one is affects the other. But often it's just easier for boys to be close to their moms, and to do their anti-authority, testing-out stuff with their dads. And, Adele, as you begin to feel that your relationship with Benji is okay—that it won't burden him—you'll begin to trust that Hy and Benji can work out their own issues, difficult though that may be. You see, the more you trust your relationship with Benji—and believe that it works *for* him—you'll worry less that Benji is so vulnerable, and that he can't manage the problems he has with his dad. You just don't need to make it all right for them—they can do that themselves. [*Adele visibly relaxed after this exchange. For the very first time in the session she sat back in her chair, raised her head and was able to look at Hy and at her sons. It lightened the whole atmosphere in the room.*]

MW: [*To dad*] So, tell me, Hy, do you and Benji ever have the opportunity for . . . well, like an ordinary conversation—just talking together about things that happen, or how you react to something, or the news, or something that interests both of you—or just everyday stuff?

BENJI: [*Mumbling*] I can talk to her—not him . . .

HYMAN: No . . . we growl at each other before we even say good morning! Seriously, Marianne, I'm not able to . . . or at least I find it hard to move off the anger and the fights and have just an ordinary, normal conversation with Benji. For Adele it's easier. She can put aside the disrespect, the violence—the mean things that happen—and talk with Benji—they talk.

MW: If you and Benji were able to have a comfortable, ordinary conversation together—what would it be about?

HYMAN: Oh, God . . . I don't know . . . but it, it would be a . . . miracle!

MW: So, what would it be about?

HYMAN: We-ell, we both like to tinker with cars—and then there's food . . . oh, boy, we both like our food!

The remainder of the session was directed at engaging Benji and his dad in conversation together. It turned out to be about food—a subject they could both really chew on! What was useful in the choice of this subject was the opportunity it gave me to monitor Hyman's tendency to moralize and thus play into Benji's negativism. I checked Adele's "pulse" regularly as she watched this process, assuring her that they could manage and get over the rough spots, that she didn't have to make it okay for them—she could just enjoy the fruits of her labor! In this context I could encourage Adele to monitor Benji's running commentary on her marriage in the week ahead, suggesting that Benji's interest in the relationship between her and her husband, and his belief that she needed him as her ally, was too great a strain on a kid who needed all his wits about him to manage his own life. Adele had no difficulty being convinced of the wisdom of this approach.

Ongoing Therapy

Therapy with this family continued for several months, using and expanding on the themes that had emerged in the initial session: the value of the mother-son attachment; the capacity for dad and son to engage constructively; the avoidance of direct confrontation with Benji when he "acts out," while holding him responsible for the results of his actions (they had agreed in the initial session that the police would be brought in if there was any physical violence, but this never happened); highlighting the "universal" aspects of the mother-son and father-son relationships in families so that old assumptions about family roles could be reconsidered; keeping Benji out of the marriage— never, in fact, discussing the parents' relationship in his presence; and relying on their sense of humor.

Following two months of family sessions, Benji's miserable behavior cooled down considerably. He was then seen separately for a few sessions while Adele and Hyman were seen together around their couple issues. Sessions with Benji focused on some of his difficulties at school and with friends, with choices about future education and other personal concerns. Seeing him separately served to underscore the idea that he could indeed be held responsible for some of his own behaviors, and could use some of his own resources in changing them. For Adele and Hyman, our couple sessions produced a lot of anger and accusation, replacing the sadness and resignation about their marriage that had been so evident in that first session, and that had been "put on hold" during our family sessions. With the more direct expression of anger about their disappointment, the way was opened and the energy released to struggle with some of their conflict and misunderstandings and feelings of failure in their marriage.

When we gathered for the final family session, Adele, who'd been hitting her psych texts again, wondered jokingly if Noah might become symptomatic now that Benji was in better shape! Hyman said if that happened he was off to the nearest tropical island. Instead, they settled for a two-week cruise together, with Adele protesting, to the end, that they couldn't possibly manage alone, without the boys, and that she'd checked the cruise ship for ship-to-shore telephone capability before signing on!

5

Peggy Papp

Couples

Questionnaire for Marital Therapists

Questioning the Unquestionable

According to a survey by Prochaska (1977), the selection of potential dates and mates among college students is still highly restricted by traditional sexist acceptance of the supremacy of the male. Two-thirds of the 150 females surveyed reported feeling free to marry only a male who was older, more intelligent, better paid, better educated, and taller than they were. Seventy percent of the males showed the opposite bias in selecting a wife. Given the above information:

1. Describe the effect you think this partner preference might have on the couple's daily interaction.

2. What type of behavior would be required by each partner to maintain this homeostatic arrangement?

3. Married men live longer, happier lives than those who are single. The reverse is true of women (Bernard, 1972). Speculate on the reasons for this.

4. If the symbol on a genogram representing marriage is ☐ ○ and the symbol representing divorce is ☐ ○ , what symbol represents the inequality between the husband and wife?

5. Draw a genogram of a couple in which you show how traditional sex roles have affected their relationship over time. Describe the process through which these traditional views on masculinity and femininity have been passed on from one generation to another.

6. Someone once said that power is an aphrodisiac. Do you think this holds true for women as well as for men? That is, is a powerful woman as sexually attractive to the opposite sex as a powerful man?

7. Would you advise a woman to refrain from obtaining power in order to preserve her sexual attractiveness?

8. TEST CASE
   A couple comes into your office and describes the common pursuer-distancer syndrome. The wife, typically in the role of the pursuer, constantly nags her husband to become more emotionally involved with her and the family. The husband, typically in the role of the distancer, resists his wife's attempts, experiencing them as an infringement on his career opportunities and independence. Which of the following diagnostic statements would you select on which to base your treatment?
   (a) The wife has unresolved dependency needs.
   (b) The husband fears intimacy because of an overly involved mother.
   (c) The wife had a distant relationship with her father.
   (d) Both husband and wife are following the dictates of society by assuming culturally determined roles.

9. Would you treat this couple by:
   (a) Coaching the wife to get more involved with her extended family so she doesn't notice that she has no relationship with her husband?
   (b) Trying to convince the husband that his career is not that important after all?
   (c) Suggesting that the wife help her husband in his work so they can spend more time together?
   (d) Helping the couple to understand and change their stereotypical roles?

10. Therapists who view the family system within the context of the societal system are taking a political position, and this contaminates systems concepts (True/False). Please explain your answer.

This questionnaire is meant to point up some of the contradictions and absurdities in attempting to treat couples' relationships while ignoring the social system in which they exist. To fail to examine gender arrangements in therapy is to support the traditional sexist arrangements still operating in most people's lives.

A feminist perspective in couples therapy involves paying special attention to a personal, social, and political system in which certain crucial experiences and avenues of expression are repeatedly disconfirmed, but in different ways for each sex. This requires therapists to question "normal" behavior and attitudes that are sanctified by tradition and to become sensitive to the manifestations of gender conditioning in daily interactions.

The time has come to explode the sham of the "neutral" position, the clinical myth that it is possible for therapists not to introject their own values into therapy. Every therapist carries prejudices, beliefs, values, attitudes, and judgments into every session. These color everything that happens in a session from the kinds of questions that we ask to the hypotheses that we form and the interventions that we make. It is important that we hold our own values up to scrutiny.

In her book, *The Future of Marriage* (1972), Jessie Bernard points out that in order to examine the institution of marriage, one must consider *her* marriage separate from *his* marriage because the nuptial state is experienced differently by each spouse. Bernard documents a considerable body of research that reveals that men gain physically, socially, and psychologically from being married; but this is not true for women, for whom marriage poses a mental health hazard. Married women, as compared with married men or single women, tended to suffer more from inertia, insomnia, nightmares, headaches, dizziness, heart palpitations, and various other pains and ailments. Married men, on the other hand, showed fewer signs of psychological distress than either single men or married women. Despite the fact that men traditionally refer to marriage as "a trap," statistics show that it is twice as advantageous to men as to women in terms of survival. Women start out with developmental advantages that marriage then reverses.

Although some of the major social movements in the last several decades, such as the women's movement and the sexual revolution of the sixties, have produced a marked impact on traditional views of marriage, many of the old attitudes still persist.

Gender Expectations That Influence Intimacy

It is impossible to discuss love, marriage, sexuality, or intimacy without taking into account the vastly different ways in which men and women are taught to experience intimate relationships. The very way we conceptualize masculinity and femininity is determined by the culture in which we learn how to think and feel about ourselves and each other as men and women. From very early on, family and society collude in feminization and masculinization programs that shape attitudes and expectations involving these intimate areas of life. Implicit in these attitudes and expectations are contradictory intentions and goals that give rise to conflicts when a woman and a man attempt to establish a close relationship. Although both men and women genuinely desire intimacy with one another and spend much of their lives seeking it, they are socialized in ways that make that intimacy difficult to achieve.

Feminization Program

Women are raised with the expectation that their main goal in life is to take care of others, and thus their lives are centered around activities that lead to the enhancement of others rather than themselves. Their sense of self is deeply embedded in affiliations and personal relationships, requiring the development of interpersonal skills and qualities of nurturance, emotional expressiveness, and empathy. These attributes prepare them for the roles they serve in families as the soothers, the peacemakers, the facilitators, those who mediate the conflicts of others and adapt to family interests.

As Jean Baker Miller (1976) has observed, a great deal of women's self-worth is associated with giving to others. Women constantly ask themselves "Am I giving enough?" "Should I give more?" "If I had given more would this have happened?" The consequences of not giving enough when others are dependent on them are too frightening to consider.

Responding to the needs of others can provide women with a sense of gratification and pleasure as they help those around them to develop and grow. However, the price they pay is that they are left to rely on others, particularly their husbands, for their sense of power, status, and authority outside the home. If they are also financially dependent on their husbands, they do not develop the skills needed to deal with the outside world. Since these skills are more highly prized in our culture than those involving home management and child rearing, a woman's important talents for nurturance, empathy, and interpersonal relationships are devalued and often discounted. This inequitable recognition of male-female contributions in the larger society is a vital component of the marital relationship, and therapists should become aware of the ways it is interwoven into daily interactions.

Masculinization Program

Unlike that of women, men's sense of self is based primarily on achievement rather than personal relationships; thus, giving to others is not part of their self-image as it is for women. Instead, their self-image is connected with doing. Although men are interested in being husbands and fathers, their definition of masculinity comes predominantly from their roles outside the family and from their positions of leadership. Success in the working world often requires repressing personal feelings, learning to master passion or weakness, and developing controlled, guarded, and calculated behavior. Mastery of these skills often results in men closing off large areas of their own sensibilities, and inhibits their responsiveness to the needs of others. Intimate relationships are situations to be contained and are often experienced as impediments or traps. But although men defend themselves against the threat posed by love and intimacy, their need for it does not disappear, and they ask from women what they are afraid of giving and receiving.

Our current media version of the strong, independent man is personified by Clint Eastwood in the movie *Pale Rider*. Eastwood plays a Christlike figure with supernatural powers. A widow and her four-teen-year-old daughter fall under his magnetic spell and offer themselves to him body and soul. He ends up abandoning both of them and riding off into the cool distance as detached and uninvolved as ever. According to a recent poll, he was voted the most admired man in America.

Some women are enamored of this kind of invincible but unavailable hero. Since they fear their own ability to survive as an independent being, they are attracted to his strength, courage, and independence. He provides them with a sense of someone strong to fight their battles for them, to defend and protect them from danger. However, his invincibility depends on his remaining unencumbered by emotional paraphernalia, so he must always ride away from commitment. Both sexes are then deprived of the experience of interacting with equals.

The Dependency Trap

The mutual dependency of men and women is the basic building block of couples' relationships, but each gender struggles with it in a different way. Women are reluctant to ask for what they need, since they don't feel entitled to have their needs met and are afraid of appearing selfish. Men, on the other hand, are reluctant to acknowledge any emotional needs for fear of feeling humiliated or rejected (Stiver, 1984).

What we see in our clinical practice are women who have difficulty making independent decisions, becoming self-sufficient, acting in their own behalf, and claiming private and psychological space. They have difficulty letting others know what they want since they often don't know what they want themselves.

There is a tendency for women to expect that their needs will somehow be fulfilled in return for their services, but unfortunately this usually doesn't happen. Rather, men feel resentful and trapped by obligation. But while objecting to the demands of women's dependency, men at the same time often encourage it as an ego-bolstering device. Women sometimes present themselves as more helpless and dependent than they really are as a way of attracting and keeping a man. Their display of dependency then serves a protective function in a relationship by making the man feel strong and competent (Lerner, 1983). The woman is afraid to move out of this dependent position for fear of upsetting the relationship and being perceived by the man as too aggressive. Not being able to negotiate from a position of strength and self-confidence, she develops disguised and indirect methods of communicating her needs such as crying, acting helpless, becoming defensive, withdrawing, or, when all else fails, developing a symptom. The man, confused by this indirect communication, resorts to labeling the woman "emotionally unstable" or "manipulative."

Men have never learned to ask for what they want because within the traditional structure of the family, they have come to expect that a woman will take care of their physical and emotional needs: cook their meals, clean their clothes, run their home, and provide a haven to which they can return after a long hard day of work. Even many "liberated" men have difficulty giving up this notion entirely. However, when this caretaking is interrupted by events such as the arrival of a child or a wife going back to school or work, many men experience intense jealousy and feelings of abandonment. Since these men hate that part of themselves that is dependent, they try to disown it and react either by withdrawing or by becoming aggressively demanding. The expression of feelings of loneliness, fear, sadness, or helplessness might undermine their sense of themselves as strong, independent men. Rather than show any sign of longings, they wait for the women in their lives to read their feelings. If the women fail to read them accurately, these couples end up fighting over other issues.

Clinical Implications

Reciprocity Revisited

The crucial question for therapists is how to translate this awareness of gender behavior into effective clinical practice. Systems therapists often allow their concepts of reciprocity and complementarity to stand in their way of challenging traditional sexist arrangements. They see their alternatives as either throwing systems concepts out completely and resorting to polemics and lectures, or retreating into a neutral and nonjudgmental stance.

The Preacher and the Parishioner

Following is a way of viewing the reciprocity in a relationship as the result of an unequal distribution of authority and responsibility, and of rebalancing it.

A couple who had been separated for many months was trying to decide whether or not to get back together. They were mistrustful of one another and complained of a lack of communication and a great distance between them.

When asked to have a fantasy about their relationship (a technique that I use routinely as a diagnostic tool), the wife pictured her husband as a preacher, up on a pulpit delivering a sermon to her. She saw herself as a little girl, a captive audience, totally helpless in relation to this dominant, overpowering authority figure. In acting out the fantasy within the session, she showed herself reacting to her husband's sermonizing by covertly rebelling, falling asleep, coughing, or, finally, withdrawing to her room and closing the door. When asked what the greatest problem was for the little girl, she replied, "He won't let me speak my mind."

In his fantasy, the husband saw his wife as a Hawaiian dancer on a beach where he was lying in the shade watching her dance. He enjoyed being entertained by her but suddenly, for some reason he could not understand, she would stop dancing and disappear. He would then pace the beach, missing her and waiting for her to return. He would never go and look for her for fear of not finding her or having her refuse to come back. That would make him feel worse and so he continued to pace up and down, hoping for her return.

This metaphorical picture revealed the wife in the stereotypical position of the helpless female—feeling powerless, lacking authority, and resorting to covert means of expressing her resentment. The husband was in the stereotypical position of the pedantic male—attempting to reach his wife through lecturing, passively depending on her to provide the pleasure and emotional connectedness, and afraid of facing his own feelings. The physical enactment of the fantasies revealed the point at which the behaviors and beliefs of each spouse interlocked to form an impasse. The husband waited in vain for a wife who would never return because she was locked in her room waiting in vain for him to stop sermonizing.

Working within the framework of their personal metaphors, I broke this impasse by ordaining the wife a minister. I suggested she join her husband on the pulpit and preach with him on the premise that there should be two spiritual leaders in the family, not just one. I then gave her the task of writing a sermon about what she considered to be the beautiful life between a man and a woman. She was to bring it to the next session and deliver it to her husband.

I suggested to the husband that instead of waiting for his wife to return when she disappeared, he should go and look for her and bring her back. He should then find a way of dancing with her on his paradise island so that she would want to stay.

The core of the reciprocity in the relationship was defined as centering around unequal power and responsibility, which the intervention rebalanced. The wife was taken out of her helpless-little-girl position, placed in a position of equal authority with her husband, and given the responsibility for assuming that authority by writing her own sermon. The husband was asked to share his pulpit by accepting his wife as a co-leader and at the same time was given equal responsibility for the emotional connectedness and pleasure in the relationship.

The Pursuer-Distancer Syndrome

Another reciprocal arrangement that therapists often encounter is the pursuer-distancer syndrome, in which the wife pursues for emotional closeness and connectedness and the husband distances to protect his privacy and independence. Systems therapists tend to ignore this pursuing and distancing as part of the couple's gender development and focus on changing the reciprocity in the relationship without taking into account the social nature of the reciprocity.

One of the most common ways of intervening in the pursuer-distancer syndrome (as mentioned in Chapter 1) is to instruct the woman to "pull back" and make fewer emotional demands on the assumption that the husband will then automatically move closer once she has stopped pressuring him. As a result, the woman is made to feel ashamed of her need for closeness, and her sense of isolation is reinforced.

Another common approach is to launch a frontal attack on the man's emotional shell in an effort to persuade him to "open up" and express all his feelings. This disregards the protective function of the shell and is likely to result in greater resistance and further withdrawal on the part of the man.

An alternative way of dealing with the pursuer-distancer syndrome is demonstrated at the end of this chapter in Walters's case,

"Does Strong Have to Mean Silent?" Using a direct approach, Walters defines the different meaning of each partner's experience and relates it not only to their unique personal histories, but to their separate gender conditioning. By generalizing the couple's problem to include the wider context of their cultural backgrounds, she reduces their sense of failure and helps the wife to feel less "crazy" and the husband to feel less inadequate. Walters explicates and puts into context the couple's shared belief that the wife's intense emotionality prevents her from thinking and acting rationally, and that the husband's logical approach prevents him from developing nurturing skills. Walters holds the husband responsible for claiming and expressing his own feelings, and rather than inhibiting the wife's need for relatedness, she validates it by helping her to make it more functional. She defines both the wife's emotionality and the husband's rationality as assets that each can benefit from and teach one another.

There are many different ways of dealing with these problems, depending on a therapist's orientation. A therapist may choose to confront the issues directly as Walters does, or to work more indirectly through the use of reframing, metaphors, paradox, or humor. The particular approach is less important than the way in which the problem is defined. A reframing seemed appropriate with one couple I was treating when it became clear that the only time the couple connected was during the wife's intense emotional outbursts. These occurred when all other efforts to break through her husband's shell failed. The husband, a scientist who spent long hours in his lab, admitted he had a problem communicating and blamed this on his family of origin who "were like zombies and never expressed any feelings. Everyone lived in isolation and loneliness." As a result he confessed he had a tendency to withdraw "from human contact." When his wife's tolerance reached the breaking point she would let loose a torrent of rage and tears necessitating the husband to engage with her. He would emerge from his shell long enough to call her "hysterical," fight with her briefly before again retreating, and the cycle would begin all over again.

I reframed the wife's behavior positively by telling the husband that every time his wife had an outburst, instead of calling her "hysterical" he should thank her for bringing him out of his shell. She was doing him a great favor by humanizing him and saving him from the isolation and loneliness of becoming a "zombie" like the rest of his family. The wife was told that she should graciously accept her husband's appreciation of her efforts, and since his out-of-shell time would probably be brief, she should take advantage of it and make hay while the sun shone.

This validated the wife's efforts to connect by defining these efforts as serving to humanize her husband. It gave the husband a different perception of his wife's intentions and, at the moment of crisis, provided them with a different way of connecting with one another.

Domestic Responsibility

The Little Red Hen and the Helper

Despite the continuous demands by working wives for domestic parity, it seems they have made little progress in changing the old order of things. Although statistics show that the majority of wives are now in the marketplace, there are no corresponding statistics that show the majority of men are in the kitchen participating equally in home management and child rearing. The two-paycheck family has resulted in women doing double duty. When it comes to the home front, many men still view cooperating on domestic chores as demeaning and as detracting from their main purpose in life.

The point for therapists in dealing with domestic issues is to avoid becoming bogged down in trivial discussions over whose turn it is to do the dishes. What needs to be dealt with are the basic attitudes and beliefs that each partner brings to the situation. Both men and women still tend to think of the house as the wife's domain. It is often as difficult for the woman to give up this idea as it is for the man. Like the Little Red Hen, she finds it easier to do things herself than to take the time and trouble to insist on the man sharing the workload. Or, if she does ask her partner to "help" her, he is apt to be resistant to what he perceives as taking orders from her, and may complain that she always wants it done "her" way. When this happens, the most common response of therapists is to point out to the woman that if she wants her spouse's help she has to let him do it "his" way.

What needs to be questioned here is the concept that a man cannot take instructions from a woman in an area that she knows more about than he does. Most wives, during the course of a marriage, take instructions from their husbands on many different subjects, from changing a flat tire to the complexities of a fluctuating financial market. The husband's knowledge in these areas is seldom challenged on the grounds that he has to let her do it "her" way. Since women are generally the experts in running a home, it should be permissible to teach men what they know so that men can share equal responsibility in the domestic arena.

Therapy that is focused on making only small accommodations or behavioral changes rather than altering basic attitudes and assumptions openly or inadvertently stabilizes an oppressive system.

Prohibitions against Anger

Taming of the Shrew: Revised

In order for couples to achieve any level of intimacy they must be able to openly express disagreement and conflict. Yet the social prohibitions against the direct expression of anger, especially for women, have a stifling effect on their ability to engage in the kind of exchange necessary to resolve differences.

In her paper "The Construction of Anger in Men and Women" (1983), Jean Baker Miller postulates that living in a weak and subordinate position continually generates anger in women. Yet women have been told that the expression of anger is destructive to themselves and to those around them who depend on them. They are given the message that the image of a caretaking person is incompatible with an angry person.

Women's anger is also threatening to others because, as Harriet Goldhor Lerner points out in *The Dance of Anger* (1985), it is an agent of personal and social change and it challenges the status quo. As long as women remain self-critical, guilty, and depressed, there is no danger of their rocking the boat. Consequently, it is not uncommon for women to convert their anger into a symptom, or into irritating and ineffectual nagging and complaining. When a woman does express her anger openly, because she anticipates she will not be heard it often emerges in unfocused outbursts, and she is then labeled "irrational" or "emotionally unstable." She ends up hating herself for having behaved like a "shrew" and negates her right to feel angry. But her anger remains unabated.

Another barrier that prevents women from the direct and open expression of their anger is the risk of disrupting a relationship upon which they are economically dependent. Most women are still supported financially by the men in their lives.

It is more permissible for men in our society to express anger than for women. A "towering rage" or a "wild fury" can be viewed as a source of power or potency in a man, whereas in a woman it is seen as unattractive and unacceptable. However, men also have difficulty in expressing anger constructively in personal relationships, but for a different reason. Miller describes the hierarchical ranking of men in our society as precluding the expression of anger in a productive interactional mode. The majority of men live in positions of subordination to other men based on race, class, religion, or seniority in the work world. Whatever rightful anger men have had in response to that subordination has had to be suppressed. Men, in their own situations as subordinates, have not been allowed to express anger at the source and at the time and place when it might be appropriate. Instead, they often deflect this anger onto others, usually those in subordinate positions in the work situation or wives and children at home. In its most extreme form this can result in wife and child abuse.

When confronted with a woman's anger, men's characteristic response is avoidance and withdrawal. They abhor emotional "scenes" in which they fear they will either lose the battle and feel humiliated and defeated or win the battle and lose the woman's affection. Their avoidance of open confrontation further frustrates and enrages the woman, who often ends up expressing the anger for both of them.

Emoting for Two

Many therapists share the general population's aversion to an "angry woman," and experience her desperate attempts to be heard as "ranting and raving." The characteristic male style, being more controlled, more logical, and less emotional than that of women, is not as susceptible to all the above derogatory terms. Therapists often get sidetracked into reacting negatively to a woman's emotive style rather than understanding or validating the problem that is causing her to emote. This response only supports the shared belief of the man and woman that it is her angry outbursts that are the problem. This characteristic pattern is graphically illustrated in the following case.

The wife opened the session by discussing a fight she and her husband had over the weekend, and the husband complained his wife had again blown up over a trivial matter. The wife admitted she had lost control and overreacted, which a previous therapist had defined as the major problem in the relationship. In recounting the events prior to the blow-up, the wife said she had felt her husband had been withdrawn and cold toward her all weekend. The husband denied this, blaming his lack of engagement with her on his being bedridden with a bad cold. In exploring the situation further, however, it was discovered that the husband had been disappointed in his wife's caretaking. He had expected her to know that he needed a vaporizer and had wanted her to go out and buy one without his having to ask her. If he had asked her, she might have refused and then he would have felt hurt and angry. Instead of risking open confrontation, he expressed his resentment through distancing and coldness. Instead of questioning his coldness, the wife expressed the anger and tension between the two of them by exploding over an inconsequential event. The husband then became angry over her explosion, and the wife felt guilty but still angry.

My therapeutic focus in this case was on divesting this pattern of any individual pathological inference. I defined the response of each spouse as a "lifelong habit" that could be overcome through practice. I then suggested daily exercises that would help the couple overcome their "habits."

The husband was told that in order to break his habit of avoiding confrontation, he should make a request of his wife at least once a day that he was sure she would refuse. This would give him practice in either accepting her refusal or in expressing his reaction to it.

In order to help the wife resist the temptation of emoting for the two of them, every time she felt herself about to blow up over a trivial issue she should first ask her husband if he was angry about something. This would give her practice in checking out his inner emotional state before she expressed it for him.

These exercises gave the couple a way of paying special attention to the signals of anger that warned them that important emotional issues were being compromised. At the same time it provided them with practice in dealing with their anger in a less stereotypical fashion.

Violence: The Power-Helplessness Equation

Men's anger can be more frightening and destructive than women's when it takes the form of physical violence. It is more common for men to resort to physical violence when enraged than it is for women, and when they do so it is more threatening because of their superior strength and size. In cases of wife abuse, old concepts that held the wife responsible for the abuse such as "masochistic" or "collusive" have been challenged and discarded by most therapists, and there is a general consensus in our field that the husband should be held responsible for the violence. This sometimes involves crisis intervention and the use of outside social and legal controls. In less extreme cases, when men limit themselves to verbal abuse, their rage can still paralyze women because the potential for violence is always present.

A case was brought to me for consultation in which the husband went on rampages whenever he became frustrated, yelling, cursing, throwing things, and making threats that frightened his wife. The husband saw himself as having no control over his anger, stating, "It is an automatic response—it's mechanical. All my life I have been mechanically inclined to become angry." Being a lawyer, he was experienced with words and confessed, "I use my mouth to whip people." He had now reached the point where he was afraid he might become physically abusive with his wife, and he wanted to be able to handle his anger in a different way.

In tracing the pattern of his tirades against his wife, it was clear that they had become more frequent and more intense since the birth of their new baby. The husband reacted violently when he felt his wife was unavailable to him. "I need constant reassurance that she loves me. When I feel abandoned by her I feel devastated and can't function. So I keep waiting for her to show me that she loves me, and when she doesn't I feel totally helpless and I go crazy."

The wife admitted she had been less available to her husband because of the demands of the new baby. "I used to coax him out of his bad moods but I don't always have the time and energy to do that now."

The first important step in treating this case as I saw it was to challenge the husband's idea that his rage was "mechanical" and that he had no control over it. The second step was to give him a way of controlling it. In order to do this, the source of his feelings of helplessness needed to be redefined. It was not his wife's unavailability per se but his *reaction* to it that placed him in a helpless position.

I, therefore, suggested to the therapists who were treating the case that they express their amazement over how much power he had given his wife, that it was no wonder he felt helpless because he had put himself in a one-down position. By passively waiting for his wife to move toward him when he needed love and affection, he had become totally dependent on her every move. If she failed to move in the right way at the right time he felt powerless, and that, of course, made him angry because everyone feels angry when they're powerless. The solution was for him to claim power. Every time he felt abandoned by his wife, instead of waiting for her to reassure him of her love, he should take charge of the situation by finding a way to reassure her of his love. Since he had a tendency, as he put it, to "run off at the mouth," he should do this without words. Being a new mother, his wife needed the kind of reassurance and love that only a husband could give.

Defining the husband's rage as self-perpetrated rather than "mechanical" required him to take responsibility for it. The intervention gave him a way to turn his helplessness into power, and it made him an active, rather than passive, participant in the family scene. It also opened up the possibility for his wife to give him more of the love and affection he craved.

On Becoming Liberated: Reactivity versus Assertiveness

A common crisis that brings couples into therapy nowadays concerns women striving for more equality and independence in their relationships with men. This often occurs at the point when women decide to make major changes in their lives such as returning to school, obtaining a job, or seeking therapy for themselves. Stimulated by new actions and ideas, they may begin to regret the years of missed opportunities or become angry at themselves for having remained in what they now view as subservient positions. Rather than channeling their anger into constructive action and taking clear, strong positions, they sometimes lash out with global accusations and unfocused complaints that only serve to confuse and alienate those around them. They fail to distinguish between taking an *assertive* versus a *reactive* position.

Recently, a wife entered my office unleashing a torrent of accusations and complaints against her husband as though a dam had burst. The husband sat stonily observing his wife while casting long-suffering glances at me as though to say, "See what I have to put up with."

Having returned to school and gone into therapy for herself, the wife had discovered she was "a person," that she had allowed her husband to treat her like a doormat, that she had been a fool to put up with it, that she wasn't going to stand for it any longer, that he was impossible to live with because he was dominating, demanding, grouchy, irresponsible, critical, distant, cold, rigid, and, to top it all off, disrespectful, because underneath he hated women and this was because he had a bad relationship with his mother which he should go into therapy to get help for, because otherwise he would be incapable of giving any woman anything, ever, besides which he never expressed his feelings because, of course, he had none and that's what made him behave in such an insensitive way, but if he thought he could continue to get away with it he was mistaken because she intended to stand up and fight for her rights.

Turning to the husband, I asked, "Does she always let you off the hook this way?" I presented my reason for this unexpected question by pointing out that the wife's combative and defensive stance released her husband from any obligation of having to take her seriously. As long as she wasn't specific about what she wanted him to do, he could continue to dismiss her outpourings as "premenopausal agitation." I then questioned the wife as to whether or not she really believed she had the right to ask for anything different from her husband. When she had convinced me that she did, I helped her to channel her anger into specific requests, and to state them with the conviction that she deserved to have them met. Her husband was then compelled to respond to concrete issues and could no longer dismiss her as having "gone off the deep end."

The Sexual Charade

Sex is seldom an act of simple mutual pleasure. It is heavily laden with symbolic meanings imposed by the feminine and masculine mystiques. Sexual relationships epitomize the battle between the sexes since it is in this area more than any other that the social and psychological arrangements of gender are manifested in their most intense and palpable form. Sex can be, and often is, used as an instrument in the subtle and complex negotiations around power and control. It can be used to regulate closeness and distance, to bestow pleasure, wield power, curry favor, withhold affection, humiliate, appease, or repair.

Until recently, the meaning of the sexual act was vastly different for each gender and complementarity was dependent on fixed rules. The traditional heterosexual experience involved the eroticization of the dominant male and submissive female. Sex for women was an act of surrender, sublimation, and abandonment. For men it was an act of conquest and power, a test of their virility and sexual potency.

In the male mystique, power and status have always been closely identified with sexuality. Men have boasted of conquests and "scoring," joked about the prodigious size of their sexual organs, and told tales of legendary sexual prowess. In barrooms and men's clubs they gained admiration from their colleagues not by having sexual relations with their wives, but from the number of reluctant women they had pursued and seduced.

The *Hite Report on Male Sexuality* (1981) concluded that sexual intercourse for men was satisfying not only because of their attraction to their sexual partner "but also from the deeply ingraved cultural meaning of the act. Through intercourse a man participates in the cultural symbolism of patriarchy and gains a sense of belonging to society with status/identity of 'male.'"

For many men, desire is detached from emotional need. Deep feelings are experienced as a threat to their carefully developed controls. For other men, the sexual experience serves as a pathway to intimacy. The bedroom is the only setting in which they can allow themselves to feel close and connected. But while men believe they are expressing love, warmth, and affection through the sexual act, the tender aspects of love are not always understood by women unless verbalized. Verbalization of feelings is a more important part of intimacy for women than for men, and this can lead to misperceptions in the sexual area.

In order to please men on whom they are dependent for emotional (and often financial) security, women have focused more on giving pleasure than receiving it. Sex initially became a symbolic act undertaken in the name of duty, obligation, and responsibility for the sake of marriage or motherhood. This attitude prevented a full appreciation and experiencing of their own sexual desires. Women often resented fulfilling men's sexual needs when their own needs for involvement and intimacy had not been met, and they sometimes reacted by withholding sex. Men failed to read this withholding as a sign that something was wrong in the relationship and instead experienced it as a reflection of their ability to perform sexually, which was tantamount to a rejection of their manhood. Their most common form of retaliation was to accuse the woman of being "frigid." This was anathema for the woman because in our society being called a "frigid woman" is as bad as being called a "bad mother." The woman generally accepted this label and felt guilty, which further diminished her sexual desire.

Barbara Ehrenreich, in her latest book, *Remaking Love, the Feminization of Sex* (1986), sets forth persuasive evidence that the motivating force behind the sexual revolution of the sixties was women's sexual discontent more than men's. Men's attitudes and behavior changed very little during this period, while there was a dramatic change in the meaning and practice of sex for women. Prior to feminism, women kept quiet about their sexual disappointments for fear of incriminating themselves. The pioneers of women's sexual liberation started a program for sexual reform, along with other forms of independence and equality, that included equality in bed.

However, many men found women's more assertive form of sexuality threatening. For women to insist on pleasure was to assert power and to challenge the double standard that was deeply rooted in male psyches. National surveys showed that men still clung to the old idea that women should not engage in premarital sex or have extramarital affairs. The implications of women's sexual freedom went far beyond the bedroom. It threatened to topple sacred ideas about love, marriage, commitment, and family. This created ambivalence and anxiety for both men and women and raised perplexing questions.

If sex were disconnected from love, marriage, and child rearing, which are connected with financial support from men, how would women fare economically in a world in which they were financially grossly disadvantaged? How would women fulfill their need for attachment and intimacy? Was the price for freedom and independence loneliness, alienation, and poverty?

And women were faced with disadvantages not only in the economic marketplace but also in the sexual marketplace. In a society that determines women's worth largely on the basis of their sex appeal, they rapidly lose ground as they mature. The opposite can be true for men, whose sexual attractiveness is often enhanced by the accumulated wealth, authority, and status of age. One has only to view the mass media, in which 90 percent of romantic couples are composed of men over 40 matched with women in their early twenties, to understand what our society considers the ideal couple. This cultural bias places a time limit on women's sexual freedom. A woman's biological clock also limits her reproductive years, whereas a man can raise a second family while collecting social security. Statistics show that divorced men are more likely to remarry than divorced women and that they marry progressively younger wives with each marriage. A recent headline in the *Wall Street Journal* (1986) proclaimed, "A Young Wife Saves Your Life—That's What the Researchers Say."

These demographics provide an ironic commentary on marital equality. Sexual equality cannot be obtained separately from economic and social equality. But disturbing questions arise as to whether or not equality is compatible with a good sexual relationship. Since equality makes a mockery of the dominant/submissive gender roles inherent in the traditional heterosexual relationship, does it not also destroy romance and passion? In a union between two equals, what happens with the traditional seduction rites—the thrill of the chase, the conquering and surrender?

Some therapists never ask questions about a couple's sexual relationship unless it is brought up as a part of the presenting problem. Like money, it is considered a peripheral issue. But by avoiding these topics, therapists miss important indicators of the ways in which power and control are negotiated in the relationship as well as symbols and metaphors that reflect other key issues.

In treating sexual dysfunction, it is important to understand the ways in which each partner's sexual socialization affects the couple's current problem. The myths, double standards, and traditional rules that contribute to the sexual charade of the overpowering male and compliant, passive female should be explored. Whenever men indicate that a woman's assertiveness robs them of their masculinity and their ability to perform sexually, the male mystique that defines masculinity in terms of control and power needs to be questioned. Sex without sexism involves sex between equals, in which submission and dominance are no longer sex-linked.

This means demythologizing the feminine and masculine mystiques by helping women to feel that they have the right to determine what is natural and normal for themselves, to pursue their desires and needs without shame, and to believe that pleasing themselves is equally as important as pleasing their partners; for men it means disconnecting virility and masculinity from subjugation of women so that sexual pleasure is not dependent on dominance and winning but on affection and companionship.

My case of "The 'Frigid' Wife" illustrates a way of resolving a sexual problem by realigning the dominant/passive position of husband and wife.

Money and Power

More couples fight over money than perhaps any other issue. This is understandable since money represents power and control. In their study of 150 couples, Blumstein and Schwartz (1983) discovered that the right to make and enforce decisions in marital relationships is influenced by the relative income of each partner. This economic hierarchy is usually weighted in favor of the man who is the primary financial provider. In three out of four types of couples studied by Blumstein and Schwartz, there was a direct correlation between income and power.

In heterosexual couples, wives gained greater financial autonomy and more decision-making power with a proportionate increase in their incomes. The exception concerned couples who still adhered to the "male-provider" philosophy. In these cases, greater power was granted to the husbands even when the wives earned as much or more than they did. According to Blumstein and Schwartz, "When the husband believes in his provider role, he has the greater say in the important decisions. If his wife shares the same view, then she yields to his wishes. Even if she is employed full time, and earns more money than he, she places their financial destiny in his hands, granting him ultimate control over their money" (p. 56). It is not money alone but money combined with the tradition of male dominance that establishes the balance of power.

In lesbian couples studied by Blumstein and Schwartz, the power balance was not determined by either woman's income. This was seen as reflecting the fact that women are not as apt as men to judge their own worth or that of their partner in terms of money. Historically, because women have earned less money than men, they have not been accustomed to using their wealth to "throw their weight around." Unlike lesbian relationships, gay male couples base the right to dominate on the financial contribution of each partner. These patterns led Blumstein and Schwartz to conclude that "it is men—who for generations have learned in the workplace the equation that money equals power—who have recreated this experience in the home. Wives and cohabitating women fall prey to the logic that money talks. But women seem capable of escaping the ruthless impact of money when no man is present" (pp. 55-56).

The fourth category of couple studied by Blumstein and Schwartz, cohabitors (unmarried men and women), provided the greatest evidence of the link between money and power. In these relationships, the male-provider role lost its importance and the couple's approach to money resembled that of gay and lesbian couples more than that of married couples. Both men and women preferred to be financially responsible for themselves, avoiding the financial and symbolic domination that marriage allows men to impose on women.

Money not only represents financial security, but has also come to symbolize status, prestige, and authority both in the workplace and at home. When he is deprived of his ability to earn money through illness or unemployment, a man feels emasculated and often reacts to these feelings of helplessness and frustration by becoming violent or by falling into a deep depression.

Money is used in a great variety of ways in negotiating marital conflicts. It is important for therapists to include questions about money management in their routine information gathering. Even when a couple is affluent and money is not a survival issue, it colors every aspect of their relationship and has a bearing on the nature of their conflicts. Women are disadvantaged at the financial bargaining table since not only do they have fewer financial resources than men but also no monetary value is attached to their daily tasks of running a home. Consequently, they are left feeling that they do not have equal rights in determining how money should be spent.

In helping couples to negotiate their financial problems, it is important for therapists to keep in mind the ways in which gender-based financial inequities determine the nature of their conflicts and for therapists to work with couples in the direction of equal say over money matters. Money traditionally has been addressed in therapy only in terms of its symbolic meaning rather than its real value. When this happens, the therapist invalidates the reality of a woman's financial dependency and actual impoverishment. A woman's financial vulnerability is reflected in the statistics that show women earning 68 cents for every dollar men earn for the same kind of work. Therapists can address this financial vulnerability by raising questions about insurance policies, division of assets, control over money, and marketable skills.

Carter's case at the end of this chapter is an excellent illustration of a therapeutic intervention that addresses the financial inequity between a husband and wife.

Toward an Egalitarian Relationship

As more and more women have entered the labor market and gained financial independence, their options in the marital relationship have tended to increase. As a result, a more egalitarian concept of marriage has begun to emerge, with an emphasis on comradeship, democracy, and equality between partners rather than subservience, authority, and duty. However, this egalitarian relationship is difficult to achieve, even for couples who intellectually support it.

Despite good intentions, men have found it difficult to practice the egalitarian ideal because it threatened their feelings of power. Veroff and Feld (1970) reported that women with strong power motivations felt "unrestricted, happy and free of problems" in egalitarian relationships. They reported fewer marital problems and more marital happiness than women with less power drive. But egalitarianism created difficulties for their power-oriented husbands as it challenged their positions of power and threatened to reveal their weaknesses.

Later studies, however, such as those reported in Gayle Kimball's *The Fifty-Fifty Marriage* (1983), present a more optimistic picture in which the husbands reported appreciating the freedom they gained with two wage earners in the family and the autonomy they experienced in having a partner who felt she was living up to her capabilities and who, therefore, did not look to him to shape her identity. These husbands also cited becoming closer to their children as a major benefit.

Egalitarian couples are still in the minority, but they point a hopeful direction for the future of marriage in which there would be no dichotomy between "breadwinner" and "dependent," between "dominant" and "submissive," between "passive" and "aggressive." Each partner would be permitted a wide range of activities, behaviors, and expressive styles without fear of losing his or her femininity or masculinity. This flexible marriage partnership can be achieved only by changing the basic beliefs and social structure that keep men and women the prisoners of gender.

Clinical Approaches

In my systemic-strategic approach to treating families and couples, I work on several different levels simultaneously. On the behavioral level, I examine the repetitious patterns and recurring cycles of interaction around which the presenting problem is organized. On the ideational level, I elicit the attitudes, expectations, assumptions, and beliefs that maintain these repetitious patterns and cycles. Men and women generally are not aware of their own belief systems since they are deeply ingrained. This information can only be obtained indirectly by listening to attitudinal statements or through the use of metaphors and fantasies. Based on my understanding of both the behavioral patterns and the attitudinal postures that maintain these patterns, I work to alter both.

One of the techniques I have developed that enables me to view several different levels of the relationship simultaneously is called *structured fantasy*. This technique is particularly useful as a diagnostic tool in working with couples as it elicits a metaphorical rather than literal picture of the relationship. This picture provides a holistic gestalt that reveals basic assumptions each partner holds about themselves and each other, the point at which these basic assumptions collide, and the attempted solutions of each partner that serves to perpetuate the problem. Using the personal metaphors of each spouse, I give rituals and tasks aimed at changing both the interlocking patterns of behavior and the culturally based assumptions and beliefs that maintain the behavior. This technique, along with others, will be demonstrated in my case, "The 'Frigid' Wife."

Cases

The following four cases demonstrate various ways of treating couples within a feminist perspective.

Carter's case deals with the all-important subject of money. It is one of the issues couples most frequently fight about because money is a metaphor for the dependent position of wives as well as a reality issue. In this case, the monetary disparities outside the home are reflected in the domestic scene where the wife must barter for life's essentials. In her original intervention, Carter dramatizes the way in which traditional "women's work" (upon which civilization is based) is still devalued. Both spouses come away with a different understanding of the economics of their lives and the way in which this affects their relationship.

Silverstein's case, "The Protective Pair," points up some of the differences between a homosexual and heterosexual relationship. In working with a lesbian couple, she discerns the elements in their relationship that are imitations of a heterosexual relationship. Rather than accepting this imitation and working within its limited confines, she suggests another possibility. She challenges the pair to use their womanly qualities to create a new and different kind of relationship, one based on equality and friendship.

Walters's couple come with the old refrain, "We can't communicate," and present themselves in the stereotypical roles of the "overly expressive" wife and the "closed-off" husband. As is usual in such situations, the wife pressures her husband for more relatedness and the husband continues to withdraw. Walters avoids the common therapeutic trap of assuming that the husband is incapable of expressing his feelings and that, therefore, nothing should be expected of him, or that the wife is crazy because she does express hers and that she needs to be contained. Instead she counters this shared belief system by helping each partner to understand and respect the communicative style of the other. In the process, both "feeling" and "reason" are validated and allowed free expression.

My case, "The 'Frigid' Wife," deals with a "sexual problem" as defined by the husband. Both husband and wife have bought into the common cultural assumption that a woman has a sexual problem if she doesn't meet the man's sexual needs. Neither connects the wife's lack of sexual desire to the other issues in their relationship that are creating the problem. The husband deals with his frustration in typically male fashion, by using what he considers to be his greatest asset—his analytic mind. He analyzes, criticizes, and tries to reform his wife. The wife reacts to his analysis and criticism in typically female fashion, by assuming he is right and then fighting defensively against him. The wife has difficulty recognizing and articulating her own needs in a coherent manner since, deep down, she believes with her husband that his needs are more important than hers and that she is not entitled to parity. At no point in the therapy do I accept the husband's definition of the problem as the wife's "frigidity." Rather I focus on altering the shared belief system regarding sex, power, authority, and responsibility that keeps the couple locked into their sterotypical roles.

Each of the cases in this chapter focuses on changing a sexist belief or attitude concerning some key issue in a couple's relationship. In each case the therapist illustrates an awareness of the ways in which sexist ideas are subtly interwoven into the couple's daily lives, and each case demonstrates a different way of changing these ideas. The presenting problems are related to traditional assumptions about key issues such as power, sex, money, communication, or responsibility; therapy aims at changing the ingrained beliefs that have maintained relationships oppressive to both partners.

cases

Peggy Papp

The "Frigid" Wife

The Problem

Kurt, a psychoanalyst, brought his wife, Jill, to our clinic because he believed she had a sexual problem. Jill, having resisted her husband's many attempts to persuade her to go into individual therapy, had finally agreed to accompany him for marital counseling. Kurt, dressed in a dark blue suit, stroked his beard as he stated that the major difficulty in their marriage stemmed from his wife's sexual inhibitions due to childhood experiences. He expressed his great disappointment that Jill was not more sensual in bed. Her frigidity left him angry and frustrated, but whenever he tried to engage her in a discussion of their relationship she withdrew from him and became remote, cold, and sexually unavailable.

Jill, 15 years his junior, sat stiffly in her chair, looking guilty and disconsolate as her husband spoke. She grudgingly conceded that he was probably right and that she did have a sexual problem, but she resented his trying to push her into therapy. She had bought into her husband's belief that her lack of sexual desire had something to do with her childhood, but she wasn't sure in what way. She stated that she didn't like to discuss this issue with him because he blamed her for everything and constantly analyzed her. "He sees me as a 'case' that he has to figure out. His idea of discussing our relationship is to ask me why I overreact to whatever he does. . . . He knows the answers to everything and makes up all the rules."

She blamed his attitude on his having been raised as a "prince" in a household in which all the women catered to him. Kurt admitted that as the only son he was considered someone special: "I was the intellectual in the family and it's true everyone arranged their lives around my work." But since he prided himself on being a sophisticated intellectual, he acknowledged this arrangement had gone out of style. However, he was having a hard time adjusting to a different one.

Jill, who considered herself a "modern, liberated" woman, was making a desperate attempt to stand up for her rights, but she was going about it in a self-defeating way. During the therapy session she alternately flailed around defensively, belligerently counterattacked, resorted to sarcastic retorts, or withdrew into a steely silence. Kurt reacted to her withdrawal with more criticism and analysis.

Structured Fantasy

In order to cut through this repetitious exchange, I engaged the couple in a *structured fantasy* exercise in which the medium of expression is metaphor and movement rather than words. The couple were asked to close their eyes and have a fantasy about each other in relation to the problem they were having. They were asked to envision each other in symbolic forms and to imagine the kind of movement that would take place between these two forms. Then they were asked to enact their fantasies physically with one another.

Kurt posed his wife as a "cold metallic cylinder with an interior space that is empty." He was a fireman with an ax trying to break in. After many frustrating and futile attempts, he ended up throwing the cylinder out of the window.

Jill saw herself as a beautiful, small snake curled up on the bank of a stream. "I chose a snake because it is viperish and has a flickering tongue." She saw her husband as a cookie monster. "He is warm but an overwhelming monster—well-meaning but lumbering." She saw him as having "fly eyes" and seeing a hundred million images at one time. "You are curious abut me the way our son is curious about an object," she told him. There was a small stream that ran between them, and she felt protected by the stream. If the cookie monster crossed the stream he would step on her—not because he was malicious but because he was clumsy.

I asked the cookie monster to cross the stream to see what would happen, and the snake instantly backed away from him. Kurt exclaimed, "This is exactly what happens when I'm trying to make love to her. She's always backing away." Jill replied, "I'm afraid he will crush me. Because of his hundred million eyes he doesn't see very well. He either has to be at some distant remove in order to get all the images together or he has to be literally using physical feeling."

The fantasies gave a visual form to each spouse's personal experience of their relationship, revealing their attitudes, expectations, style of relating, and manner of dealing with the problem. Kurt viewed his wife as inpenetrable. As a fireman, a man of action, he saw his only solution as the use of physical force to break through the steel cylinder. His brawn and his ax were his only resources. When they failed him, he could think of nothing else to do but throw the cylinder out the window. He was unaware that the cylinder had been erected to protect Jill from his critical fly eyes and the clumsiness that might crush her.

Jill's image of herself as a beautiful snake with a viperish tongue indicated her perception of herself as a being who must operate subversively from a lowly position. Her only weapon was her "flickering tongue." She felt unable to protect herself through her own power and had to rely on the stream that ran between them for protection. The cookie monster, although well-meaning, was clumsy and could not see those close to him. He could only feel them physically or hold them at a great distance.

Using the Metaphors

In discussing their reactions to the fantasies, Kurt voiced his surprise that Jill saw him as so threatening, but it only validated his belief that she needed individual therapy. Jill stated that she found the exercise useful since "it showed me I am capable of expressing what my concern is without getting angry and just yelling. It's not direct, so it allowed me to say calmly what I've been having a hard time saying because Kurt is always pressuring me."

The overriding issue between them, as I saw it, was authority and culpability. Kurt, as the self-defined authority, was holding Jill responsible for their problem by placing the sole cause of their difficulty on her lack of sexuality and her backing away from him. Jill, rather than challenging his view of the problem, inadvertently supported it by defensively backing away. Staying within the framework of their metaphors, my goal was to help Jill find a way to cross the stream without being crushed, and to help Kurt find a way to break through the cylinder without using force.

I then decided to see each of them separately and offer suggestions as to how they could change their positions in their fantasies. In a separate sesion with Jill, I told her that by backing away from the hundred million eyes she only invited the cookie monster to pursue her and try to analyze her further. The more she backed away, the more he pursued and probed. This put her in a one-down, defensive position. I suggested that the snake should cross the stream and take the offensive—not by attacking, as she had been doing, but by using her "viperish tongue" in a different way. Every time Kurt started to analyze her, rather than becoming defensive she should turn the tables on him and analyze his need to analyze. In a friendly and concerned way, she should become curious about all the childhood experiences that might have contributed to his need to analyze and she should ask him many questions about his relationship with his mother and father. The purpose of this approach was to take Jill out of her helpless position and put her in charge of the situation over which she felt she had no control. By reversing her position with Kurt in this humorous way she would no longer be the victim of his "fly eyes," but instead would turn them back on himself. It is difficult to remain defensive while gently poking fun at a situation.

In a separate session with Kurt, I pointed out that it was impossible to break through a steel cylinder with an ax. He agreed, and said that was why he was so frustrated. But he did not like the other alternative, which was to throw the cylinder out the window (where he had thrown his other two wives, this being his third marriage). I suggested that before our next session he should use his hundred million eyes to try to figure out a way to get through the steel cylinder without an ax—perhaps by finding a secret lock to open, the right button to push, or a way to melt the cylinder. He was asked to keep a notebook in which he recorded Jill's reactions to his different approaches and to analyze any differences he noted. He was not to share his observations with Jill but to bring them to the next session. In this way, I put his analytic skills to work in the service of becoming more attuned to Jill's feelings and desires. In order to analyze her reactions to a different approach, he first had to approach her differently.

Reactions to Tasks

In the following session Jill reported, "When Kurt made a provocative remark I got him to replay what was going on in his own head rather than reacting to it myself. It gave me a way of seeing the humor in the situation and not feeling so helpless. Helplessness is an option I've found easy to fall into. . . . At one point he caught on to what I was doing and we both started to laugh."

Kurt reported on the notes he had taken and concluded that Jill had become more available emotionally and sexually whenever he moved toward her in a less pressuring and more loving way. He described a wonderful experience they had on New Year's Eve. They stayed home alone, turned on music, danced, drank champagne, and had marvelous sex. Jill said it was because she was relaxed and the experience was surrounded by pleasure and fun. "It's sometimes hard for me to be sexual unless I have a sense of participation in which I have equal say. You must come together in some way before you have a physical union, and I can't get together with you if I feel we're not communicating about other things." Kurt retorted that she had placed so many requirements on this natural, simple act that it had become "quasi-impossible." Mirroring stereotypical gender attitudes, Kurt expressed his desire for sex to be free, spontaneous, and detached from other aspects of the relationship, while for Jill the other aspects of the relationship determined sexual desire.

Jill went on to say that she was very moved by Kurt's support of her since the last session, and Kurt again insisted it was because they had made love. Jill bristled at this, saying, "Why do you have to attribute it only to that?" Kurt couldn't understand why she was upset and recalled an earlier incident when Jill suddenly became angry when he credited the improvement in their relationship to her becoming more sensual. Jill was only vaguely aware of why this upset her and had difficulty trying to explain it. She ended up backing down and apologizing for her reaction. In the following excerpt I help them both to see that her anger and frustration stem from Kurt's continuing to make sex the main issue, thus placing the blame for the problem on Jill and ignoring other aspects of their relationship.

THERAPIST: So Jill, you are having difficulty explaining that the reason you are angry is because he just criticized you? That he just blamed the whole problem on you by saying everything is solved when you become more sexual?

JILL: That's probably where it came from.

KURT: That never occurred to me. Now you say it I see it.

JILL: I was aware of it on a secondary level, but I've never been successful explaining that type of thing to him before.

KURT: (Now blaming Jill for not explaining it to him correctly) Peggy mentioned it and it clicked right away. It is certainly easier to understand than that diffused anger of yours.

JILL: My explanations are never understood by you.

KURT: You don't try hard enough. If I don't understand you, you must keep leading the horse to the water.

THERAPIST: You think the responsibility is hers then, Kurt?

JILL: Yeah, why should it all be my responsibility. If the horse doesn't show any willingness to learn, why should I keep trying to lead it to water? You are telling me again, "You didn't try hard enough to do it the right way. You should learn to communicate better." It's my responsibility again. You're telling me my poor communication is the cause of our problem.

KURT: (*Trying to be patient*) Since it's your problem, you must take the first step and I must take the second step. I can't take the second step until you've taken the first.

JILL: Says who? Where is it written that I have to take the first step and you the second? Why don't you take the first?

THERAPIST: (*To Kurt*) What would be the first step for you?

KURT: To become more aware of potential criticism. But if I say something to make you angry I expect you to tell me.

JILL: Why don't you just stop criticizing me?

Kurt was left momentarily without words, but quickly recovered and took the offensive.

KURT: Look, I'll be perfectly honest. I'm sure Jill would be more loving and warm and sexual if I never criticized her or tried to analyze or guide her—that seems to be the gist of what is happening here. But that's impossible. Why? Well because—let's face it—I'm older, I've had more experience and I know more. There are so many things she just doesn't understand or see. I was raised in an environment where knowledge and wisdom were respected (*Laughing a little embarrassedly*). You're asking me to change myself in fairly significant ways. I don't know if I could do that. You're asking me to be a saint.

I jokingly said I thought sainthood would become him, since he certainly had the beard for it. Kurt, obviously pleased, went on.

KURT: I can make one of two decisions—either I can leave the marriage, which I don't want to do, or I can make significant changes—which I don't know if I want to do.

Jill was frightened by the threat and started to back down with "You don't have to make a significant change, just give me a little appreciation."

THERAPIST: Why are you taking him off the hook?

JILL: Because this scares me. If he can't accomplish this significant change, he will leave the marriage.

THERAPIST: So you're going to protect him from struggling with that decision? He has said he doesn't want to leave the marriage. You wouldn't want to rob him of the opportunity to change, would you?

In this way I challenged the couple's basic pattern of Jill retreating and Kurt attempting to maintain the status quo. I then explored with Jill what she meant when she said that she found it difficult to be sexual when they were not communicating about other things. She stated that although they worked at equally taxing jobs, she was expected to carry the burden of keeping their world going while Kurt was "off in academia." For example, during Christmas she ended up doing everything by herself, including cooking a large meal, inviting all the people, decorating the tree, and buying, wrapping, and mailing all the gifts, including those to his family. "It's no fun when you're all alone," Jill said. "This is the story of our life. When I go to bed I'm too tired to be interested in sex after working all day and running the home."

Kurt then began a long lecture on the importance of his work—lectures that had to be prepared, twelve hours of reading in preparation for a class that he was teaching, appointments with patients, a book he was writing. In the face of all this, Jill again began to back down. I persisted in encouraging her to state specifically what she wanted from Kurt in terms of a more equitable domestic arrangement. However, once again she asked for appreciation rather than equality. "When she's tired, try a little tenderness," the old song goes. It was clear that deep down Jill believed that Kurt's work was more important than hers and that it deserved her sacrifice and support.

Dramatizing the Dilemmas

One way to deal with deeply ingrained beliefs is to articulate and dramatize the ambivalence surrounding them. Since this case was being observed by a training group, I decided at this point to have the group take a different position from me in relation to the couple's readiness to give up their beliefs. The division between the group and me served to mirror the couple's individual dilemmas, to make their alternatives clear, and to challenge them to do something different. After excusing myself to have a "consultation with my team," I returned with the following message that presented our divided opinion about change:

THERAPIST: The group thinks, Jill, that you will not be able to make any demands on your husband or ask for what you need because deep down you believe his concerns are more important than yours.

JILL: (*Listening intently*) The group is partially right, but I want to get over that.

THERAPIST: And, Kurt, they think you will choose not to make a significant change because it would mean giving up some of your privileges, and they believe your privileges are more important to you than Jill.

KURT: They are very naïve and simplistic. They have totally misunderstood my motives and intentions.

THERAPIST: I agree with you, and I believe the group is overly pessimistic. I think, Jill, that you are perfectly capable of getting in touch with your needs and priorities and stating them clearly to Kurt. You have indicated that you're tired of being a curled-up snake on the other side of the stream, and I think you are ready to cross the stream and deal with the cookie monster. And, Kurt, you have used your analytic skills to develop many important insights about yourself and your relationship with Jill, and my guess is that you will decide that Jill is more important to you than your privileges.

During the next session, Kurt stated that he had gotten in touch with something very important after our last meeting.

KURT: I asked myself, "Why did I resent Jill complaining about my not doing enough around the house?" And to be absolutely level, it comes from my background. (*Self-mockingly*) I'm supposed to be the scholar—I'm the intellectual. Everybody is supposed to arrange their lives around my work. I think I take that as a matter of course, almost, that everybody arrange their lives so I can do this work. That's what it was like for me when I was growing up. How dare she question it!

I remarked, "The group didn't think you'd be able to give that up because the roots are deep and it's powerful stuff." Kurt countered with, "Well, they were wrong . . . I have done a lot of thinking and I have a more realistic appreciation of the situation. I've always wanted more than I've had. I kept pressuring her to be more sensual, more insightful, more intellectual—more like me. Part of my pushing and prying was to try and make her more like me. I realize now she's not going to be like me. She is more giving when I'm less demanding. But, of course, I had some help from Jill. She let me know more clearly what she wanted."

Jill smiled and said undefensively that she was willing to share half of the responsibility for the change.

Summary

In this case, I dealt with the presenting problem of the wife's "frigidity" as part of the couple's interactional system involving issues of power, authority, communication, and responsibility. Rather than focusing on the wife's psychosexual development in an attempt to uncover the source of her "sexual problem," I helped her to sort out her feelings and needs in her current situation, first through the use of fantasy and then, more directly, through verbally articulating them. By challenging her secretly held belief that her needs were not as important as her husband's, I enabled her to move out of her helpless position and take more control over her life.

My work with Kurt focused on helping him to become aware of the role he played in his wife's emotional and sexual withdrawal and helping him find ways of reaching her other than through the use of his analytical mind. In finding new ways to reach his wife, he began to take his share of the responsibility not only for the problem but also in seeking a solution to the problem. In giving up his old ideas of power and privilege, he was able to begin to see his wife separately from him and to reap the benefits of a richer relationship with her.

Olga Silverstein

The Protective Pair

The Cultural Stereotyping

I chose this case because it most clearly demonstrates the powerful cultural nature of coupling.

The gender-role assignments and designations, sometimes clearly and sometimes covertly defined by the larger context, are well documented. Women are affectively connected, are sensitive to emotional issues, and can express feelings more easily. Men are more instrumental and outside-oriented, less emotionally open, and so forth. These are the stereotypes of our culture.

It is difficult to perceive coupling without these designations. An error for a therapist might be the denial of the specialness of a lesbian couple—that is, two women in an intimate sexual and social relationship. Somewhat akin to a white liberal therapist who claims to be color blind is the therapist who claims that a couple is a couple.

In fact, two women living together might be expected to have too much of a good thing—too much communication, sharing, caretaking, and so forth. Instead, what can and often does happen is an unconscious imitation of a gendered relationship. That was the problem for Bea and Annie.

Bea, as the older, more experienced member of the pair, had taken on the "male" role, while Annie acted out the traditional "little woman."

The Couple

The first call came from Annie, who immediately asked me if I saw lesbian couples. I answered that I had, and would. She then said that she and her lover needed to see someone as soon as possible, as things were getting very difficult and she felt they were in crisis.

Annie was a thin, tense-looking 35-year-old, while her lover, Bea, was a matronly looking woman of 50. They had been together for six years—three good and three bad years. The problem was hard to define—they started out by saying they needed to learn to communicate.

ANNIE: We don't communicate. I know Bea is angry and upset with me—when I ask her what the matter is, she says, "Nothing," or, "You should know." It drives me crazy, but I can't get her to tell me.

THERAPIST: But she has communicated that she's upset, right?

ANNIE: Right.

THERAPIST: Can you tell the difference between "upset" and "angry"?

ANNIE: Most of the time.

THERAPIST: So maybe the communication is fine. Bea doesn't even need to talk, you read her so well.

THERAPIST, TO BEA: Would you say she's right—some of the time—most of the time—all of the time?

BEA: It doesn't matter if she's right or not. I'm sick and tired of her reading my mind. She "knows" I'm upset before I do. I walk in the door, and before I open my mouth she says, "What's the matter?"

THERAPIST: Then what do you do?

BEA: Sometimes I tell her. Sometimes it just pisses me off and I say nothing, but she'll keep after me until I scream. Yesterday I threw a bowl at her—luckily she ducked. I'm afraid I'm going to kill her one of these days.

THERAPIST: Annie—does it ever happen the other way, that Bea is reading your face and trying to check out her perception?

ANNIE: No, I never sulk. I was taught to put a good face on things. My mother had a little poem she'd recite to us. "Laugh and the world laughs with you—weep and you weep alone."

THERAPIST: So how would Bea know if you were angry or upset?

ANNIE: I only get upset when Bea upsets me, and then she knows.

THERAPIST: She just knows?

ANNIE: Yes.

The History

Annie and Bea met at a mutual friend's house ten years ago. They knew each other casually for some years before they decided to live together. At the time they met, Annie was involved in a heterosexual relationship, and Bea had been living with a woman for five years. "We liked each other a lot, but just as friends." Then one night Annie had a terrible fight with her boyfriend and Bea offered to drive her home. Bea stayed the night, saying, "She was so young, so unhappy—I couldn't leave her." They became lovers. It was not Annie's first lesbian relationship—she had had some experiences in high school—but then, she said, "I was trying to be straight—but then after I stayed with Bea, I knew that that was what I wanted."

Annie comes from a middle-class suburban family where the father was "king." She had two older brothers, both married and living at some distance from home. "My mother was a saint," she told me. "She anticipated their every desire. Mine, too, I guess, but not as much. I was her pal. She'd say, 'Let's get things straightened up before the men get home.' That was when my brothers were still kids. She always called them 'the men.' My father was great. He took care of everything. Every Saturday night he sat down and gave out the week's orders— 'Stewart, you do the grass, Matthew, you go to the store for your mother, and Annie, you do the dishes.' He took care of my mother. It was always, 'I'll ask your father.'"

THERAPIST: What do you think, Annie—was your mother a happy woman?

ANNIE: If you asked her, she'd laugh and say, "Laugh and the world laughs—"

THERAPIST: What do you think?

ANNIE: No, I think I'm the only one who knew. I could always tell by her voice, her face—the way she twisted her fingers. But she'd never admit it. Even now, I know it kills her that I'm living with Bea. I told her two years ago that we were lovers and she promised not to tell my father—and I know she hasn't—but she looks at me with those spaniel eyes and I could die.

THERAPIST: I guess that's where you learned to read faces so well.

Bea's story was somewhat different. She comes from a large Southern family. "Poor—you don't know poor till you've seen southern white poor," she said.

BEA: My father drank. When he wasn't working, he drank. Sometimes he beat up on us kids and once, only once, I remember he hit my mother. I picked up a poker and told him that if he touched her again, I'd kill him. He knew I meant it and never touched her again. Not that I saw.

Anyway, I got married when I was 16 and had three kids by the time I was 20. One night my husband came home drunk and I thought, no, not again. I took the kids and the car and just drove off. I had a few men, but it was always the same. The first woman lover I had was when I was 30 and the kids were getting big. She was only a kid herself but I loved her. We were together ten years. (*She sighed.*) When she left me, I thought I'd die. The kids had all gone by then. The girls got married—Georgie, my boy, is in the Navy. I was a damned good mother.

When I met Annie I was living with someone—but I didn't really care for her. It was just not to be alone—you know. Anyway, Annie was sweet and little, and she needed someone. We were real good in the beginning because I tend to be moody, but Annie is like a songbird. And she'd always cheer me up but lately I can't do anything without her fluttering around—asking, "What's wrong? What did I do? Tell me what to do, I'll do anything."

"The Marriage"

Although they came from very different backgrounds, Annie and Bea shared certain characteristics with most women. They were both nurturers and caretakers, as evidenced by Bea's good mothering of her children and of her own mother, and her response to Annie's youth and neediness when they met. But once the relationship had settled into a "marriage" it took on all the gendered division of roles that exists in a traditional marriage. No wonder they were confused and felt unable to communicate.

I challenged the two women about their inability to communicate.

The Therapy

THERAPIST: I'm really surprised. I would expect that two women who started out as friends would continue as friends even if they have become lovers. When did you start playing Mommy and Daddy?

At another point, I asked them both to write down what they thought was good and then bad about being female.

Annie's list read:

1. Women make better friends.
2. Women understand things about people.
3. Women care about others.
4. They are not as selfish.
5. Being female means you can be weak or needy without being ashamed.
6. You can cry.
7. Women are not as competitive.
8. They want things to be nice.
9. Women are not aggressive.
10. Women are more loving.

Bea's list read:

(The Positive)

1. Women are not aggressive.
2. They don't have to show how big they are.
3. They don't try to overpower you.
4. Women are on the same side.
5. They know how to take care of people.

(The Negative)

1. They get hurt too easily.
2. They don't take care of themselves.

BEA: Is that a female thing?
THERAPIST: I think so.
BEA: Well, then it's not positive.
ANNIE: I got that. (*Laughing*)

I asked them both to talk about their previous heterosexual relationships.

ANNIE: I only had one man—besides my father. Does he count? Oh, well, Billy. Billy and I went to high school together. He was not like my father. But in a way I guess he was. Always telling me what to do. We used to fight terribly, but then he'd be sorry and he'd want to make up—that always meant sex—go to bed and make up. I couldn't understand that. Still can't. How do you make love when you're hating someone? I can't.

THERAPIST: Most women can't. Women generally need to feel loving to make love.

ANNIE: Don't men?

THERAPIST: Not always. Sex has many meanings for people, but it is often different for men and women.

ANNIE: So women need to feel loving to want sex. I'm going to put that on my list.

THERAPIST: So what do you think?

BEA: My husband was not a bad man, but he liked to throw his weight around. I understood that. I didn't even care. He had a certain air—you know—"I'm cool." He was cute, but he knew shit about me and cared less. Later, when the kids came and he started drinking, he turned mean. I think because he didn't know how to give us things—I don't know. And I hated the sex. That was a big thing. I know that now, but we could never talk about it. I'd try to talk to him and he'd walk out, slam the door, come home drunk. It was too much like home. He never hit us or anything, but still . . .

Later I was with other men but it never worked for me. George—George was good to my kids and I loved him for that, but he wouldn't talk to me—I guess he couldn't. I wasn't very understanding, I guess. I'd try to drag things out of him. Finally, I left because I was just making us both miserable. Maybe I should have been more understanding. He was a good man, I guess.

THERAPIST: Would you put your female tendency to take responsibility for relationships on the positive or negative side of your list?

BEA: Do I do that?

THERAPIST: It seems so.

BEA: I don't know. Shouldn't I?

THERAPIST: Well, it does leave the other person out.

BEA: I don't know if it's negative or not.

THERAPIST: It depends on whether you're taking responsibility for your part or the whole thing. Is it possible to have an equal relationship—two adult women with loving respect for each other—or would that be too much of a good thing?

Gender Issues

As the gender issues became more explicit, and the idea that they were indeed two women in a relationship was confirmed and supported, issues other than the vague "communication" surfaced.

Annie told me that she had been working as a hairdresser ever since she had met Bea. But a few months before this interview, two of the women she was working with decided to open their own shop and asked her to join as a third partner. She said she was afraid to tell Bea because Bea was always dreaming of opening a little restaurant of her own—she worked as a waitress—but it never happened. "I couldn't do that to her," Annie said. "I'm afraid it would hurt her."

I again pointed out that she, Annie, was acting like a good little wife—putting her own needs and goals aside, protecting her mate's ego.

Bea was very upset by this, saying, "I don't want her to do that for me. I would be very happy if she did her thing."

THERAPIST: How come Annie doesn't know that? When did you stop talking to each other about important things?

BEA: I guess when I started acting as though I was the Poppa Bear.

They both laughed.

I then pointed out how Bea had gotten into a corner where she was doing all the things that men do. She withdraws from Annie when annoyed or angry. She wants to take care of her because she's "sweet and little and needed someone." She's become overresponsible for the material well-being of the pair and feels overburdened, but says little about that and broods silently.

"What a conventional arrangement!" I told them, "It's perfect!"

BEA: (*To Annie*) Are you really thinking of opening a place of your own? That's neat—that's really neat.

ANNIE: (*Annie was delighted*) How about you and the restaurant?

BEA: Well, you get started first and then maybe you can help me get started.

ANNIE: Oh, I will. I will. I'd love that.

The only existing model for partners in this culture is the complementary one of marriage. Annie and Bea had structured their lives "as if" they were a heterosexual pair. Treating this pair as though they were a conventional couple might have rigidified the "as if" quality of the relationship. Reaffirming the positive qualities of being a woman freed them to relate as the good friends and caring women they both were.

Betty Carter

The Person Who Has the Gold Makes the Rules

I chose this case because it presents so clearly the issue of money-as-power and the dilemma posed by the traditional expectation of women to be financially "taken care of" in exchange for home and child-care responsibilities. This supposedly "equitable" arrangement has a way of breaking down under stress when it suddenly becomes crystal clear that, for all practical purposes, it is *his* money, not *theirs*, and that he wields, at the very least, the considerable power of absolute veto.

"Being Taken Care Of"

In spite of the dangers for the woman inherent in this arrangement in a society that has a high divorce rate, negligible alimony, and low and/or uncollectable child-care payments, the force of traditional socialization is so strong that this is still the main arrangement practiced or sought after in the upper economic classes. The women in these families are taught to draw their own status from the wealth and position of their husbands, and they receive negative reinforcement and loss of status on all sides if they aspire to careers of their own.

In addition to the women raised in wealthy families, we read now of some of the new breed of successful young career women who decide, after a decade of "doing it all," to quit their high-powered work, move to the suburbs, and stay home with their children. These women have become exhausted because neither their workplace nor their own marital arrangements have changed enough to support their careers *and* their parental responsibilities, and so they have ended up with two full-time jobs. It is easy to overlook the dilemmas faced by these highly educated and competent women because their affluence, or their husband's affluence, disguises their powerlessness.

In addition to the pressure exerted on these women by the expectations of their husbands, it is important to recognize the influence of their own socialization, which has led some to feel insecure and unable to support themselves. The belief that one has a "right" to be supported financially is an extremely hard ideal to give up if you have not been raised to feel competent to do so for yourself and have not been trained in the necessary skills.

In this social class, the men are raised to focus on high-powered careers with large incomes and to expect that their wives will buffer them from all other responsibilities as well as actively support their careers through entertaining, social activities, willingness to relocate, and so forth. The better the wife carries out this supporting role, the more rich, important, and powerful the man becomes, and the more dependent and powerless she becomes. Alcoholism is a common problem for these wives, and a bitter divorce can devastate and impoverish them.

The wives participate in their own entrapment through their belief in the teachings of their upbringing that "being taken care of" financially is their right and their reward, in marriage or in divorce, and that working wives are, by definition, handicapping their husbands, neglecting their children, and demeaning themselves.

The Dangers of Dependency

This formulation does not consider the dangers—economic and psychological—in a life plan of dependency on others. Thus, when conflict arises, the wife finds herself without sufficient power to negotiate, and must rely on pleading, blackmail, or deviousness to pursue her goals. The financial value of her role is denied, both its own worth and its value in freeing the husband to earn. It is *not* an understanding between them that he earns *for their partnership* while she tends to other equally important functions. Rather, both husband and wife tend to view the money he earns with her help as *his*, to be "shared" with his wife and family out of duty or kindness. This view requires his good will and acquiescence in financial decisions and gives her no financial autonomy or power to negotiate. She may believe that she has a "right" to some of this money, but if there is a conflict, personal or legal, she will soon feel the limitations of that belief.

Unfortunately, the power of their socialization is so strong that many middle- and upper-class women fail to see the basic threat to their autonomy and maturity inherent in the system of "complementary" roles, and blame their difficulties on personal failings of their husbands or themselves.

For the purpose of making my point, I present in the following case only the nuclear family and the first phase of the therapy. When the problem presented here was resolved, I said to myself, like the therapist at the end of *Portnoy's Complaint*, "Now we can begin," and we proceeded with the other issues that were identified by the couple.

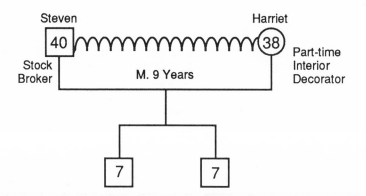

See page 96 for an extended definition of the genogram.

Presenting Problem: "We Don't Communicate"

Harriet said that she had asked for the appointment because of her complaints about the marriage. Steven did not think they needed therapy but was willing to "come along."

Most of the couple's arguments with each other focused around money: how extravagantly she spent and wanted to spend; how tight and stingy he was. No matter how I tried to shift to emotional issues, they came back to their arguments over money, so I decided to use this power issue as a way to start work with them. Their situation is not unusual, but their candor is.

STEVEN: This is not "our" money; it's *my* money. I work my ass off and I am not going to permit wild expenditures that throw my money away. She has a full-time maid; she has a stable of baby-sitters for our sons; she works only when a particular job or client turns her on; and she thinks I'm some kind of sugar daddy. I feel exploited.

HARRIET: (*Bursting into tears*) What do you think it takes to manage *your* household and raise *your* children? I don't work more than I do because *your* children need me. And even if I worked full-time, I couldn't earn anything close to what you earn. Why do I have to beg, plead, or trick you out of every penny I need for myself, the boys, or the house?

Steven's father had ruled his household with a firm hand, granting and denying requests from his wife and children on every conceivable issue. Steven thought this structure had worked fine, and he was trying his best to duplicate it.

Harriet described herself as a "daddy's girl," saying that her father had given her whatever she wanted but she had never asked for anything "unreasonable." She was reluctant to work out a regular budget because Steven then went over it and crossed out many of the expenditures she thought were important for their house or for herself and the children. She had no position from which to negotiate with Steven, tending merely to react defensively and rebelliously to his position.

Every attempt I made to translate "money" into other emotional meanings failed. Nor could I interest either of them in further investigation of any issues with their parents.

Finally, Harriet cried rather histrionically: "How can we, as master and chattel, discuss *anything*?" Steven said: "I wouldn't go that far, but I certainly do think as far as responsibility for money goes, we *are* parent and child."

Negotiating for Change

Their phrases rang in my ears: "master and chattel," "parent and child." How, indeed, could two such unequal partners negotiate anything that could not be rescinded at the whim of the more powerful one? How could I get Steven to see the actual financial worth of Harriet's contribution to the family? What would it take to get Harriet to stop emoting and start thinking through to a position?

What had I done about such dilemmas in the past? Simple. I had scolded the wife (in a nice way, of course) for being irresponsible about money and had urged the husband to give her a "household allowance" and "delegate" to her the authority to manage it within an agreed-upon framework. This solution removed the nuisance of financial arguments without requiring any change in the power balance of the relationship. Unfortunately, it usually lasted only until he disapproved of some particular expenditure. "It would be easier if they were getting divorced," I thought, "then they'd have to work out a more equitable financial agreement." That's when the idea came to me: I said that I would not work with them any longer unless they first settled their financial arrangement with a mediator, exactly as they would do in a divorce. Harriet agreed immediately and Steven, feeling himself to be in an impervious position, "went along."

About four months later, they made another appointment with me. With considerable help from an advisory accountant, and a mediator, Harriet had demonstrated that her contribution to their partnership was worth a considerable amount per year, in addition to support for the boys, giving her legitimate claim to a large share of their net income and assets. She said that if financial quibbling continued to be a problem, she would insist on actually collecting the money and keeping it in a separate account to spend when and as she wished.

Steven doubted that would happen since they had finally agreed on a budget during mediation. He said that the experience had shaken him and had changed his view of the financial value of his wife's role. Harriet said that once she realized that she was *entitled* to part of the family income, she was able to stop crying and start thinking about what she really needed for personal and household expenses. When she saw that a budget could reflect her priorities, as well as Steven's, she became interested in developing one. Most of all, she said, she now felt that it was unsafe as well as childish to be so dependent on money earned by someone else and she planned to change drastically the priority of work and financial earning in her own life. "I kept thinking—suppose this was a divorce and Steven was furious and uncooperative; where would that leave me?"

Conclusion

In this case, I had acknowledged Harriet's feelings of powerlessness by sending her to an arena where her inequality would be addressed and where she would be taught the skills necessary to begin to handle money competently and to value financial independence. Ironically, Steven was so relieved by her new attitude that he said it "almost" made up for the loss of control he was experiencing.

Marianne Walters

"Does Strong Have to Mean Silent?"

Couples who have communication problems often experience their relationship as one in which the woman is endlessly seeking more conversation and information, greater relationality, support, emotional intensity, and fuller expression of feelings; and the man is endlessly protesting and withdrawing in a haze of confusion about what more is needed, wanted, required—feeling that no matter what he does it is never enough, and not even sure that he would know what to do if it ever became clear what she wanted him to do. And both feel failed.

But experiencing conflict and feeling failed in a couple relationship have different meanings for each partner, meanings that are connected not only to their unique personal history, life conditions, and emotional makeup, but also to broader, generalizable conditions rooted in a gendered culture. Her social approval is more dependent on maintaining a successful marital and family life; his on maintaining a successful work or public life. She has a greater stake in feeling competent on the interpersonal level; he, on the problem-solving level.

And yet it is interesting to consider that although this prototypical couple (pursuer-distancer) presents conflict, they have a shared belief system: that men do not have personal skills to nurture relationships and that women do; that women are overinvolved in their relationships and men too distant; that a man needs a wife and a woman needs a relationship; that women need intimacy and men fear it. This shared belief system makes men feel incompetent in relationships, and makes women feel crazy because they are constantly seeking to get what *both* of them believe is not there to be had. So, in their coupling, he feels inadequate, and she feels disappointed. Moreover, since he feels inadequate, he expects her to take care of those family matters that require relationship skills: his and/or her parents, his and/or her siblings, their children, social arrangements, and the like; and she feels put upon, burdened, and unpartnered in having to carry primary responsibility for these family affairs. And so the couple maintains a socially acceptable system, even though in conflict with it. If he "can't," she will protect him, even as she presses him "to do." Her emotionality protects him from having "to do" what he "can't do." If she "can," it seems only reasonable for him to expect her "to do," with or without his help. Thus, the ship stays afloat: he rows and she bails water!

Within this context, I seek a direction in couple therapy that helps each partner to be more aware of the experience of the other as not only reactive, but also gender differentiated, generalizable as well as particular; a way of being that has deep roots in cultural forms and foundations. If awareness of their shared belief system remains obscured in their conflict, it will undermine the relational competence that both partners need in order to couple successfully. Acknowledged and understood as part of their gender development, and thus common to many couples, it can be used to reconstruct their efforts to couple in ways that are not defined as simply particular to their couple system but socially prescribed as well. This removes some of the sense of failure for each of them. And it widens their vision beyond each other, expanding the possibility for each partner to explore new repertoires of behavior that are not contingent on the repertoire of the other.

A feminist perspective in couple work does, I think, need to include the concept of the "social individual" as well as the concept of "we." This will be particularly empowering for the female partner whose self-identity is typically organized by her relationships. For the male partner, the benefit will be in providing a context within which he can risk behaviors he had previously assumed were not in his domain. In the following case discussion, I have included an excerpt from one of my early interviews with a couple that illustrates the ways in which social and gender messages can be woven into one's interventions. It is an example of process that helps to extricate the woman from feeling primary responsibility for change, and that holds the man to an ownership of his feelings and reactivity. This sets the stage for her to feel more in charge of her emotions, and for him to trust that he can translate his emotions into effective interpersonal behaviors.

Becky and Jim

Becky and Jim came to see me in great distress about their marriage. I had known them for about two years prior to their seeking help with their own relationship. Previously they had come to The Family Center around severe problems with their 14-year-old daughter, Sara, and were seen by a therapist under my supervision for about a year. With Sara's running-away and acting-out behaviors improved and under control, Becky and Jim had turned their attention briefly to their 13-year-old son who was underfunctioning in school. In both of these circumstances Becky and Jim, despite differences, were a source of strength and support to each other. Now, they complained of growing alienation between them—that is, Becky complained, while Jim sat stony-faced and silent.

    Becky is a very bright, volatile, expressive Jewish woman. Jim is a steady, solid, very intelligent, laconic gentile man. Becky has strong, complicated, emotional family ties. Some would describe her extended family as enmeshed. I would describe them as deeply involved with one another. Jim seldom sees his extended family, but their relationship is cordial and nonconflictual. Some would describe them as distant; I would describe them as not very deeply involved with one another. (I think it helps if we use words that denote ongoing activity rather than words that can serve as labels—but I diverge.) When Becky is upset, both agree she "carries on." When Jim is upset, they both agree he withdraws. In previous family sessions, Becky would sometimes burst into tears and run out of the room, particularly if she felt the therapist had "misunderstood" her, that is, wasn't sufficiently supportive. Jim would just ride out the storm, steady and concerned, but not drawn in by her "outbursts."

    Becky and Jim have been married for fifteen years, since she was 17 and he 21. Essentially, they ran away together. They have three children, Sara, 14, Michael, 13, and David, 6. Jim is a construction crew supervisor and Becky is a nursery school teacher. She has two sisters with whom she is very close, a brother they all adore, a mother she struggles with, and a father they all cater to. Jim has a younger brother he helped to raise. They were close when they were younger, and drifted apart as each pursued his own life choices. Jim's mother is a high school teacher, and his father is retired on a disability pension. He was a tractor plant manager. Jim thinks his father is pretty authoritarian and his mother long-suffering, but he respects them both. Although he stirred things up a bit in this quiet and respectable family when he married a Jewish girl, things have settled down and his parents enjoy seeing their grandchildren on their infrequent trips home. On the other hand, Becky's parents, who run a summer camp, went "berserk" when she married a gentile boy, but now they are crazy about him and wild over the grandchildren. Obviously, both Becky and Jim enjoy being a bit nonconformist, at least in their choice of marriage partners.

Couple Process

Becky began our first couple session describing the breakdown in their communication, and her increasing sense of desperation about the viability of their relationship. She complained of a growing sense of alienation between them, of loss of affection and support. Where before they had hung together, now they seemed to be always on opposite sides of any issue. She wanted more from Jim in the way of relationship, support, communication. She was afraid they were losing all of the passion. And whenever she wanted to talk about their relationship, to discuss her feelings and concerns, he refused, accusing her of being "off the wall," hysterical, and upsetting the whole family. Jim agreed that they had a communication problem, but felt it was getting blown up out of all proportion by Becky's hyperbole and endless dissatisfaction. She never seemed happy any more, the way she used to. Becky was beginning to act out of control at times, and his only recourse was to back off, to get out of the way. She worries all the time about everything, and gets angry with him if he doesn't accept her constant anxiety—about him, the children, everything—and then denies her the support she wants. She worries about their relationship, the house, his work, her work. She never lets up. She even worries about his not worrying, seeing it as a sign of his lack of commitment and concern.

BECKY: I'm tired of having to walk on eggs with him, Marianne. Why should I have to? I can call my sisters and act like myself. He makes me feel like I'm the odd man out. I've been furious with him for the past three years. I want him to understand that I'm *not* an unreasonable person, that my emotions are *not* crazy, and that if I feel like crying right now it doesn't make me a nutty person . . . (*She begins to sob and cry*) . . . and I'm angry with you, Jim . . . and just because I'm emotional it doesn't make me wacko . . . and the kids do not perceive me as wacko . . . that's just you putting it into their heads . . . I love you, but you're so reasonable . . . I think I've seen you cry once, once . . . and I'm not like you, Jimmy . . . you think the whole world should be like you . . .

MW: Becky, Becky . . . I wonder when this happens, and you're feeling so upset and so alone . . . is there some way Jim can help you?

BECKY: (*Sobbing harder*) No, no, no . . . because he doesn't understand me, Marianne. He doesn't understand any of my feelings . . . they're alien to him. He doesn't know what I'm about at all.

MW: (*Holding her hand and handing her a tissue*) Oh, Becky . . . that's just not possible . . . all these years . . . all that's happened to the two of you . . . you know when you say that . . . it kind of wipes him out . . .

BECKY: It's not what I mean to do . . .

MW: I believe you . . . but it's like you think he doesn't have any understanding . . . that he doesn't feel things . . . I hope that's not the case . . . it would be sad . . .

BECKY: (*More in control of herself*) Yes . . . sad . . .

MW: What do you think, Jim? Is there a way you can help Becky when she's this distraught? I tell you what . . . you move over here, Jim . . . sometimes the farther away one is from the "scene of a disaster" the more insurmountable it seems . . . the more powerless one feels . . . (*We exchange seats so Jim is closer to Becky and I'm across from them.*) 'cause you know, Becky needs some help and you're the one that can . . .

JIM: It's not that I think you're unreasonable, Becky. It's just that I think that sometimes what you feel and the way you say it is so strong . . . it, well, it blots out other people. That's what I think. (*His finger tentatively crosses her hand.*)

BECKY: Well, but Jimmy . . . how else can I . . .

MW: Now wait a sec, Becky, that's an interesting idea that Jim is trying to express. But I don't think he's quite finished his thought. So, Jim, when Becky is like this . . . you feel blotted out?

JIM: Well, not here. But I think that sometimes when she's really raising a storm it sets me on edge.

MW: You feel on edge . . . or you feel blotted out? You see, Jimmy, you said something very interesting . . . a way you feel, a reaction you have, that makes you very critical of Becky . . . what was it?

JIM: Oh, yeah . . . I said that sometimes she feels things so strongly that it blots out other people's feelings . . .

MW: Does it blot out yours, or other people's?

JIM: Well, maybe that's how I see it is for me and the kids.

MW: You and the kids?

JIM: (*Tentatively*) Well, me . . . sometimes . . . well, me . . . a lot of the time.

MW: Okay, Jim . . . I think Becky can handle that . . . she needs to hear what you're saying . . . that sometimes you don't feel you have a place to be . . . but all she experiences is your criticism. Jimmy, it's so tough for you to say, "Me too, I have feelings too!" So, instead, you criticize Becky for having strong feelings.

BECKY: (*With great intensity*) Jimmy . . . I want to know that you're human . . . sometimes I don't think you're human . . . I've told you that before. I just sometimes think that you're like . . . I know that you can show joy, that you can show love, but you can't seem to show any other kind of feeling . . . I have trouble knowing that you can feel other things . . . for yourself . . . for me . . .

JIM: That's because you never keep quiet long enough to listen.

MW: And now you get critical, Jim. You see what happens? The funny thing is that I think Becky was actually trying to protect you when she got all worked up just now . . . I think she felt things were getting a little tough for you here, and so she jumped in. Maybe she thinks she can "take the heat" better than you. Maybe that's what you both believe. Well, anyway, let's get back to what you were saying, Jimmy . . . so, do you think you feel blotted out because Becky feels things so strongly . . . or because you're not sure you know how to handle strong feelings . . . maybe even your own?

JIM: I don't know, I don't know . . . I always thought it was her always getting so worked up . . . so, so much feeling . . . I'm not sure what it is . . . I guess I feel there can't be two on stage at the same time. And maybe I resent that she doesn't appreciate my subtlety, that she doesn't attempt to operate on my wave length . . . because your way, Becky, is filling the air waves whereas mine isn't; and so what kind of room do you leave for others to grow?

MW: For others?

JIM: Well, for me, I guess.

MW: So you don't feel you have room to grow?

JIM: Well, if Becky fills the space, the only way to make some room is by shoving . . . and I don't like doing that.

MW: You know, men often avoid confrontations with their wives, Jim. I think Becky can understand what you're saying . . . in fact, this kind of contact makes her feel close to you.

BECKY: Jimmy . . . I want to hear how you feel. I want to make room . . . to know you have feelings too. What do I do to stop filling up all the space? Where do I begin?

MW: By not worrying about what to do . . . by not assuming you have to take the next step.

BECKY: But . . .

MW: No, no . . . Becky, let it be. Jim, it may be hard for you to say what you're feeling . . . but you sure have a lot in there (*heart*) and in there (*head*) . . . a lot. And Becky, when he gets tentative, or even brief, you fill in. I think you both believe that Jim doesn't know how to deal with emotional things . . . so Jim backs off and Becky . . .

BECKY: (*Interrupting*) So what do we do to change it?

MW: Oh, hush . . .

JIM: (*Holding Becky's hand*) Becky, I can communicate . . . it's just different . . . it's not like you do, it's not all over the place . . . wild . . .

MW: So now you begin to get critical, Jim, because you feel you have to defend yourself. It's hard for you to express your thoughts and emotions, and so Becky fills the space, like you say. But, Jim, it's not that you don't have those skills . . . you're just out of practice. You didn't have those sisters like Becky had to work out on! And maybe, like lots of guys, no one ever expected you to talk things over when you were worried or in trouble. That's something people expect more from girls than from boys when they're growing up.

BECKY: Oh . . . Jimmy . . . I didn't know . . . you never said . . . I thought you didn't . . . that none of it mattered to you. You're so strong. You know . . . I wonder . . . do you think, maybe, that you have to be silent to be so strong?

JIM: It's not like I don't think about all that stuff . . . just maybe not as much as you . . . but a lot. It's moving around in my head . . . (*They sit quietly while Jim plays with Becky's hand, strokes her shoulder. They are both staring straight ahead, not able to meet each other's eyes.*)

MW: You're filled with a lot of emotion, Jim . . . looking every which way but at Becky . . .

JIM: Yeah, I feel like . . . well, it's different. Not that there isn't good reason to be critical sometimes . . . but why should her stuff stop me?

BECKY: It's so overwhelming . . . I never thought he . . . I can't look at him either . . . I never knew he even had strong feelings about anything . . . you always act so reasonable . . . oh, Jimmy . . .

MW: So, maybe Jim, you need some help in talking about your own worries, feelings. Becky, now that you know that they're there, maybe you can take the time to ask, dig around, wonder . . . When you're afraid they're just not there you push and fill in . . . You're afraid of the open spaces . . . they might just stay empty.

JIM: I guess I figured there wasn't room for both of us on center stage . . . and I'd have to be bumptious, pushy, if I wanted to initiate anything. And anyway, I figured I'd have to have my own shit together if I wanted to get some of the action.

MW: You see, Becky, Jim isn't sure he has those skills you take so much for granted . . . he . . .

BECKY: (*Interrupting*) Skills! skills! but, Marianne, I thought they were crazinesses . . . not skills . . . I never thought they were skills . . . my God!

MW: So, Becky, you were wrong, and now you know better!

Reflections

Such an encounter in therapy provides a context for change that builds on a connection between couple conflict and the different experiences, expectations, and roles of men and women, wives and husbands. Hopefully, it gives each some appreciation and respect for the experience and perspective of the other, not just as one's complementary other, but as a person whose social experiences and psychological development have fundamental roots in a highly skewed, gendered culture.

We could speculate that this couple was experiencing conflict that had previously been detoured through their symptom-bearing children, or that Becky had not separated emotionally from her family of origin, or that they were playing a reciprocal game that obscured their mutual fear of intimacy; or we could stick with the familiar thesis of the complementary interactions of her pursuit and his distance. We have many frames in which to fit this couple. The one you choose will have implications not only about what you think "will work," but about the message you intend to impart.

If Becky had continued to believe that her emotionality was "crazy" rather than a valuable personal skill, then even positive change in those behaviors that were dysfunctional in their relationship would leave her with the awful sense that if one feels strongly and is emotional one can't behave rationally. And it would not be sufficient to remain neutral about such a belief; if it is not revised in therapy, then the mental health of women is at risk.

And so for Jim: If he had continued to believe that he had no voice because Becky's voice was so strong, then he would have remained committed to the belief that his relationship skills were dependent on Becky's restraints, and even positive change in his dysfunctional behavior would leave him believing that strong feelings endanger reasonable behaviors.

This reason-emotion split is often at the base of couple conflict. It is also a widely accepted premise among therapists. That is, many therapists try to operate on the assumption that objectivity and reason depend on the reduction, if not the absence, of emotion. When one remembers that in our society "reason" is male-identified and "emotion" is female-identified, one can easily imagine the implicit, if not explicit, effect of such a belief system on the male and female members of a couple. The beliefs of a therapist will inevitably be reflected in her/his choice of words, behaviors, and interventions. The issue, of course, is to struggle toward a synthesis of reason and emotion that does not endanger either member of the couple by reproducing behaviors and attitudes in our therapy that merely reinforce cultural biases.

Conclusion

Jim and Becky worked with me for about three months, during which time Becky struggled with gaining more control of her emotionality without feeling she needed to diminish its intensity, and Jim got engaged in exploring ways he could expand his taciturn nature into subtleties of expression. As Jim felt more secure in his communication skills he did not try to avoid confrontations with Becky, and we had some real showdowns in my office! In the course of therapy both Jim and Becky began to experience her emotionality as less threatening, so her behaviors naturally became less volatile. Similarly, as both of them became more sure of Jim's emotional resources, he gradually became less critical of Becky and she of herself.

Interestingly, their complementary behaviors didn't change all that much, nor did they ever practice rituals or performances with each other designed to change their interpersonal transactions. Becky remained the high-tension wire in their relationship and Jim the grounding element. They just gradually came to value each of their own ways of functioning so that neither had to overdo it.

Family Transitions

6

Divorce: His and Hers

The Changing American Family

THE AMERICAN FAMILY has changed drastically in the past twenty years or so. In spite of the upset reactions of those who decry these changes as a "breakdown" in traditional moral values, it needs to be understood by mental health professionals that these changes are the result of long-term social, economic, and demographic trends affecting the basic structure of American society. They are not the consequence of some current social fad, and they are not going to be reformed or deflected by the exhortations of politicians and clergy to turn back to "traditional" values or by the efforts of therapists to "hold the family together." To be helpful to people, therefore, a clinician must be sensitive and responsive to the many needs of families as they *are* rather than as some would like them to be.

According to a recent publication of the U.S. Bureau of the Census (Glick, 1984), the population base for baby boomers' first marriages peaked in 1982, and their divorces will peak in 1990. Recent dips in the divorce rate are just that—little dips in a long-term upward trend. Ninety percent of this population will finally marry, and 50 percent of them (45 percent) will divorce. Sixty-five to 70 percent of those who divorce (33 percent) will remarry, and 60 percent of the remarried (20 percent) will redivorce. Thus, one-fifth of all persons in their thirties in the 1980s can expect to experience not one, but two, divorces.

So, the paradigm of the secure, uncomplicated American middle-class family, the ideal standard against which most families still compare themselves, is substantially a myth left over from the 1950s. One of the most important tasks of family therapists is to help people to let go of these outdated blueprints for a functional family, and to help them develop new ways to function successfully—emotionally, socially, and economically—within the various structures available to the contemporary American family. To do this, we must first change our own thinking.

The Meaning of Marriage

Actually, the meaning of marriage is undergoing a radical redefinition in our lifetime. This redefinition is the result mainly of three factors: (1) advances in contraception, which make it possible for women to control their own reproductive choices; (2) the women's movement, which makes having fewer or no children psychologically possible; (3) increased longevity, which has added 24 years to the average American's life since the turn of the century, as well as an average of 15 to 20 years together (or not together) for a married couple after their children have departed—a new and problematic stage of the family life cycle (McGoldrick and Carter, 1980). Today, less than half of one's life need be devoted to parenting, and so there is much more intensity of focus on the quality of marriage. And since women have been able to regulate pregnancy and childbearing for the first time in history, we now have options, for the first time ever, to consider paid work careers in addition to, or instead of, marriage and parenthood.

Until this generation, women were still handed directly from their fathers to their husbands. Women have always been taught that marriage is the solution to their problems of living, and were not taught to develop autonomy or to identify personal life goals other than marriage. Therefore, they have traditionally looked forward to marriage tremendously, only to become disillusioned and depressed when they discover that often they are not taken care of in marriage and family life, but rather are expected to take care of everyone else.

Whereas for men, career and family goals are independent, parallel, and unconflicted, these two areas come into severe conflict for women. Working mothers, especially those with babies and young children, find themselves with two full-time jobs on their hands, no matter how much help they have, and many have inadequate help or no help at all. The decision to have a baby, for a middle-class American woman in her mid-thirties, is difficult as she tries to weigh the option of currently disrupting her own career against possible future regret about not having children. She is usually correct if she thinks that having a baby will affect her life and career more than her husband's.

The Financial Consequences of Divorce

Divorce also affects a woman's life more drastically than it does her ex-husband's. Ninety-two percent of children are in their mother's custody after divorce; 75 percent of child support payments are not fully paid; 50 percent are not paid at all. Court monetary awards to women at the time of divorce are made on the basis of the judge's incorrect assumptions that the woman will (1) soon remarry, (2) be able to get a decent-paying job, or (3) find affordable child care. Thus, the wife is seldom awarded more than a third of the couple's financial assets for herself and the children, while the husband is allotted two-thirds for himself. In the year after divorce, a man's income continues to rise, whereas a woman's income drops drastically (Weitzman, 1985). Nevertheless, welfare mothers, working mothers, and mothers who give up custody of their children are all thoroughly disapproved of in our society, and a large segment of the population still advocates teaching daughters to become financially dependent wives. An editorial in a recent issue of the journal *Social Work* (Hopps, 1987) commented on the irony that equality of the sexes should be an assumption of no-fault divorce law: ". . . for if men and women are effectively unequal before and during marriage, how can they be equal at its termination?" The no-fault divorce laws are an excellent example of a well-intentioned attempt to be fair, based on a false assumption. If a wife has no income, no skills to earn sufficient income, and bears all or most of the responsibility to raise the children as well, then any arrangement that does not take these facts into account can never be remotely fair or equitable, much less equal. As Weitzman puts it: "To grant equal rights in the absence of equal opportunity is to strengthen the strong and weaken the weak" (p. 213).

Thus, women of all classes have become the nation's new poor. In the year 2000, virtually all American poor will be women with dependent children. The failure of many men to support their children financially, even those who can easily afford this support, can be seen as a reactive move to counter the moves of women toward greater independence. Furthermore, at the level of the larger system, we are one of the few industrialized Western nations that makes no adequate social provision for child care or for paid maternity leave with job security. It is not surprising, then, that women with the lowest incomes are among the first to remarry, since marriage is still the main "solution" to social and economic insecurity that our society offers to women.

The Rate of Divorce and Redivorce

The current (1985) rate of divorce for first marriages is 47.5 percent. The divorce rate is highest for couples with young children since divorce typically occurs after an average of 7 years of marriage. However, the divorce rate for couples married more than 20 years has been rising dramatically. Contrary to popular opinion, second marriages are not usually more successful. The divorce rate for second marriages is currently 49 percent and is projected to rise to 60 percent by 1990 for those now in their thirties (Glick, 1984). And second divorces come sooner, after an average of only 4 years of marriage.

Divorce as a Phase of the American Family Life Cycle

Let me now turn to the basic conceptual framework within which I view the emotional process of divorce and remarriage. This framework was developed during a three-year clinical study of remarried families by myself and Monica McGoldrick (McGoldrick and Carter, 1980) following our work on the family life cycle.

Briefly, we came to view divorce as an interruption or dislocation of the family life cycle, which produces the kind of profound disequilibrium in the family system that is always associated with shifts, gains, and losses in family membership. In this view, we conceptualize the need for families who are undergoing divorce to experience one or two additional phases of the family life cycle in order to restabilize and then proceed developmentally at a more complex level.

Thirty-five percent of American women who divorce do not remarry. These families go through one additional phase of the family life cycle and may restabilize permanently in so-called single-parent families. During this transition, all the members of a post-divorce family must do the emotional work of mourning the loss of the intact family and giving up fantasies of reunion. The marital partners need to accept their own part in the breakup and work out custody, visitation, and financial arrangements that are as functional as possible for all family members. Obviously, this process is often aborted or avoided, as documented in all current literature on the subject. The poor handling of these emotional and financial tasks hurls vast numbers of divorced women and their children into poverty and may create bitterness and strife that complicate future relationships for all family members.

Sixty-five percent of American women and 70 percent of American men who divorce do remarry (Norton and Moorman, 1987), and these families require the negotiation of a second additional phase of the family life cycle, in which they adequately work through the emotional process, before restablization occurs. In this additional phase, family emotional process consists of struggling with everyone's fears regarding a new family; dealing with hostile and upset reactions to the new marriage; and trying to discover or invent a new paradigm of family that will allow for the complex new roles and relationships.

The Emotional Process of Divorce

The heart of the emotional process of divorce is to retrieve one's self from the marriage, that is, to give up as finished the hopes, dreams, and expectations that one had invested in the spouse and the marriage, and to reinvest these hopes and expectations in one's own self. This degree of self-direction goes against the grain of everything that women have been raised to believe about themselves.

Men and women inevitably have made different kinds of investments in marriage and will thus have different emotional experiences as they seek to disengage. In helping women through the emotional process of divorce, the therapist must keep in mind the fact that women have been taught to invest their entire identity in marriage; they have been given the major responsibility for the success of the marriage; and they have been taught to look toward others, not themselves, when setting life goals. Because of women's socialization and the economic and physical realities they face, a woman client during or after divorce may present in a state of extreme guilt, anxiety, and uncertainty, regardless of who it was that initiated the divorce. It is crucial that the therapist *not* assume that the chief solution to the divorcing woman's problem is remarriage, but rather be able to help the woman connect with her strength, competence, and ability to go it alone until she chooses otherwise.

It cannot be overemphasized that throughout the entire cycle of marriage, divorce, single parenting, and remarriage, women—the emotional and physical caretakers of the family—are taught to bear the major responsibility for seeing that it all works out happily for their husband, for their children, for their parents, for their ex-husband's parents, for their new spouses, for their new spouse's children, and for their new spouse's parents.

If these transitions in the process from marriage to remarriage don't go smoothly—and they cannot—women blame themselves, and are often blamed by others, for their supposed failure.

When the Man Initiates the Divorce

Generally, there are two basic configurations for couples on the verge of divorce. In the first, the man is threatening divorce and the woman is unprepared financially, emotionally, and occupationally to take charge of her life and her children's lives. If this woman is also poor, uneducated, and unskilled, her problem is primarily social and political rather than emotional. Psychotherapy alone is not the solution, although there are ways a therapist can be helpful. However, prior to this generation, women in general, not only poor women, have not been permitted to experience the first phase of adult development, which is to identify for themselves personal life goals that lead to economic independence and emotional maturity. In the recent past, emotional maturity for women was defined entirely on their ability to nurture others. Now, women are beginning to claim a self-definition that includes economic independence. Nevertheless, even if a woman is not poor, is well educated, and has a career, she will still tend to suffer the emotional distress of feeling unprepared to go on alone because of the pervasive influence of the female socialization process that trains her for dependency.

The Task of Self-Definition

The main task of the therapist in working with divorcing women is to help them to use the crisis of divorce as an opportunity to redefine themselves. The creative possibility in this crisis is that it provides a chance to do now the personal developmental work that may have been skipped earlier. Therapists can help women undergo this development through the work of the emotional divorce, that is, by helping them to relocate within *themselves* the hopes, dreams, and plans that were previously invested in marriage and spouse.

It is extremely important that we do not leave our women clients stuck in the victim position during this process, but, instead, fully support their ability to take charge of their lives and to develop a personal identity in which marriage is a choice, not a requirement. Clinical work of this nature, in my framework, will include work with the family of origin as well as with the ex-spouse. One young woman, Kathy, provides us with a clinical example.

The Case of Kathy: A Clinical Example

Kathy was well-educated, upper-middle-class, 29 years old. Her husband announced after ten years of marriage that he was leaving her to marry another woman. They had no children and no financial problems. Nevertheless, she came into treatment shocked, devastated, confused, and feeling unable to go on alone.

Following are a few excerpts from a letter she wrote to her husband after a year of what I call "divorce therapy," which consisted of helping her to gain perspective on the divorce, to extricate her identity from the marriage, and to develop personal life goals for herself that neither excluded nor required another marriage. The process of writing the following letter helped Kathy to take charge of herself in the relationship with her former husband for the first time since her marriage and to emphatically remove herself from the victim position in which she felt stuck when he departed. It had the effect of a separation ritual.

Dear Michael,

I have spent a good part of this past year trying to put our marriage and divorce into perspective and trying to recover from the shock and devastation I felt when you left me, even though I now think I had actually given up on us as a couple before you did.

I can now acknowledge that we did not have a perfect marriage or even a good one. I realize that I contributed to our poor marriage, but it was not entirely my fault, which is how I felt when you left.

The things I blamed you for that I now realize had little or nothing to do with you, were: my leaving music school; my taking a job I hated; my depending on you to manage our money; my thinking that my future depended on what you chose to do and where you chose to live.

However, I do think you had a lot to do with the fact that I felt I had to do all of the cooking and most of the housework; and that what I was doing always seemed much less important than what you were doing. Still, I was afraid to even think of leaving you and managing on my own. We never got around to having children, even though we kept pretending we'd do so as soon as our careers were settled. I think we got married when we did because your father had just died and I wanted a good way to leave my parents' house and in those days we couldn't just live together.

Despite all of this, it was probably the best marriage I was capable of at the time. I'm not sorry about it, and I don't think I ever will be. There were many very special things about us together that I know I will not be able to repeat exactly with anyone else.

Anyway, I just want you to know that although this has been the "worst year of my life," it has also been one of the best. I feel better about myself than I ever have. I like myself and I'm proud of myself. I've actually made friends with my brothers and am able to talk more openly with my mother than I ever believed possible (I know you'll have trouble believing that one!)

I'm concentrating now on my real life problems, like becoming a better musician, figuring out how to make a living without giving up music again, working out a lifestyle that keeps a balance between work and play, and resolving those old problems with my family. I have decided not to waste any more energy blaming you for ending our unsatisfactory marriage.

> **I'll always care about you and I truly wish you a happy marriage this time.**
>
> **Love, Kathy**

When the Woman Initiates Divorce

Today, it is much more common to find that the woman is the one precipitating the divorce. These are often middle- and upper-class or professional women who think they can financially afford being divorced. Or, regardless of finances, they are women who feel they have tried in vain to change a now untenable traditional marriage contract and must leave.

Some women may not actually want the divorce but may be using a divorce threat—rather like a suicide gesture—as a way of getting their husbands to recognize the seriousness of their discontent. It is important that the therapist explore carefully whether a woman wants to leave the marriage or wants help in learning to confront her husband and negotiate with him. In either case, the family therapist can help these women through the decision-making process, but should not get involved in giving advice or opinions concerning the actual decision.

The therapist will have to pay particular attention to directing the woman toward clarifying her own position rather than permitting her simply to react to her husband's position. This is a key aspect of all therapeutic work with women, whether focused on the marriage or on the process of divorce. Women are often so emotionally expressive and so willing and able to articulate the emotional problems in the couple and family that no one, including the woman herself, may notice that she almost never says directly what she wants. Pleading, defending, criticizing, placating, demanding, crying, hinting, or complaining is not the same as stating, from a position of entitlement, what one wants. In life, women have been taught not to define or negotiate directly for what they want; we hope that in family therapy they can be encouraged and taught to do so.

Problems for Men in Divorce

The emotional threats for men at the time of divorce have implications for women as well, and also illuminate dysfunctional patterns that both women and men tend to perpetuate reciprocally post-divorce.

For divorcing men, there is the serious possibility that they will lose their children in one way or another. Unless fathers take concrete steps to stay connected with their children, all of the forces at play during divorce and remarriage act to increase the emotional distance between father and children. It is now that a heavy price tag is handed to the fathers who pursued traditional family roles that prevented them from learning the skills necessary to conduct their own relationships with their children. An extremely useful component of divorce therapy with fathers may be discussing with them such concrete issues as having available adequate space for their children to visit them; being able to relate to children of various ages; and managing their relationships with children without excessive reliance on grandmothers, aunts, and girlfriends. Divorcing men need help in first acknowledging and then managing their hurt and grief at the loss of home and family; their guilt at leaving their children; and their lack of understanding about their own part in the failure of their marriage. Too often, the chief emotions divorcing men experience and express are anger, outrage, and desire for revenge. These emotions lead to outbursts and behavior that may intimidate their spouse and children, and the therapist as well, and lock the man into an escalating power struggle that isolates and alienates him. To be helpful, a family therapist must tap into the more tender feelings that are hidden or sealed off by the anger. The release and integration of the more tender emotions that men have been trained to disavow and to blot out will obviously be useful to the man not only in obtaining a decent divorce but in pursuing all of his relationships more satisfactorily in the future.

Similarly, a man's unacknowledged emotional dependency on his wife may leave him without the personal resources or support network to deal with the stress of divorce, and he may become immediately involved in another marriage or intense relationship. This tendency to treat divorce as a legal, logistic, and economic event rather than an emotional process leaves the man without the time and emotional space to fully experience his losses, to grieve, to reflect on the marriage, to change accordingly, and to move on to new relationships in a more grounded and connected way. Before a divorcing man seeks refuge and forgetfulness in another intense relationship, I try to interest him in the rewards of improving his relationship with his children, parents, and other family members and in expanding his social network and its level of intimacy and support. I am sometimes not successful in engaging divorcing men in this way, but those men who are willing to go through such a resocialization process frequently find that they can experience closer relationships with their children and other relatives and friends after divorce than they did during their marriage. The skills acquired in pursuing and conducting one's own emotional life enable the man to remarry when and if he chooses to rather than because he has to find another caretaker as quickly as possible.

The following excerpt from an interview with a divorced man in Lillian Rubin's book *Intimate Strangers* (1983) gives us a vivid snapshot of American marriage and divorce:

I understand now that women have been a stand-in for men's emotional life. I'm not just talking about other men, I mean for me, too. In a thousand ways, my ex-wife, Amy, lived out my emotional life for me. I could count on her to take care of all the things in life that required having feelings and acting on them— even with my own kids. And when she wanted to stop because it got to be too much of a burden, it destroyed us. It was as if she'd abandoned me in her most important function. So I wound up having an affair with a woman who made me feel alive again. Of course, Amy found out and that did us in. But, Jesus, why did it have to take a divorce and three years of living alone and two years of therapy (with which I'm not finished yet) for me to get it; I feel like a fool sometimes (*with a short, ironic laugh*). Well, that's what Amy said about me, only I didn't know what the hell she was talking about then. (pp. 259–260)

The Outcome of Divorce

It is not possible to fully analyze the meaning of a process of great magnitude while it is still unfolding. And so it is with respect to the impact of divorce on the American institutions of marriage and family. The negative aspects of an eruption as painful as divorce are, of course, immediately obvious in the turmoil that it produces in the lives of children and families. And for many years, "respectable" women didn't feel entitled to initiate such turmoil, especially if their husbands didn't drink or abuse them. If her marriage was unhappy or oppressive, well, that was bad luck, or woman's lot, or a cross to bear. The prerogative to initiate divorce was the man's, and he often made responsible financial arrangements for the wife and children he left behind.

Today, since women's expectations for themselves have risen to the level where many are not willing to adapt permanently to marriages that they find untenable, more women than men initiate divorce and, in response, many men have given up responsibility for financially supporting their children. In the final analysis, it may be found that the wholesale exit of women from their marriages as soon as they had a little financial independence is not so much a commentary on these particular women and their husbands as it is a damning statement about the traditional form of marriage.

And so, in some ways, this painful emotional process has a hopeful side, and we as family therapists can work to maximize the positive aspects of divorce, such as the development of a more self-reliant identity for women and the learning of more nurturant and interpersonal skills by men. To move divorcing spouses immediately in a useful direction and to avoid the major negative fall-out of divorce, I believe that as soon in the process as possible therapists need to talk to women in detail about their specific financial plans and to men about the concrete arrangements they are making to stay connected to their children. It is harmful to our clients to ignore the reality of their social context (which they are often unaware of) and to proceed as if the emotional outcome for the family were not directly related to the economic and logistic arrangements they make for themselves and each other as they change their family structure.

Clinical Dilemmas

Talking about therapeutic directions at the time of divorce is a lot easier than actually being able to carry them out. The explosiveness of the emotional process during and after the divorce decision makes orderly planning on behalf of both spouses virtually impossible for the therapist as well as the couple.

When marital therapy arrives at a decision to divorce, is the therapy finished—with spouses referred individually to other therapists? Do they switch as a couple to "divorce therapy" (however that may be defined)? Are they both likely to want to remain with the same therapist? And in what format should the therapy then proceed?

Often, one of the spouses comes to marital therapy wanting to do the "decent thing" even though the decision to divorce has been secretly made. Another objective on the secret agenda is to deposit the rejected spouse with a therapist to help cushion the blow. Rejected spouses thus deposited with therapists were, until recently, almost always women, producing for the therapist the familiar dilemma of helping the woman to assume the major responsibility for achieving a decent divorce for her family while her husband made unilateral economic and logistic decisions. How does the therapist help the wife in this crisis without encouraging the extremes of "unilateral disarmament" (letting her husband and his lawyer run over her) or "massive retaliation" (using the children and the legal system for vengeful escalation of hostilities)?

Although, today, there is more possibility than before that the rejected spouse will be the husband, it nevertheless remains more likely to be the woman who stays in therapy or seeks it out because of women's greater understanding of divorce as an emotional process, because of their feeling of responsibility for the emotional impact of divorce on their children, and because women still find it easier than men to ask for help. In most divorce cases, whoever is the initiator, the therapist often faces the dilemma of helping the woman without the therapy's becoming isomorphic to the problem, and the further dilemma of what stance to take vis-a-vis the absent husband. Should he be left out there as a "loose cannon"; defended against as a hostile force; or, if engageable, how can his participation be most helpful to himself and his family?

In the following cases, the thorny issues of therapy with post-divorce families are approached in different ways, without losing sight of the different issues and specific vulnerabilities of each gender at the time of divorce.

cases

Betty Carter

"Something Has to Change"

I selected this case because the couple's initial adherence to traditional family structure and sex-role functioning provides such a clear view of the inevitable problems of that structure and the futility of trying to view those problems within the sole context of the nuclear or extended family systems. Such a limited view exacerbates personal blaming, a process that had already exploded in the couple's relationship before they got to me.

I also selected this case because it shows the potential for mean-ness in even the "nicest" people as they get caught in the whirlwind emotions of divorce. At one time or another, she nags, screams, rages, evicts him, and won't let him see his children; he stonewalls, withholds money, intimidates, bullies, demands to see his children and later distances from them, reluctantly entering and finally withdrawing from therapy. In other words, this is a typical divorce scenario.

The Presenting Problem

Janice and Michael arrived for their initial appointment with me the day after Janice had "kicked Michael out" of their home because she couldn't go on with "such an unsatisfying marriage." Janice said that unless things between them improved she would get a divorce.

They had been married for eight years. They were both in their early thirties, with a boy aged 6 and a girl of 4. Both extended families were extremely traditional, working class, second-generation East European Catholic. Janice was an only child; Michael was the oldest of three, with two younger sisters. His parents had always had a highly conflictual marriage, for which Michael blamed his mother. Here is a diagram of their nuclear family:

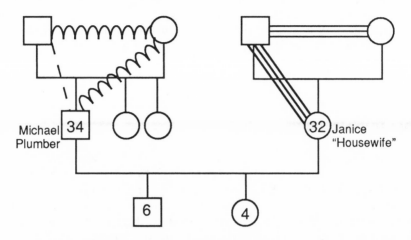

See page 96 for an extended definition of the genogram.

Janice explained that she had started to feel depressed after the birth of her daughter, and had gone into individual therapy two years ago because the depression persisted. She had felt "crazy" about needing a psychiatrist, she said, but now realized that she had been reacting to the boredom of her routines of housekeeping and child care, and had felt that Michael did not provide enough excitement or social life to "make her life more stimulating." She felt she needed more from life than he "gave" her. Michael didn't want her to work and she agreed that she should stay home while her children were young, but she had warned him that *something* had to change.

Janice's individual psychotherapy had put her in touch with her discontent about her life, but did not challenge her family's adherence to their traditional roles. She still held her husband responsible for doing something about the quality of her life, and assumed that it was his job to "make her happy." She was fulfilling *her* role—why couldn't he perform *his*? If he didn't shape up, she would have to divorce him and find someone who would "make her happy."

Janice was quite bewildered when I asked her what specific changes she wanted in her life, and what she wanted from Michael. She said she wanted Michael to rethink what *he* wanted from marriage and from her, and then she'd see if it made her happier. No matter how I rephrased my question, she didn't grasp the notion that *she* needed to develop goals of her own for which to negotiate. Janice cried on and off through most of the session and spoke mostly in vague terms of her need for "love" and "happiness." Michael alternated between the desperate frustration of not understanding what was happening and an angry coldness at her "refusal" to be happy with the "ideal life" he had "provided" her and their children.

This scenario contains both the traditional expectation of the dependent young wife that she should be taken care of emotionally as well as financially and the hurt bewilderment of the traditional husband who works hard to provide material things, as he has been taught to, and then can't understand the cause of his wife's dissatisfaction.

Therapy Strategy

Because this couple was so locked into their conflict and couldn't gain any perspective on their situation, I decided to see both sets of parents (in separate sessions). Both families were in close contact with the young couple and were involved in trying to hold them together. From talking with the in-laws I learned a lot about family attitudes, including the following message, about sex roles and therapy:

- That Michael had such a distant relationship with his father that he was unable to turn to him for advice or support with his marital worries. He would have liked to talk things over with his mother, but regarded it as "unmanly" to do so.
- That Michael's parents thought therapy was only for the "weak" or the "mentally ill" and were not interested in further sessions.
- That Janice's father, when he learned of her marital problems, had gone out for a beer with Michael and told him to take a "firmer hand" with Janice if he wanted a good marriage.
- That Janice's mother had a highly ambivalent attitude toward a woman's role, having first indoctrinated Janice with the value of education and ambition and then blamed her for getting depressed in her role as homemaker.
- That Janice's parents both thought Janice should "take charge" of the family, but that she should do so "diplomatically," making the adaptations necessary for harmony without openly opposing Michael.

In a mixture of individual and joint sessions with Michael and Janice over the next year, and in coaching each of them to disentangle themselves from conflicting parental messages, I tried to guide the process through the following stages: (1) helping Janice to think through for the first time what she wanted for herself in life and what she wanted out of marriage (which took a long time); (2) helping Janice to tell Michael what she had decided she wanted (which was even harder for her); (3) helping Michael to distinguish between what he had been taught were "proper roles" and what he might actually want (a distinction he found extremely difficult to articulate); and (4) helping Michael to hear Janice's wishes as her *wishes*, not as complaints or threats against him (which he wasn't able to do).

The Wife's Dilemma

When Janice married at age 24, she, like so many brides before her, had been under the spell of the romantic ideal of living "happily ever after." Having been taught by her family and society that marriage was the key to a woman's happiness, she had vague expectations that marriage and family would make her "happy" and no notion at all that she might need to participate actively in the process.

Since she expected Michael to "make her happy," she was profoundly disillusioned with a life structure consisting of tasks and roles that didn't "make her happy." However, mindful of the spoken and unspoken rules against stating her wishes and needs *directly* to a man, she felt able only to express doubts, complaints, and dissatisfactions, and to defend herself angrily against the belief, shared by both of them, that there was something wrong with her for being so unhappy. The following exchange in therapy illustrates this dilemma:

JANICE: I've told him over and over again that I'm not his mother and I'm not his maid, but nothing makes any difference.

THERAPIST: What do you want him to do?

JANICE: Well, talk to me, for one thing. He comes home every night, gets a beer, and plugs himself into the TV. He says he works hard all day and wants some "peace and quiet." What does he think *I* do all day? Lie around?

THERAPIST: I guess he doesn't realize what a job it is to wrestle with two small kids all day.

JANICE: That's right! That's right! And it isn't as if I'm the "homebody" type, and he knows it. You know that? He *knows* it, and still he does nothing.

THERAPIST: What do you wish he would do?

JANICE: Huh? (*Not comprehending that she might address the issue*)

THERAPIST: I mean, you might present Michael with ideas about what changes you'd like to make in your . . .

JANICE: Why should *I* have to figure this all out? Aren't they *his* children too?

THERAPIST: Sure, they're his children, but it's *your* life. I'm not sure you believe you're entitled to have a few ideas about your own life.

JANICE: Well, am I? I married him, didn't I? I wanted a house and kids, too. I can't help it if I'm not *really* laughing and dancing all day as I go from the sink to the stove to the store.

THERAPIST: Do you think you're supposed to be? Do you think getting married makes women love doing laundry?

JANICE: (*Laughing*) Well, he sure acts like there's something wrong with me for not being . . .

THERAPIST: (*Joining laughter*) . . . like the millions of women, all over the world, who really *adore* doing laundry.

After much more of this kind of exchange, and long conversations with her mother about her mother's unsatisfactory solutions to this dilemma, Janice finally agreed that it was *her* job to think about how she wanted to live her life, and not Michael's job to "make her happy." However, it took quite an additional period of work before she decided that she could try to negotiate directly with Michael about some changes without giving him angry ultimatums or, at the other extreme, pleading for permission.

Trying to Negotiate Change

The specific issue around which their negotiations failed was Janice's decision to return to graduate school and then to work, at a slow but steady pace, beginning when her daughter entered school full time (in about a year). Michael was categorically against the idea of Janice's working outside the home until the children left for college, "at which time the extra money might be needed." He took his wife's interest in a career as a personal affront.

My attempts to involve Michael more in discussing this or other issues with his parents were largely unsuccessful. I believe he wanted to save his marriage, but only on his own terms. He was unable to overcome the traditional ideas of his upbringing that gave him no flexibility in role functioning, no access to his own emotional life, and no permission to acknowledge vulnerability or a need for help. After the initial crisis, he refused to ask his parents to come to additional sessions, and he neither carried out successfully any suggestions about changes he might make in his relationship with his parents nor his own unthinking fulfillment of family messages about marriage and the life of a man. Michael dismissed his family programming as "irrelevant," or he conducted therapy tasks in a perfunctory manner designed to fail. He insisted that he was not the person with the problem.

After trying to discuss her career impasse with Michael for a period of months, Janice took a stand. She said in a clear, nonhostile way that her personal decision to return to school and then to work was not negotiable and that if Michael couldn't accept that, they couldn't remain married. At that point Michael left therapy in a huff and threatened Janice with a "divorce she would never forget." He refused to give her money any longer and said he would hire a divorce lawyer called "the shark." I phoned Michael and asked him to return to therapy to discuss this new turn of events, but he refused on the grounds that the therapy was clearly "not working."

Many factors influenced Janice's willingness to question her belief system and Michael's inability to do so. For one thing, outwardly she had the most to gain from a change and was experiencing the most discontent with the status quo. Conversely, Michael felt he had the most to lose since he couldn't grasp the supposed benefits to him of "creating chaos at home." He also felt so strongly that his self-respect and identity were linked to "providing for his family" that he couldn't let in alternative ideas. Most important of all, I believe, was the problem that, as a male in his emotionally closed, rigidly traditional family, he felt unable to have the kinds of personal discussions with his parents that might have shed some light on his programming and its antecedents in the "old country" ways of his parents. Instead he scorned "psychological" approaches to life and blindly followed what he called "simple, old-fashioned values." Michael was up against patriarchy in one of its purer forms and his ethnicity, his sex, and his sibling position (oldest son) all militated against his making the changes called for in his marital situation.

Negotiating the Breakup

I encouraged Janice to get good legal advice and to be as nonreactive to Michael's threats as possible. She borrowed money from her parents, took charge of the children, and maintained contact with the children's paternal grandparents, in spite of their coldness toward her.

As a result of our work, after seven months Janice wrote a firm, nonangry letter to Michael that appealed to his personal decency and his love for his children, and reflected thoughtfully and evenhandedly on their marriage and the finality of its demise. After several meetings over dinner, Michael dropped "the shark," agreed to go with Janice for divorce mediation, gave her temporary support money, and together with Janice and the children came back to see me for two sessions of therapy focused on the family breakup. I believe that Michael's acceptance of the finality of the divorce decision and his turn-around willingness to cooperate in making it a less destructive experience for everyone resulted from Janice's ability to stick to the position that she and I worked out when Michael bolted: She would instruct her lawyer to block Michael's legal intimidations and threats firmly but without escalating to counterthreats; and she would cooperate fully in giving Michael, his parents, and sisters visitation rights and access to the children. In pursuit of the latter goal, she initiated and maintained contact with Michael's parents, and remained fairly nonreactive to their barely disguised anger and blame. Janice did not find this plan easy to carry out, and sometimes said she wanted to "give him back some of what he's dishing out." But, with occasional outbursts and much raging to friends, she stuck to the plan partly because, as she said, "If we go for a free-for-all, he'll win." I agreed with her, although I didn't call it "winning."

When Michael participated in two sessions of therapy designed as a joint parental attempt to reassure and listen to the children, I tried again to interest him in further sessions alone or with the kids. Again, he gave me many "reasonable" reasons why that wasn't necessary. He also rejected my offer to refer him to a male therapist who specialized in divorce work or to short-term groups for divorcing people. I gave up the idea of engaging him further in therapy.

Janice continued to meet with me periodically during the following year as her divorce came through and as she made plans to return to part-time school and work. She said it was all much harder than she expected, but she didn't regret it. She reported that Michael visited and supported the children regularly and that he now had a live-in fiancée. I made mental note of that typical "solution." She wondered if he would "allow" his new wife to work after their marriage. Then she corrected herself: "I mean, I wonder if she'll allow him to dictate her life to her."

We returned to our discussion of her plans for her future.

Gains and Losses

Adding up the gains and losses after a major transition like divorce requires a lot of bookkeeping. You have to go back to "his" and "her" marriage to review what was at stake for whom. Janice certainly lost her innocence and a life of being financially supported. She gained a new sense of self-reliance, a career interest, and more adultlike relationships with her parents. She does even more of the kind of household tasks she hates than she did before, but she allots much less time and emotional energy to such work. She's often pressed for money. She's more tired, but less depressed; she's exhilarated, but scared and sometimes lonely. She says it was worth it, and she'd do it again. I hope she doesn't have to.

It's harder to make a case for the children's gains. They're unhappy about the divorce and wish it hadn't happened. They went through a year of anxiety symptoms that abated when their parents stopped fighting. Now they're flaring up again as they try to avoid dealing with their father's fiancée. I tell Janice that they'll do better with happy separated parents than miserable parents staying together. I believe this in general and I hope, as I look at the children's unhappy faces, that it will be true for them.

On the surface, Michael certainly seems to have gained the most—or lost the least. He lives in a new condo instead of an old house; his car is a much later model; he has found a new woman to take care of him and be his companion; he has more available spending money than previously; and he sees his children on schedule. He's not unhappy.

However, he has learned the least about himself, grown the least, changed the least. His relationship with his parents remains the same—distant and dutiful. He seems to be pursuing the same goals as before with the new woman in his life. He sees his children less often now that he's "involved" and usually takes them to his mother's house or out with his fiancée, who tries desperately to win their favor.

One's evaluation of the gains and losses for each of them, and for the family as a whole, depends on one's definition of what's important in life. Janice declares a large net gain; she says she never could have developed herself to this point within that marriage even if Michael had been willing to change. Michael still doesn't know why it had to happen but he's accepted it and says he has recouped and "moved on." The kids turn thumbs down. They want both parents—together. Period.

Although I consider the outcome "fairly successful," still I would have been more pleased if Michael had been willing to risk the changes that beckoned in either his marriage or his divorce. But that was for him to choose, and he made his choice.

Peggy Papp

On Golden Pond Revisited

When a marriage breaks up because of the husband's relationship with another woman, the wife often directs her anger and bitterness toward the other woman, blaming her rather than dealing with the painful issues with her husband. The two women then end up fighting each other while the husband withdraws from the crossfire.

In the following case, the wife's resentment toward the other woman not only prevented her from severing the bond with her husband five years after their separation but interfered with her mothering ability, which had been a source of great pride and comfort to her. Eventually, the symptomatic behavior of her son motivated her to seek therapy. During the process of the therapy, I reframed the wife's bitterness toward the other woman as being protective of her husband and suggested ways of using it as a resource and thus turning it to her own advantage. This released her from the last vestiges of attachment to her husband and permitted her to request what she needed most from him—a cooperative arrangement regarding their son.

Presenting Problem

The wife, Martha, telephoned our agency for help in controlling her 17-year-old son, Tom. She reported that he was disobedient and defiant, that he lied, provoked fights, and was "unmanageable." I learned that Martha had separated from her husband, Charles, five years earlier and that Tom's two older sisters, Ellen, 23, and Beverly, 21, had moved away from home and were living on their own, leaving mother and Tom alone together. I requested that Martha bring the entire family in for the consulation, including her husband and the two older daughters.

The First Session

Martha began the session by pouring out her feelings of failure and despair over not being able to cope with Tom. Being a good mother had always been a great source of pride to her, and she felt she had been an especially good one up to this point. Now she found she simply couldn't handle Tom and she didn't know what had happened.

In gathering background material, I learned that the parents had separated because of Charles's relationship with another woman, Gloria. This relationship had been going on for many years prior to the separation, and Martha reported it had had a devastating effect on the whole family. Charles could not make up his mind whether to stay or leave his family, and his ambivalence created havoc with family relationships. Finally, he left the home at Martha's request and moved into an apartment with Gloria.

After the affair was discovered, Martha, who was described as being energetic and high-spirited, sank into a profound depression.

"We were a very close family and when Charles disappeared twice a week it was such a rejection for me. I had felt like a strong capable mother and wife—cooking, cleaning, minding the store, I did everything—and then I collapsed. I was the healthiest, strongest woman in the world and I collapsed. I realize now I had a nervous breakdown. I lost 35 pounds and cried all day. It took several years of individual therapy before I was able to pull myself together. Now I blame myself for staying in the marriage too long. Five years of taking abuse and loneliness before I was able to stand on my own two feet."

Charles sat looking guilty and said apologetically, "It was wrong what I did. I should have just left but I was confused. I couldn't make up my mind and it was terrible for everyone. I loved this other woman but I also loved my family and didn't want to leave them."

Two years earlier, he had asked Martha to give their relationship another try, and they had dated for six months but had both come to the conclusion that it couldn't work out for them. Despite their mutual agreement that they were better off separated, neither had filed for divorce, each waiting for the other to legally terminate their relationship.

Although Martha claimed to have resolved her feelings regarding the separation through her individual therapy, she continued to harbor tremendous bitterness toward Gloria, with whom she had fought continuously. She claimed Gloria had treated her abominably, and consequently she had forbidden the children to see her. The oldest daughter, Ellen, refused to abide by this ruling, and this disobedience had caused a rift between herself and her mother. Martha was deeply hurt by what she considered to be her daughter's "disloyalty" to her. Tom and his other sister, Beverly, respected mother's wishes and were fiercely loyal to her, causing tension between them and Ellen.

During the years the children were growing up, Martha had assumed major responsibility for raising them, while Charles maintained a distant position, retiring to the library on the few evenings he was home. "He never liked to have his peace and quiet disturbed," Martha declared ruefully. This pattern still continued, with all the children coming to Martha whenever they had problems of any kind. Since the separation, Charles's contact with the children had been informal and unscheduled, on a catch-as-catch-can basis generally initiated by the children. In exploring the way in which the parents currently dealt with Tom's behavior, it was revealed that they never communicated with one another except in a crisis and had no agreed-upon plan of action. Although Martha suspected that Charles often undermined her disciplinary measures, she never confronted him since she refused to call him either at home or at the office (where Gloria worked) for fear of having to speak to Gloria on the telephone. Charles confessed that he bent over backwards to give Tom everything he asked for as a way of trying to win back the love and respect that he felt he lost as a result of his leaving home. It became clear that in indulging his son, he often unwittingly contradicted many previous decisions made by Martha. Tom took advantage of the rift between his parents by playing one against the other. He openly admitted, "If I ask my mother for money and she says no, I ask my father and he gives it to me."

Reframing the Symptom

In deciding how to intervene, I considered the common strategic approach of reframing Tom's symptomatic behavior as serving to keep his parents connected. For example, I might have said that Tom's behavior was serving to bring his father and mother back together and thus was his way of trying to reunite the family. Or that by misbehaving he was trying to distract mother from her grief and fill up the emptiness in her life. Or that his immature behavior served to keep him from growing up and leaving home, since he knew mother would be lonely without him.

All of the above could serve as the basis for a valid hypothesis to explain the symptomatic behavior since they connect Tom's behavior with family transaction and challenge current perceptions of the problem. However, I discarded each hypothesis as placing the responsibility for the problem on Martha. They all imply that if only Martha were not grieving or lonely or in need of a father for her son or still clinging to the relationship with her spouse, Tom would have no problems. I chose instead to define the problem as a continuation of Martha's pattern of protectiveness toward her husband.

At the end of the session I told her I thought she was directing her bitterness toward the wrong person, and I was amazed at how, after being separated for five years, she still managed to be so protective of her husband. By not permitting the children to have any contact with Gloria, she was allowing Charles to continue his romantic illusion that he could have a relationship with Gloria undisturbed by interference from his children. This also protected him from having to assume any responsibility for the children, leaving Martha to shoulder the entire burden.

Martha was taken aback by this unexpected point of view, explaining that it was certainly not her intention to protect their relationship. I said it might not be her intention, but it was certainly the result of what she was doing.

I then raised a series of hypothetical questions aimed at underscoring the protective nature of her actions. I asked her what she thought would happen if she were to send Tom to spend a weekend with Charles and Gloria while she went away with friends to the country? How did she think Charles would handle that? What did she think Gloria's reaction would be? What effect did she think Tom might have on the relationship between Gloria and Charles? If all three children began visiting them regularly, did she think it would disturb Charles's peace and quiet? Which child did she think would cause the most problems?

In attempting to answer these questions, Martha became increasingly aware of the way she was helping to preserve a romantic ivy-covered tower for Charles and Gloria in which they never had to confront the reality of Charles's children. Not only was she depriving herself of a source of relief and help in parenting, but she was permitting Charles to undermine her parental control over Tom.

She asked me what I thought she should do. I told her I thought she should use Charles as a resource to give her more time for pleasure and relaxation. "If only you could stop protecting Charles by continuing to fight with Gloria, both of them could be a great asset to you." Martha said she needed to think about what I was saying, and I made an appointment to see her and Charles alone together to discuss the situation further.

Subsequent Sessions

Martha began the following session by saying, "I was stunned by what you said last week about my protecting Charles and Gloria. I've been doing a lot of thinking and I've decided I don't want to do that anymore." I then explored Martha's and Charles's current feelings about one another; they agreed the separation was best for both of them and that they had no desire to resume their relationship. They did, however, express a desire to work out a joint plan of action for dealing with Tom. We then proceeded to establish some common ground rules and ways that each parent could check with the other. Since Martha was the primary caretaker, Charles was to check with her before making any major decisions; Martha agreed to swallow her pride for Tom's sake and call Charles whenever she felt it was necessary. The parents resolutely put the plan into effect and Tom, no longer able to play one against the other, began to abide by the rules.

At the following session, on month later, both parents reported there had been a marked improvement in Tom's attitude and behavior. Charles was checking with Martha about major decisions and Martha stated, "I feel free now to call Charles any time I need to. After all, he is Tom's father! And I've told all the children they can do whatever they want to do about Gloria. That's their problem now." Tom observed that his mother was in a much better frame of mind and said, "We're improving together."

Commenting on the changes that had taken place, Martha stated, "It did a tremendous thing for me to realize how I was working against my own best interest. And, ironically, as a result I made a commitment to myself as to how I want to live my life." She went on to say that last week she and Tom had been watching Henry Fonda and Katherine Hepburn grow old together on television in *On Golden Pond*, and at one point Tom turned around and said, "Does this make you feel sad?" And Martha replied, "No, Tom, not at all." "And for the first time I didn't think of Charles. I'm going to grow old alone. But that's what Tom meant—'Mom, you're going to grow old alone.' And that's when I knew I was cured! I didn't think of Charles. Five years we've been separated and for the first time I felt separate. It was a wonderful night for me."

In a follow-up call eighteen months later, which took the form of separate telephone calls to each parent, both reported Tom was still doing well and their respective relationships with him had greatly improved. They were in the process of getting divorced and both were making plans to remarry. Martha had met a "wonderful man" and had changed her mind about spending the rest of her life on Golden Pond alone. She ended the conversation by saying, "I hope Tom will adjust well to his new stepfather."

Summary

This case described the resolution of a triangle between a husband, wife, and other woman that remained active for five years after the husband left home. This triangle typified a situation in which the most intense animosity existed between the two women rather than between either of the women and the involved man. It also typified the wife's continued pattern of protectiveness toward her husband at her own expense. When she was able to stop shielding her husband from the children and request what she needed from him, she was able to extricate herself from the marriage and establish her identity as a separate person.

Olga Silverstein

Rescue Operation

Given the almost sacred attributes with which we endow marriage, it is not surprising that for many women their own unhappiness is not justification enough for leaving. If there are children and the husband in question is an adequate father—and certainly if he is a good economic provider—the wife will find very little support for leaving the marriage from her family or friends, or even from many therapists, were she to seek professional help. The socially supported reasons for leaving a "good" man and thereby breaking up a family are few but well-defined. Unhappiness is not on that list. If, indeed, the husband is truly a good man and not an abusing husband, "falling in love" with another man is often the only option. Leaving one man for another is less of a threat to the social structure that decrees that women define themselves in terms of the man to whom they are connected.

The Call for Help

In this case, Cassie had been married for 12 years, quite unhappily, and was the mother of three children.

I received a frantic telephone call from a man who rather incoherently told me that his wife had run off with the delivery man—that she had been gone for three days—that he was alone with the children and that someone had to talk sense to her.

With some effort I was able to ascertain that she called daily to check on the children, that he had alternately ordered, begged, and threatened her to come home, but at that point she always hung up on him. I suggested that the next day when she called he was to suggest that they meet in my office to try to figure things out and to make some plans for the future. I gave him an appointment for the next day.

They arrived at the appointed time almost at the same moment. They came up together in the elevator silently. Bill was a small, tense man in his late thirties, Cassie a small, deliberately plain woman a few years younger.

Presenting the Problem

He entered the room talking. She followed silently and sat at the edge of her seat like a young child waiting out the parental lecture.

Bill kept up a ten-minute tirade directed at his wife, totally ignoring my presence. Obviously, he was using my office as a meeting place. The notion of therapy had not occurred to him.

I decided not to interrupt (I don't think it would have been possible), but I watched Cassie, who sat with downcast eyes; every once in a while she would look up, catch my eye, and look down again.

Finally Bill ran out of breath, turned to me, and ordered, "Tell her! She has responsibilities—she has three children, for the love of Christ! Tell her!"

"I don't know what to tell her," I said, "I have no idea about what's going on, just that you're very angry. That Cassie cares about the children since she calls every day to check on them. And that's all. So let me get the story."

BILL: I don't believe it, it's like a bad joke. My wife ran off with the delivery man. The little jerk seduced my wife. It's humiliating.

CASSIE: I can't stand it any more. Nothing I do is right—it's not Bill's fault. Would it be better if I had an affair with the president of your company?

BILL: Damn right!

CASSIE: (*Wavering*) It's not Bill's fault. He works very hard and he's good at everything. Everything . . .

THERAPIST: Everything?

CASSIE: (*Half-smiling*) Almost.

THERAPIST: So?

BILL: Damn right I work hard—It takes effort to support this bunch—look at her—(*He turned to me*) she looks like a damned sixties jerk.

Cassie was dressed in jeans, sneakers, and a big man's shirt. Her fingernails were bitten to the quick. Her hair was caught back in a ponytail with a rubber band.

CASSIE: (*Resigned*) He doesn't like anything about me.

THERAPIST: Is that why you left?

CASSIE: No—Jack is wonderful. He used to finish work on the street and then I'd make coffee and he'd sit and talk to me. I—(*She started to cry*)—I don't know why I left.

BILL: That jerk seduced her—she's such a little ninny—she's gullible. Come home—goddamn it. I can't stay home with the kids any longer. My work is piling up. Come home! Cut out this crap!

CASSIE: (*Barely audible*) No, I can't.

I arranged to see Cassie alone the next day.

She arrived looking much more pulled together and informed me that she had called her mother, who lived out of town, to come look after the children. "It wasn't fair to expect him to look after the children," she explained. Away from Bill she appeared more mature and spoke with more conviction. "Believe it or not, I used to think of myself as an okay person."

Cassie's Story

Cassie and Bill met during their first year at college. "We slept together on our first date and a month later I was pregnant. I wanted to have an abortion. Bill wouldn't hear of it. He said he would take care of me and he did. He was terrific. He arranged everything! He told my father. He reassured him that he was going to marry me. And he did. He did. He even arranged for my clinic visits. Anyway, I never went back to school. But I don't think I wanted to. Bill worked after school and on weekends and I had babies—three beautiful babies."

Cassie was bullied by Bill and her parents into marriage. Her attempts at refusal were halfhearted, as in fact she was confused and ambivalent. No great student, she took the opportunity to leave school with a legitimate excuse. She was getting married. She was going to have a baby. An immature young woman (she was 20), she had been infantilized by her parents and saw marriage as an opportunity to declare herself independent. Once married to a take-charge man who alternately took care of her and bullied her, she remained frozen in her childish posture. At 30 she was still a child-wife, but she was growing increasingly unhappy. However, with no financial resources—Bill handled all the money and the house was in his name, as was the car—she felt trapped. But, most important, she explained that she could not find a legitimate reason to break up the family.

I decided to see Cassie and Bill separately initially, in order to reassure her that I was not joining the forces striving to bring her home.

Bill's Story

When I saw Bill alone he told me pretty much the same story: "I had to do everything—Cassie is a big baby. Don't get me wrong—she's a good mother—but that's it."

I then saw Bill and Cassie twice together, Bill insisting magnanimously that he was willing to have Cassie come home, Cassie whimpering "I can't."

Helping Cassie Work It Out

I asked Cassie to bring her mother in, for several reasons. On a practical level, I knew that if she were to go through with this separation she would need parental support until she could function on her own. By now, I was pretty sure that Jack would not figure too prominently in the picture. I also felt it was time for Cassie to begin the process of behaving like an adult woman with her mother.

I saw Cassie alone with her mother. Mother very much supported Bill. "Cassie has always been immature. I was very relieved when Bill married her (sic)—I knew he would take care of her, but now she's off with that bum, that trash . . ." She wept; Cassie wept. Then Cassie said, "It's not Jack. I never wanted to marry Bill. I wasn't ready to marry anyone. I don't think I'm ready now."

It was not easy for Cassie to talk to her mother directly. She was used to taking a one-down childlike posture with all the adults in her network. Only with her children was she her competent, mature self.

But during the four sessions she met with her mother in my office she noticeably grew in stature. One day she said to her mother, "I realize now that you let Daddy bully you as I let Bill bully me. I don't believe that you ever thought Bill was the right husband for me, but you wouldn't go against Daddy. But Daddy is dead now—you're free. I don't want to wait until Bill dies to be free."

I then saw Cassie alone for the next four sessions. We explored her feelings about herself, her marriage, her children, and her goals for the future; they clearly did not include Jack.

CASSIE: I can't live with Bill—I just can't. He won't let me do anything—I mean anything. Can you imagine—I'm not allowed—allowed to drive with the children in the car!

As she talked it became clear that Jack was Cassie's way of leaving her marriage.

THERAPIST: How long have you been looking for a rescuer?
CASSIE: (Smiling) I guess all my life.
THERAPIST: I guess I'm a little puzzled—why would an intelligent, capable woman—I know you're that because everyone says you're a terrific mother—need to be rescued from one man by another?

Cassie was silent.

"It's a puzzle," I continued. "You mean the only reason for leaving a relationship where you are so unhappy is another relationship? I can see why Jack is having such a good time—he gets a chance to play "knight in shining armor"—but what's different for you? You've been damsel in distress for years. Perhaps we could set up a duel and the winner can ride off with you into the sunset."

For the first time Cassie laughed at that absurd picture, and we were able to move into making some concrete plans for her future. She was able to first confront Bill directly and tell him that she wanted a divorce. At first he wouldn't accept it as her decision, but insisted on blaming Jack. Cassie, also with a little help, confronted her mother and asked openly for her support. "Yes," she said, "I think I'll even need some help financially till all that gets settled with Bill and I'm working."

The Outcome

When Cassie came to the realization that she was using Jack as an excuse to terminate her marriage, she was ashamed and upset. He was, in fact, very angry, and dealing with that was hard for her.

I pointed out to her that avoiding anger had led to some difficult situations for her. "It's not just that, but I've never been alone. I don't know if I can manage," she said.

It's indeed hard to be a single mother. I pointed out the difficulties in as much detail as I could. I reminded her that Bill could make it very hard for her financially.

It is always important to help a woman appraise the situation realistically. Cassie had never acted with forethought and consideration for her own best interests. If she had, she might not have succumbed to fears about her father's anger and Bill's refusal to accept an abortion. She had gone passively and thoughtlessly into a future not of her own choosing. Now, it was important that she look realistically at her options.

"Well, I guess it's time for me to grow up," she said.

When Bill understood that Cassie was serious, he relaxed. He agreed to come to one last session with Cassie. We discussed the practical details of separation. They both agreed to try divorce mediation rather than the more adversarial legal route.

Now, three years later, Bill has remarried. Cassie is finishing a social work degree and working three mornings a week. The children are doing well. "You didn't tell me how hard it would be," she said on the phone. "Oh, yes I did." "I guess you did, but I'm glad I didn't believe it because I might not have done it, and Bill and I would have gone on and on, miserable together."

Marianne Walters

"For Your Sake"

The following case is about choice—or the lack of it—and one of the ways in which therapists can create a context in which choice can be experienced, even in situations not of one's own making. Most often for divorcing couples the decision to divorce is not a mutual one, and one of the partners feels he or she has had no choice in the decision. Of course, choice is central to the experience of being in charge of one's own life. For women going through an unwanted divorce, the experience of loss of control over one's life is exacerbated by practical, as well as emotional, circumstances. Women, as Betty Carter has pointed out, usually have more to fear in the aftermath of a divorce in relation to social, financial, child-rearing, and work conditions. So, particularly in working with women, it is important to help them to experience choice even while going through an unwanted divorce. This is some-times a rather subtle process, not having much to do with real alterna-tives in the sense of social and economic needs, but rather having to do with the very process of coping with an unwanted, unchosen, reality. Often, it is necessary, as in the following case, first to go after the interactional processes that obscure the vision of choice before we can begin to reconstruct the act.

The Presenting Problem

Robert and Linda came to see me because their marriage was falling apart. It would be hard to imagine two people more devoted to each other, two people more in love. Yet, their sadness was palpable. Robert had, several months before, "come out" to Linda, owned his homosexu-ality, and admitted that he had had several affairs with men. Linda was devastated. But she did not want to end the marriage. She loved Robert. He was her best friend, the most important person in her life. Robert felt he could not continue in the marriage. He loved Linda and could not continue to inflict such pain on her. He hated the duplicity. They had been agonizing about their situation for weeks, going round and round, seeking every alternative. They were exhausted, emotion-ally drained.

Robert and Linda had met and fallen in love with each other in college. But they were each pursuing pretty demanding careers, Linda in public relations and Robert in economics, and chose not to marry until they had both completed graduate school. After their wedding—a big Italian affair—they moved to Washington, where Linda took a job on Capitol Hill and Robert went to work for a public policy think tank. They had been very happy for most of the eight years of their marriage. In addition to demanding, but very satisfying work, they have an active social life, a circle of close friends, and they travel and enjoy many of the same cultural and intellectual interests. Only recently, when Linda began to want to talk about having a family, did serious tensions begin to develop. Before that, conflicts or disagreements between them would result in passionate arguments that were resolved with equally passionate "making-up." Now there is either a lot of accusation, blame, and denial or, for Linda, the even more disturbing scenario of Robert withdrawing, walls growing up between them, dead ends and despair.

Robert comes from a close-knit Italian family of six—two brothers and a sister. His parents have been married for over forty years. They own a grocery store in "little Italy," which after years of struggle has become quite successful. His mother was able to retire from the business about fifteen years ago and be a full-time housewife and mother. Linda comes from a fairly affluent WASP family who live in a suburb of Boston. Her father is a lawyer, and her mother is deeply invested in volunteer work. Linda's only sibling, a sister, is married and has two children. She is seven years older than Linda.

In our first session together, Linda still seemed to be traumatized by the realization that her husband was homosexual, and Robert was almost desperate to have some resolution of the agony between them. They moved from comforting and being gentle with each other to anger, accusation, and tears. Their emotions ran the gamut of what would be expected under the circumstances. Linda felt betrayed, humiliated, abandoned, insulted, angry, sad, unbelieving, and fearful. She vacillated between believing he "could change" to believing they could live "this way." She could not imagine life without Robert, and she could not imagine how she could have lived with him and loved him for so long and not known. She was furious with him for not telling her, and equally furious with him for telling her. She felt their life together had "been a lie," and that their life together was the most real thing she had ever known. Robert was sad but sure that, despite the terrible cost to both of them, he was gay and could not change that. In some ways he was despondent, in other ways relieved to have "come out." He was contrite about the years of duplicity—but also clear that he did not feel he had had a choice; he had been in the closet so long he did not know how to come out. He was afraid for himself, for Linda, for his family—for their whole way of life. He had tried to deny his homosexuality, and was in fact successful for the first years of their marriage, but then was drawn back to men and had some one-night stands, which led to a few affairs, the most recent of which had become important to him. He loved Linda too much to continue living this way, hurting her this way.

Their Dilemma

The most significant feature of their beginning therapy was the difference in their goals: For Linda, it was a last, desperate effort to save her marriage; for Robert, therapy was to help him find a way to effect a decent, honorable, and least painful dissolution of their marriage. The following sequence occurred in our initial session.

ROBERT: I just can't bear to see Linda suffer so. It's not fair. None of this is her fault. She keeps trying, and I can't seem to find a way to help her understand. Darling . . . (*Robert puts his arm around Linda, and they just hold each other.*)

LINDA: But, Bobby—I love you. What do you want me to do? Just give up on all we mean to each other?

ROBERT: It's hard for Linda not to believe that the strength of our relationship—all we've been—well, that it won't, over time—well, make things different. I understand that feeling. That you think—if you try hard enough you can change anything. But it's unrealistic, and I want to help Linda be able to let go of that idea—to help her come to terms with the way it is.

MW: Oh, Robert—I think, I think maybe that's the crux of the problem you two have now.

ROBERT: You mean that Linda keeps hoping we can—that she thinks it's possible for our marriage . . .

MW: No, Robert—I mean that the problem, or the issue for the two of you now, is that you continue to believe that it is up to you to find a way to convince Linda—that you need to help her to give up her hope that your marriage can be saved—that you need to hang in there until she lets go.

ROBERT: I'm not sure I understand.

MW: Robert, your concern for Linda—your protests that you can't continue to hurt her this way—you're drowning her in your—well, in your altruism.

ROBERT: Oh, my God—that's the last thing I want to do.

MW: I know that. Your concern for Linda is real—it's loving and honest—but what happens is . . .

LINDA: What happens is I keep hearing that he feels he has to leave for my sake. I think he wants to stay—but, Bobby, you think you're being fair by insisting you have to leave. No, no—being fair is our trying to work this out together, to keep what we've got.

ROBERT: Linda . . . Linda, that's not possible.

MW: Robert—I still don't think you've got it. I don't guess Linda has either. Or maybe Linda gets it partly; but Linda you're so confused and hurt at this point that it's like—well, maybe like huge waves rolling over you—and you keep coming up at different places in the ocean, gasping for breath.

LINDA: You got it—and I always feel like I'm treading water. Maybe I don't even know how to swim anymore—I used to be a good swimmer. Marianne, what did you mean—what don't I get?

MW: That Robert's wanting so hard to make it all right for you— trying, God knows, in good faith—to help you accept where he is—his putting his need to leave the marriage on not wanting to keep hurting you. Well, this continues to cloud—to obscure—the real issue. That Robert needs to leave the marriage because he needs to be with men, not with a woman, not even a woman he loves. When he says, even once or twice, that he needs to leave because he can't keep hurting you this way—you grab hold of that like—what do they call those things they throw out to you when you fall overboard?

LINDA: A life-preserver? I don't know what you call them—but it feels like a lifesaver, something to hold on to—I don't want him to feel he has to leave for my sake—I don't want him to leave at all—but, when he says that, I know how much he loves me, I know he doesn't really want to end our marriage—oh, oh—oh, Marianne, I see what you mean! Oh, God—I hate this whole thing . . .

ROBERT: Marianne, you mean I shouldn't try to help Linda? That's not possible—we've always helped each other . . .

MW: No, it's not about not helping her, Robert—that's absolutely wonderful—it's not hard to see why Linda loves you so very much—no, Robert, it's about helping her in a *different* way. You see, when you say you have to leave for Linda's sake, it reinforces Linda's belief, or hope, that you don't really want to leave, and so she gets caught in trying to convince you to stay, rather than beginning to turn her energy toward dealing with herself—toward coming to terms with your having to leave the marriage so you can live your life fully as the person you are.

LINDA: (*Crying*) How can I ever come to terms with our having lived a lie? With Robert cheating—with, with—

ROBERT: (*Tearful*) Believe me, I understand that it feels that way— I guess it is that way—but it was not about you, it was—it is about me. The lie was my struggle—with me, with you, my parents, work, our friends.

MW: And now you're back at the beginning—you will say all the things to each other that you have said a zillion times—and it won't change anything. Are you saying anything new to each other now?

ROBERT: No, no, no, of course not—we can't . . .

MW: You can, Robert, you can. You need to be strong enough to say why you must leave your marriage—not because it's not fair to Linda, not for her sake—although, of course, that's in it too. No, it's for your sake, so you can be free to be who you are. You need to trust that in the end Linda can handle this—you need to trust her strength and, in fact, her love. To give her credit for being able to manage a painful reality.

Of course, this sequence, in its various manifestations, needed to be repeated several times during the session for Robert and Linda to get hold of the idea that Robert's protectiveness of Linda, and especially his framing his need to leave the marriage in altruistic terms, served to keep her helpless. It was hard for Robert, a truly loving person, to understand that in wanting to make it all right for Linda he was also trying to ease his own guilt and contrition—and that, in fact, this is an especially seductive trap for women. Linda would continue acting out her part of this scenario—berating, pleading, anguishing—a part which, in fact, protects him from having to assume full responsibility for what he needs to do. And so as long as Linda is, so to speak, in pursuit, she will have no energy left to begin her own healing process.

Facilitating Choice

In the second session both Linda and Robert were very subdued. During the intervening week Robert, on my advice, had refrained from saying anything along the lines of not wanting to keep on hurting Linda, or that he had to leave the marriage for her sake. In the absence of those words, of being comforting and protective of Linda, he had little to say and a distance between them had developed—a distance that both of them found quite uncomfortable and unable to breach. I likened this distance to the symbolic dissolution of their marriage— their each needing to deal with at least some aspects of their situation alone, on their own; beginning to have to give up the comfort of always being there for each other. Their distance and discomfort had displaced the sadness and tears. Linda was more overtly angry, yet still trying to convince Robert of the two alternatives to divorce: trying together to help him "to change," or failing that, seeking together a way to live with his homosexuality. Robert, of course, pointed out that neither alternative was a viable one; but whenever he tried to convince Linda that either of these alternatives would be too painful for her, or that it would be unmanageable for both of them, I held him to speaking only for what was necessary or possible for *him*. The session was in sharp contrast, emotionally, to the previous one.

I felt it would highlight and be consistent with the direction of the therapy to see each of them separately; and the next three sessions were individual ones, within the same weeks, but on different days. With Robert, our work was primarily focused on his concerns about "coming out" to his family, which he felt would be inevitable in the wake of the divorce, and ways in which he could stay "in the closet" at work. Occasionally he would drift back to "wanting to make it all right" for Linda, but could accept my blocking this. These sessions were poignant. Despite more open, accepting attitudes in our society, the awful struggle and pain of being a homosexual in a heterosexual world was the reality that Robert had to deal with regarding his family, his work, and the everyday experiences of derision and scorn.

With Linda the sessions were volatile—like being on a roller coaster. She would chug up the hill, and then come crashing down. My intention during these sessions was to provide the context in which she could begin to experience again some choice in her life and thus begin to regain control of it. With Robert no longer clinging to the pretense that he needed to leave "for her sake," she was face to face with a reality over which she had no control, and so she saw no alternatives for herself emotionally. She was angry about the years of duplicity, but could use help in beginning to depersonalize this—to understand that it was not so simple as his lying to her; that it was a journey in which he did not have the means with which to engage her. This led to self-pity—"Why me?"—and from there to "How could I have been so unknowing, so insensitive?"—and from there to "How will I ever be able to trust my own judgment again?" Of course, the real question was, in what ways could she trust her judgment—did she still know the quality, the value of the man she had *chosen* to live with all these years? Were the pleasures, the growth, the experiences she had *chosen* to share with him any less real? Would she *choose* a different kind of man now? If Robert were not homosexual, would she have *chosen* differently?

Finally, after working through some of these processes, encountered in any loss, Linda was able to consider with me an alternative that had never occurred to her or seemed possible: to keep connected to much of what she had *chosen* in deciding to marry Robert in the first place—his warmth, humor, intellect, integrity—by remaining his friend.

Individual sessions with Linda were extended for another four weeks as we worked together to help restore her sense of choice and control within a context over which she had no control—the reality of

Robert's sexual preference. During this time, Linda proposed to Robert that they remain friends, continue to share some of the things they enjoyed together including mutual friends, and maintain an interest in each other's lives. She reported that Robert was noncommittal, and even seemed somewhat disturbed by the idea.

We met together again for two sessions. Robert and Linda were already working out some of the legal and material aspects of a divorce. The more difficult problem for this couple was what they would do about their relationship. Robert wanted to put the question of an ongoing friendship on the back burner. He couldn't manage that now. He needed to be entirely free of emotional encumbrances in order to deal with adopting a new life-style. He was afraid he would get caught up again in all that he loved in their life together. At first Linda backed down, but I kept her "on the case." She needed to convince Robert that she was ready to have a friendship with a man she had loved; that this was a choice for her, free of wanting to resume the marriage, which she now truly believed was as impossible for her as for him. It was hard for Robert; he was pretty confused about how things were going to be for him—with a new lover, his family, friends. Linda began their friendship by helping him sort some of this out, confining her help to those areas in which she felt some knowledge and competence, and staying clear of those areas that could no longer be between them.

I saw Linda and Robert separately on an as-needed basis for the next year. A few weeks ago Linda called to ask if she could drop by with her husband and introduce me to her three-month-old baby boy. Robert is the godfather.

Concluding Note

A note about this case in relation to the threat of AIDS. I saw this couple in 1982, when I had only the vaguest awareness of AIDS as a health issue. Robert assured me, as he had assured Linda, that he was always careful. Obviously, what we know today about the epidemic proportions and major health risk of AIDS would have seriously complicated, if not altered, my work with this couple.

For instance, we would have needed to consider, at the outset, the decision for both of them to be tested, and to confront the issue of trust within a context when not knowing a partner's sexual history can be life-threatening. My intention, of course, in presenting this case is to illustrate principles and techniques of an empowering therapy for women who are divorcing. No longer, however, can we ever work with gay men and their partners without being painfully aware of the terrible shadow being cast over their lives by the specter of AIDS.

7

Marianne Walters

Single-Parent, Female-Headed Households

HOUSEHOLDS HEADED BY a single parent have become a common variation on family life in contemporary America. Over 6 million families with children under 18 living at home are one-parent households headed by a woman. About 20 percent of all mothers in America today are raising their children alone, that is, in father-absent households.

The statistics are compelling. Based on Census Bureau reports for 1984, experts predict that *one* of every *three* families will be headed by a single parent by 1990; that a quarter of the now-married mothers and fathers will be single parents sometime in this decade; and that approximately half of the children born in the 1980s will spend part of their childhood living with one parent. Since 1980 there has been a 13.2 percent increase in the number of female-headed households; since 1970 a 100 percent increase. Between 1970 and 1984 the number of single-parent families of all races has more than doubled. Although the rate of increase of such families among blacks has been less than the national average, the female-headed family currently accounts for 42 percent of all black families.

The rise of teenage "out-of-wedlock" pregnancies and births, with more teen mothers choosing to keep and raise their children, has swelled the ranks of mothers raising their children alone. Contrary to popular belief, the actual rate of adolescent pregnancies has declined since 1960. But pregnant adolescents are much less likely to marry than was the case twenty years ago, so that now the majority of teens who bear children do so out-of-wedlock. If present trends continue, demographers estimate that fully 40 percent of today's 14-year-old girls will be pregnant at least once before the age of 20. For 51 percent of black teens and 19 percent of white teens, these pregnancies will result in non-marital births.

The economic consequences for women raising children alone, either due to divorce or to a teen birth, are indeed profound. Only half of those young women who give birth before age 18 complete high school, as compared with 96 percent of those who postpone childbearing. On average, they earn half as much money and are far more likely to be dependent on welfare. There is a sharp decline in the standard of living of many, if not most, women and their children following a divorce. One study (Weitzman, 1985, p. xii) claims that "on average, divorced women and the minor children in their households experience a 73 percent decline in their standard of living in the first year after divorce. Their former husbands, in contrast, experience a 43 percent rise in their standard of living." While these figures appear to be overstated, it is nonetheless true that the proportion of poor persons living in female-headed households has increased dramatically in recent years. Over half of all children living in poverty are in households headed by women. With disadvantage begetting disadvantage, this phenomenon has come to be known as the "feminization of poverty" (Rix, 1980).

Despite the severe social and economic consequences of single parenting, such families continue to appear at every level of American life, among the rich and the poor, in rural counties and urban centers, in suburbia and exurbia, within all religious groups and ethnic populations. It is becoming familiar. The single-parent family cuts a swath across middle America as well as among the poor. Female heads of households are housewives, lawyers, typists, factory workers, nurses, businesswomen. They are divorced, widowed, never married; they are lesbian and heterosexual; they live alone, with extended family, or in shared households; in apartments, private homes, and farms. Some have never worked, some have careers, some are itinerant workers, some are on welfare. They are large families and small ones, with children of every age. Single-parent families come in a variety of sizes, shapes, colors, and reflect the spectrum of social and economic change that has characterized family life in the past decade. The one unchanging characteristic is that the vast majority of these families, despite new divorce and custody laws, remain female-headed (92 percent). The social, economic, and psychological contexts and conditions for single-parent families is a women's issue.

Liabilities and Labels

Despite the numbers and the social and psychological diversity of single-parent families, they continue to be seen as an anomaly, and societal attitudes remain largely disapproving. The female-headed household is perceived as deficient regardless of economic or social status. Even a relatively stable single-parent family is regarded as psychologically at risk, and any rumblings of trouble within the family will be viewed as the product of an incomplete system or a deviated social unit.

The labels used to describe single-parent families—divided, broken, fatherless, torn—are generally pejorative. The message repeatedly received by members of single-parent households is that something is wrong, your well-being is at risk, healthy development is highly unlikely. The way these messages are delivered can be subtle. In the recent issue of a large metropolitan daily, two stories about local teenagers appeared on the same page. One reported the receipt of a large scholarship for academic honors by a graduating high school senior. While her parents were named, the fact that they were divorced and that she had been raised in a single-parent, female-headed household since the age of six was not mentioned. The other story reported the break-in of a small grocery store by two high school boys. Both were reported to be from "broken" homes, the implication being, of course, that their antisocial behavior could, at least partly, be attributed to that fact. It is highly unlikely that any reportage would imply that the academic success of the young woman could be attributed, at least partly, to her having been raised in a female-headed, single-parent family.

In an anthology of the essays, articles, and poems of single parents entitled *Momma*, one young mother wrote: "We call our homes 'single mother' homes. We think that we're single-parent families. First year psychology texts say we're pathogenic families. To us, our children are special, as they are to any mother, but not that much different from other kids in the neighborhood or at the child-care center. To social scientists, our children are 'culturally deprived'—the victims of a broken home. In our daily lives, we and our children suffer the consequences of the researcher's findings. . . ." (Hope and Young, 1976, p. 43).

Psychological research on single-parent families has been primarily focused on the effects of father absence, especially on the male child. Since maternal custody is the most common social pattern, and the difficulties of growing up with an opposite-sex parent are believed to be greater than growing up with the same-sex parent, there is particular concern for the effects on males of being reared solely by females. Psychological research has typically relied on male subjects and male behavior to establish modes, models, and norms. Consequently, the list of problems attributed to father absence for boys is quite long and very grim—everything from homosexuality to lowered intellectual ability. The list of outcomes for girls is shorter, but not much more promising. The underlying assumption is that two parents in a single household are necessary for the successful development of a child and that no parent, especially a female parent, can singlehandedly raise a well-adjusted child, most particularly if the child involved is male. The net effect of most research on single parents is the representation of the single-mother home as a deficit mode of family life. The nuclear family continues to be considered the social ideal and the most viable family model. The increase in single-parent families has generally been perceived as the result of a breakdown in the moral fabric of our society, a breach in traditional family values, and thus a threat to adequate child rearing.

Although much has been written about latch-key children, absent mothers, and deteriorating family ties, in fact, according to a 1982 Bureau of the Census survey, about 60 percent of working mothers with children under five reported that their children were cared for by a family member, most notably grandparents. Only 15 percent of all working mothers in the 1982 survey reported that their child attended a nursery school or day care center; 22 percent reported that their child was cared for by a non-relative outside of the home; and 2 percent relied on ex-husbands for child care. Of course, such care decreases as children get older and, certainly, more children are left on their own than is desirable. But the economic double-bind for single mothers seems to be intractable. If they work full-time to support their children they will earn 68 percent of what men earn in similar occupations; 70 percent of them will work in low-status jobs in which three-quarters of the employees are female; over one-third of them will do clerical work; and, lacking seniority and advanced training due to their recent entry into the marketplace, they will be the first fired. Furthermore, the scarcity of low-cost, publically supported day care is legion, with the majority of mothers needing to secure independent, private arrangements for the care of their children, much of which is financially out of reach. If they work part-time in order to be at home more with their children, three-quarters of them will be in the lowest paying sales, clerical, and service occupations within which they will receive virtually no fringe benefits, such as health insurance, and where the opportunity for advancement is virtually nil. In either case they face work situations that do not allow for absences related to a child's illness or accident, in which flextime is a rare commodity, and where career ladders will dead-end for them far from the top.

If, on the other hand, they choose to stay home with their children they must be dependent on child-support payments (which only 49 percent of divorced mothers received in full, and 28 percent of whom received nothing), on help from family and friends, or be forced to go on welfare. If they go on welfare in order to stay home with their children, they will be subject to accusations of laziness, dependency, and irresponsibility. Even if given some job training they will likely return to the lowest paying jobs, and the cycle will repeat itself. In recent years we have witnessed such families swelling the ranks of the homeless, working poor. The median income of the female-headed, single-parent family is one-third that of the two-parent family, despite the fact that expenses are similar. One-fourth of white single-parent families and nearly one-half of black single-parent families live in poverty. According to a 1986 Census Bureau report, a staggering 33.5 percent of single-parent families were living below the poverty line compared with 8.9 percent of all families with children.

Despite these repressive social attitudes and oppressive economic realities, single-parent families have continued to survive and to multiply. And this is not just due to the rising rate of divorce or of teen pregnancies and births. More parents are choosing to be and to remain single parents. There is a substantial rise in the number of individuals maintaining single-parent households permanently. And several emerging subgroups are creating new visions of single parenting. For instance, there are significant increases in single persons adopting children, or using artificial or natural means to have children, while remaining single. These mothers, and some fathers, are making active and responsible choices to raise children alone. Some have never married and some have been previously married. They are usually on the older end of child-bearing years and have established careers and economic independence.

Whatever their origin as single parents, there is a continuing struggle to find their place in the larger society, to position themselves in a social limbo in which there are few rules or traditions or rituals to guide them, and little help from schools, religious and social institutions, or government agencies. Left largely to their own resourcefulness they are creating their own sociology, their own rules and rituals, their own family traditions, their own child-rearing practices, their own self-help groups, communities, and networks. This struggle itself has created a kind of cohesion both *within* and *between* single-parent families. Single parents have formed nationwide organizations, have lobbied together for improved child-care facilities and work conditions, and have sought ways to create systems of support for each other. And despite the dire predictions, many children are growing up and flourishing in such families, with no conclusive evidence that their emotional development or intellectual potential is more at risk than that of children in two-parent households. Clearly, the overriding issue that differentiates the potential for children growing up in single- and dual-parent households is poverty itself.

Myths, Images, and Realities

Single parenthood has become the subject of public debate, media exposure, popular journalism, investigative reporting, documentaries, books, and stories. While some view the advancing tide of single-parent families as part of the flood of social change that is "drowning" traditional family values and morals, others see it as a legitimate redefinition of the family, a conceptual and physical restructuring that is congruent with changes in contemporary life.

Being a single parent in a female-headed household is an unpleasant reality for many, a rewarding way of life for a growing number, and a considered choice for some. Before it became a choice for women, being a female single-parent had many negative consequences, among them the following: (1) becoming a social pariah; (2) having your children labeled "illegitimate"; (3) having your children described as the "product of a broken home"; (4) finding it difficult, if not impossible, to obtain credit; (5) finding it difficult, if not impossible, to obtain a real-estate loan; (6) finding it hard to obtain employment even within an occupation for which you are qualified; (7) discovering that your child's behavior, when problematic, is always due to her/his membership in a single-parent home; (8) being told you've failed; (9) being told your children are at risk; (10) being pitied.

Such consequences have, of course, not been entirely eliminated. But the very familiarity of single parenthood on the social and cultural landscape of America has made life easier for such families. Changes in social attitudes, and the challenge to discriminatory legal, fiscal, and employment practices brought about by the women's movement, have made conditions for female heads of household, and their children, less debilitating. And the fact that single parentdom can actually be a viable *choice* for women has not only empowered all female single parents, but has also had a profoundly unsettling effect on ideas about what is socially acceptable. The very notion that a woman can raise children and manage family life without a male partner is a challenge to the basic premises of patriarchy (that is, entitlement and power through men). As a *choice*, it still stirs controversy, even among those who are committed to maintaining such choices for women, and it is a risky choice. But the very fact of its existence is a profound step forward in legitimizing female-headed households.

Of course, single-parent households existed long before the women's movement of the '70s, the sexual revolution of the '60s, or the postwar migrations of the '50s—all of which have been blamed by various social commentators and critics as causes of the erosion of traditional family life. Women of color, women belonging to ethnic minority and new immigrant groups, and women on the dole have been heads of households and sole custodians of their children for decades.

But their experiences in building families, and coping with the prejudice and discrimination they encountered along the way, went largely unnoticed and unrecorded except when it was used to explain crime, delinquency, poverty, and other social ills. It was not until the ranks of such families swelled with women whose membership lay in the white, Protestant, middle-class of this country that demographers, social theorists, and family experts took notice. Now single-parent families are studied and analyzed in professional circles, and their experiences reported in the popular media.

It is interesting (but somewhat disheartening) to note that in some respects the popular media has latched onto a more positive view of the single-parent family than that which prevails in our professional fields. For instance, on television there is the popular sitcom of the single mom and her two daughters ("One Day at a Time") and the even more radical departure of a prime-time show about two moms and their kids sharing a life together ("Kate and Allie").

Some years ago when *Newsweek* first featured an article on single-parent families, the magazine cover depicted the torn photograph of a family, with parents glaring at each other over the somber, blonde, blue-eyed child caught in the middle. Inside, the story focused on the current crisis, with dire predictions of worse to come. More recently, on the cover of the July 1985 *Newsweek*, which featured a story on "The Single Parent," there is the picture of a smiling mom teaching her youngest daughter how to bat a ball while her older daughter plays catcher. Inside, the article presents the problems, the struggles and setbacks, but also suggests "single parents and their children are . . . in the process of midwifing . . . the birth of a new kind of family . . . and many of them are discovering that the new family has its own claims to legitimacy . . . . The nuclear family has split and divided itself into many possibilities . . ." The March 1983 issue of *Working Mother* featured an article on "The Blessings [yes, the blessings!] of Being a Single Mom." In March of 1982 *Good Housekeeping* published an article, "When Women Raise Families Alone," on the successes of single parents, on which I collaborated with my friend Nonny Majchrzyk. And despite the fact that the movies needed to make a man the hero of their single-parent saga, *Kramer vs. Kramer*, the story and its characters contributed to depathologizing this kind of family. (Yet it is a telling commentary that the first film featuring a single parent cast that parent as a man, presumably to legitimize the subject and increase its popularity.) Nonetheless, with increasing frequency, single parents are being characterized on the big screen as well as for the home audience; they are the subject of talk shows and docudramas. They appear in current novels and human-interest articles. And every such popular exposure contributes to rendering female-headed families more familiar, and thus less threatening and more acceptable in the minds of the general public.

Research Models and the Single Parent

Research models that shape both our theory and our practice are typically organized by traditional social expectations and norms regarding family functioning, family structure, and the role of women in society. The prevailing assumption that a single-parent family deprives children of role models and childhood experiences necessary for the acquisition of appropriate sex-role behaviors, an assumption profoundly influenced by psychoanalytic theory, has never been countered in the family therapy literature. Moreover, much social science research, embedded in this family-deficit model, supports the belief that women cannot manage social, economic, and psychosocial tasks outside of the context of marriage—a belief that is implicit, if not explicit, in much of our practice with single-parent families. In fact, much of the family research on which we rely for definition and explanation of the characteristics and functioning of single parents has done little to help depathologize such families.

Even the critically acclaimed work of Wallerstein and Kelly (1980) studying the long-term effects of divorce on the emotional well-being of children, while clearly intended to generate improved social attitudes, policy, and services for such families, has, in fact, often been interpreted in such a way as to highlight the negative outcome of divorce and single-parent family life on the growth and adaptation of children. While the researchers make the crucial point that the attitudes of the parents about themselves and their life situation both before and after the divorce, their level of emotional satisfaction and adjustment, is, as in all families, central to the healthy development of their children, this point seems to get lost in the broader interpretation of their findings. For instance, in an article in the January 1980 issue of *Psychology Today*, Wallerstein and Kelly review the results of their research. The article is headlined with the news that "five years after the breakup, 34 percent of the kids are happy and thriving, 29 percent are doing reasonably well, but 37 percent are depressed" (p. 67). While the headline also states that "what counts most are the two parents' attitudes," the "but"—the depressed children—clearly claims the attention of the reader.

Yet, such statistics pretty much reflect the state of affairs for the population in general; that is, about 30 percent of children do very well growing up, about 30 percent do reasonably well, and about 30 percent have trouble (here labeled "depressed"). In fact, if one looks behind the study's statistics to the actual numbers, you get a rather positive picture of the outcome for children following a divorce. One hundred thirty-one youngsters were studied by the researchers. That amounts to 44.5 kids happy and thriving after the divorce, 37.9 kids doing reasonably well, and 48.4 kids depressed. Considering that they've all been through a major family upheaval, that makes the odds pretty good. Only four more kids are unhappy than are happy (after the divorce), and if you add the first two categories, 82.4 kids in 60 families are OK! That is certainly a finding worthy of the most extensive investigation, application, and dissemination, since it directly addresses the crucial need to depathologize the single-parent family.

Unfortunately, as with most such studies, the gendered norms that devalue mother-headed families are not factored into the investigation of outcomes for such families. The findings are correlated primarily with conditions, issues, relationships, structures, attitudes, and interactions that exist *within* the family.

Study after psychological study, by virtually ignoring such factors as income, lowered standard of living, geographic dislocation, and lack of child-care facilities, or by not taking into account the critical and pejorative social attitudes that surround the single-parent family, confirm the concept of this family as a deficient, handicapped social unit. A few studies have attempted to expand the context of investigation of single-parent families, and recently there has been an emergence of new perspectives based on integrative reviews of the literature. This meta-analysis has allowed some look at the assumptions that organize the process of research and theory building. For instance, Marotz-Baden and colleagues, in an examination of the deficit family model that has organized research on divorce and the single-parent family, conclude: "There is little evidence suggesting that divorce is directly related to negative developmental consequences for children. Rather, circumstances associated with poverty and conflict between parents in any family form seem to be contributing factors" (Marotz-Baden, Adams, Bueche, Munro, and Munro, 1979, p. 28). They go on to suggest that it appears to be more fruitful to consider the social-interactional dynamics that lead to a given outcome than to focus on the structure of the family as the critical independent variable.

In a review article that focuses on using the strengths of single-parent families during the divorce crises, Peterson and Cleminshaw (1980) state that three primary factors determine the resolution of the divorce situation: (1) the objective stress of external conditions; (2) the pre-existing attitudes and coping skills of the individuals involved; and (3) *the definition of the situation that the individuals impose on the experience.* In summary, they state that social norms define, and social attitudes organize, the degree of respectability or stigma the single parent and her children internalize. Internalizing less negative attitudes functions as a major source of strength and stability for the single-parent family. When the marital dissolution and the new family form are viewed and internalized as less deviant, both parents and children have greater access to their own personal and emotional resources. This framework provides the family therapist with a significant point of entry in working with single-parent families.

Clinical Implications

General systems theory as applied to models of family therapy held out the promise of contextual sensitivity, but absorption with the structural and systemic characteristics of the family unit itself has often dimmed that promise. Moreover, this concentration on the internal, on the family system *qua* system, has created a context that is so organized around the "medium"—the systemic properties of the technique, the intervention, the strategy—that it has frequently desensitized us to the "message," particularly as it carries traditional, gender-defined social norms and assumptions.

Perhaps a clinical example will illustrate my point. In a consultation group, a family therapist discussed her work with a single parent whose son was having many school problems. This mother constantly called her ex-husband to talk about the son's problems, to seek his involvement, to get his advice, and to try to come to some agreement on what needed to be done. She felt frustrated in her dealings with the school and angry at her ex-husband for giving advice but refusing to become involved. Almost daily she would get calls from school about her son's behavior; she'd then call dad, he'd make suggestions, she would argue with him because "he didn't really know what was going on" and couldn't "understand" since he "wasn't there." He'd tell her, "Then go ahead and do it your way," and she was left "holding the bag," feeling failed with school, son, and dad.

The therapist chose the following course of action as a way to empower the mother: the mother was directed to stop asking her ex-husband for advice and to turn over to him sole responsibility for negotiations with the school. She was then to instruct the school to contact dad with regard to any future complaints or issues regarding their son. The therapist worked with the mother to abandon her dependent behaviors and to take a clear, independent position of her own with both school and ex-husband. The therapist used ideas of complementarity in framing the intervention: "To the degree that you pursue, he distances; to the degree that he distances, you pursue." To break this dysfunctional cycle she suggested mom should back off from the pursuit and take a stand on how *she* will "be there," thus allowing dad to operate in a less reactive way.

Another therapist in the group suggested that mom could be directed to pretend that she was totally unable to manage the school problem, had no ideas on what to do, couldn't even think about it anymore—in other words, to feign total dependence. A third member of the group suggested a counterpoint: one therapist could deliver the message that the son's symptom functioned to keep parents engaged with each other, and that if he behaved mom would get depressed, so she should continue seeking her husband's counsel; the other therapist could insist that mom would not get depressed and that she should disengage so dad could take more responsibility. A fourth therapist suggested that the hierarchy in this family would need to be restored: Mom should establish clear expectations with her son with regard to school performance, set rules, and enforce appropriate sanctions. The therapist would help her set goals and organize more effectively around family management tasks. Since her interactions with dad are undermining for her son, more appropriate boundaries should be structured between the parents, with rules established for telephone contacts and the like.

Clearly these interventions would "work" and are systemically grounded. The task of the consultation group was to analyze each of the interventions for the message (or metamessage) it might convey that could, implicitly or explicitly, reinforce sexist cultural norms or gender stereotypes. Since the therapist was working with the mother-head-of-household family it seemed obvious that the major pitfall was in conveying messages that mom was the problem.

Gender-biased Metamessages

In the first intervention, the therapist instructs the mother to turn the management of their son's school problem over to the dad. The danger is that mom will "hear" in this intervention not the empowerment intended by the therapist but the message that if, left to his own devices, dad can "do it better." Will she be empowered by delegating (or relegating) authority to her ex-husband in an arena in which she feels failed? Furthermore, in critiquing the reciprocal-loop concept of "pursuer-distancer" the group cautioned on the need for sensitivity to a cultural context in which dad's distance is more acceptable than mom's pursuit, and does not arouse the same fears of incipient pathology. Images of distant fathers simply don't conjure up the demons of pursuing mothers, so that despite its reciprocal formulation the impact of the message is more pejorative for women than for men. (We still live in a world where dad's attendance at *one* PTA meeting is applauded, while mom's missing *one* meeting is cause for alarm.)

The second intervention suggests that mom do what women have been counseled to do for eons—fake it, pretend you "can't do" in behalf of getting him "to do," or, more crudely, act "dumb" so he'll feel "smart." Other than serving to improve mom's acting skills, this intervention conveys the gender-stereotyped message that "artful" manipulation of a relationship is what is expected of women, and that getting her own act together is of secondary importance to finding a way to improve his.

The third suggested intervention is congruent with societal assumptions that attribute a child's behaviors directly to the dynamics of parental interaction—in this instance, to the divorce and continued conflict over authority. The metamessage is blame—in this instance, with mother in therapy, blame falling on the mother. Further, although each therapist takes a different position, the message conveyed by all three reinforces the idea that a woman's primary sense of well-being is to be found in her relationship with her spouse or children, without reference to other sources of self-esteem.

The fourth intervention, regarding structures, rules, and sanctions, reinforces the prevailing social standard that hierarchy rests on power and being in charge, and conveys the message that mother's need to "understand" and "be connected" are not valued. Moreover, with female single parents such standards of hierarchy, especially when teenagers are involved, may simply be impossible to achieve, if only by virtue of size and strength.

The group struggled with alternative interventions intended to decrease the potential of sex-role-stereotyped messages, and which might even go counter to such cultural biases. With this in mind the following course of action was developed.

The therapist would suggest to this mother that her efforts to engage dad in their son's school problem, however well-meaning and surely worthwhile, are just not, at this time, going to work—for whatever reason. Probably the reasons are too loaded with past history to sort out at this juncture. What does matter is that in trying so hard to get her husband to take more responsibility she is depleting the very energy she needs to manage the problem. It is therefore self-defeating and keeps her in a position that is either oppositional (with ex-husband) or protective (with her child). This position restricts her ability to utilize her own knowledge and skills as a parent. Moreover, it generates feelings of failure and of alienation from her son, so she forgets what she knows, and perhaps even what she likes, about her son. Within this framework the therapist would direct the mother's attention to what has worked for them in the past, what the son does well, what they do well together—the sources of their *connection*. The therapist might suggest that the mother think of one thing, *outside* of his school performance, that her son could do to make her feel better, and work with them on achieving this. She would coach mom on ways of dealing more effectively with the school, using role play and strategizing on "what if's." And she would offer to participate in a joint conference with the school if mother felt such was needed. She would help mother to gather information from the school and from other sources (such as testing) about what is contributing to her son's poor school performance. Becoming better informed about the nature of her son's difficulties would help mother to feel more in charge, and enable her to get "tougher" with her son if that should prove appropriate. The therapist would encourage mother to reassure her ex-husband that she's "on the case" if he should inquire about his son's school situation. And the therapist would explicitly reassure mom that her son's behavior is not her fault and has nothing to do with a "broken home"; at the same time assuring her that interventions on her part can indeed be of help to her son. Working within areas that are manageable, providing "at home" tasks while helping mother within the sessions to experience new ways of connecting with her son, will not only increase her parental skills but will improve her self-esteem—a necesssry prelude to more autonomous behaviors.

Strengths That Characterize Single-Parent Families

Several years ago the Family Therapy Practice Center, with the help of a foundation grant, designed a project to explore the strengths of single-parent families. Discouraged by the dearth of professional literature on the characteristics of well-functioning single-parent families, and the volume of literature describing their problems and pathology, we set out to pursue a positive definition of this family life style. Through single-parent self-help groups, churches, schools, and informal collegial networks, we advertised our interest in interviewing and videotaping single-parent families who perceived themselves as functioning successfully. The volume of response was far greater than our expectation, but funding constraints allowed us to interview only the first 25 families that responded. Interestingly, 5 of these families were male-headed households, representing 25 percent of our "subjects," as contrasted with the less than 10 percent of such households in the general population. Nothing about our "study" was objective or available to quantification. We had no criteria for success; they were self-defined and therefore subjective. Our purpose was to see if we could come up with any useful generalizations to counter the deficit model so widely internalized by both therapists and the single-parent families with whom they work.

The parents and children we interviewed helped us to identify the following characteristics of their single-parent households as contributing to positive family functioning: (1) a single "line" of authority that simplified family decision making and decreased conflict born out of the splitting or triangulation of parents; (2) the opportunity for one parent to combine and integrate nurturing (caretaking) and managerial (executive) functions, rather than having these functions divided by gender-defined expectations and roles; (3) flexibility, or permeability, of generational boundaries, permitting the expansion of opportunities for companionship between parent and children; (4) a reduced hierarchical structure with respect to household organization and management, resulting in a greater sharing of family tasks and the assumption of multiple roles for individual family members; (5) increased expectation for the quality of family membership; and (6) a heightened awareness of the family as an interdependent unit.

As a social unit, the single-parent family is both more affected by, and responsive to, extrafamilial systems. Thus, attitudes and conditions of school, church, or workplace reverberate with more intensity within the single-parent household, creating waves that wash over it with greater power to heal or hurt. Single parents tend to develop friendships that are *utilitarian* as well as social, with friends assuming functions *within* the family as well as outside of it. There is greater proximity between family and the world of work, with the employment life of the parent often regarded as an extension of the family system. Children tend to be more knowledgeable about their parent's work conditions and responsive to the effect of those conditions on parental functioning in the family, and on the parent's general sense of well-being. Family tasks are set with respect to real, rather than preconceived, needs; tasks that actually need doing as opposed to tasks that are assigned or created to teach one "how to do." The single-parent family, conditioned by experiences of transition, change, and redefinition of family roles, rules, and functions, develops an expanded repertoire of coping skills with which to respond to new developmental tasks or external requirements for change.

The families we saw, families who defined themselves as successful, were not families without problems. They presented the whole gamut of problems with children that we encounter every day in our offices—acting-out adolescents, poor school performance, withdrawal, somatic symptoms, delinquency, conflict—but they all reported that having weathered these storms they felt stronger as a family, more prepared for new "turbulence."

Most felt they had been poorly prepared for the dislocations triggered by separation, divorce, or death of a spouse, or for the need to reestablish themselves while "under assault" by all kinds of unfamiliar and unforeseen circumstances. They passed through a time when few things—income level, employment status, living situation—could be taken for granted. For most of the single parents we interviewed, this was uncharted territory, with no map to mark their course.

An unmistakable element in the approach our interviewees took in coping with the changes in their lives was in defining what was happening to them as a *family* issue. The parent's preoccupation with her own turmoil was balanced by a concern with the family's need to restructure itself. By necessity they had to pay attention to the "whole"—and to identify resources both inside and outside of the family that may have previously gone unnoticed. The tasks of everyday living presented an area in which the family could demonstrate and exert control over its own destiny. For most families, living together was no longer an overly familiar "given" to take for granted, but a shared accomplishment. Our interviewers often heard comments like, "We got through the bad times *as a family*, which really surprised us." One teenage daughter commented, "When my father left, there were a lot of things we didn't know about each other. There was the stress for my mother—her husband was gone. And Dad's going was particularly tough on my brothers. It was as if the four of us banded together. It took effort, but in the long run we gained a lot because we began to know more about how we fit together."

While single parents and children often seemed like partners in survival, there was rarely confusion about where final authority rested. Now one adult had primary responsibility for keeping the family together, providing care, and maintaining order. Far from seeing this as a disadvantage, the families we interviewed, parents and children alike, considered the single line of authority simpler and more streamlined than before. Contrasting the present system with the old, our interviewees seemed to savor the freedom of sole authority. One summed it up in saying, "I can be the captain of my ship. When I say no, it's no. I try to be fair, but I admit I like being at the wheel."

Among the families we interviewed, there was a greater expectation that everyone, including young children, contribute to the maintenance, well-being, and welfare of the whole family. As one single parent told us with both regret and pride, "In these kinds of families, kids have to grow up faster, take on new roles—like learning to wear different hats for different occasions. Sometimes they can't be 'just a kid.'" As Robert Weiss (1979) has noted, "Although these youngsters may regret not having a more traditional family and a more carefree youth, they often respect themselves more for having been able to respond to what they recognize as their family's genuine need for their contributions" (p. 110).

As in any family, some responsibilities were explicitly assigned (as when a teenager is asked to look after her infant brother on weekends when she and her siblings stay with her divorced father); some are assumed without formal assignment (it is understood that someone, other than mother, will do the dishes before the family goes to sleep). But whatever the approach in a given family, chores take on a particular importance in many single-parent homes. The children in our study knew that not only were their contributions to the family valued and needed, but that their independence and ability to care for themselves were also genuinely prized. With the family less structured along lines of provider/parent and consumer/child, the children in these families are more sure that they have something else to offer their parent besides completing their chores, staying out of trouble, and getting good grades. More opportunities arise in which a child may be called upon to nurture a parent. Some of these may be a matter of logistics; when mother is sick, her small son may have to tend to her. Others are more subtle and suggest possibilities for parent-child intimacy and emotional reciprocity. While the dangers of child parentification, invasion of privacy, and breakdown of generational boundaries was not lost on these families, they described, through many anecdotes, the heightened sense of competence that came with knowing what to do for each other.

Young children's efforts to take care of their parents produced some memorable family vignettes. One mother recalled the time she secluded herself in her home to work on her thesis as her dissertation deadline loomed ominously before her. She instructed her children, "If you break a leg, dial 911 because I absolutely cannot come out of this room." She emerged several hours later to find that a pipe had burst in her home. Her three children, ages 9, 7, and 4, had formed a bucket brigade and were busily bailing out the bathroom!

One mom described the evolution of the successful single-parent family this way: "I remember one time, right after the divorce, my oldest boy had to wear a bow tie to his confirmation and I didn't know how to tie it. I went out and bought him a pre-tied one. Then I cried all night, thinking, that's how it's going to be with us—never the real thing. So I learned how to tie a tie real quick! Now all three boys seem to have an addiction to bow ties."

Perhaps the most potentially creative opportunity found in managing female-headed, single-parent homes is in the adaptations these parents have created, and will continue to create, for integrating in one person the typically gender-differentiated parenting functions—to nurture and to manage, to provide care and to function in an executive capacity, to give leadership and promote well-being, to foster autonomy while encouraging interdependence, to provide the means of support while preparing the young to support themselves. One of the most basic threats to the successful functioning of female-headed families is the deeply ingrained belief that these functions are, and must continue to be, gender-defined and differentiated. The means, modes, and styles that women will develop as heads of household in interdigitating, weaving, and integrating these functions should serve as a model for all families in the future.

Shaping a Therapeutic Context

In each of the following cases of work with single-parent, female-headed households, the therapist has clearly rejected the deficit model imposed on such families and focuses the therapy on creating a context in which the parent and her children can internalize more positive images and definitions of their family. While the interventions of each therapist remain specific to and consistent with her particular methodology—as illustrated throughout this book—the rejection of a deficit perspective enables the therapist to reference herself to a belief system encompassing the viability, choice, normalcy, and creative possibility in single parenting. Of course, we are all dealing with dysfunctional systems and problematic behaviors, and none of us believes single parenting is an optimum solution. Neither, however, do we believe that this family form is pathogenic. But therapists will need to pay more than lip service to such a belief. The pervasive influence of the deficit perspective that attaches to single parents, and the fear that their dependency, disorganization, and neediness engenders in therapists will need to be consciously and consistently countered.

Peggy Papp in her case discussion takes on the crucial issue of choice. The element of choice with respect to single parenting, particularly for women, though it is an option assumed by only a small percentage of people, is central and crucial to a nondeficit model of single-parent family functioning and to the empowerment of all female heads of household. Single parenting as a choice, an elected family structure, serves to legitimize this family form; the absence of choice pathologizes it. In her own struggle with this issue, Peggy illustrates the significance of the therapist's own attitudes and beliefs on the directions of therapy and, of course, on the therapist's choices of intervention. In this case, Peggy deals not only with a challenge to traditional values and biases, but also with a therapist-client relationship that expands each, creating a context in which the client's experience and life situation are validated.

Olga Silverstein's case illustrates the creative use of a gender context to enable a divorced mother to understand her dysfunctional behaviors toward the men in her life in a new way. In the process of helping her client "to see things differently," Olga enables her to seek behaviors that are more personally satisfying and productive. She avoids the clinical clichés of the overinvolved, intrusive, overbearing mother, or the stereotyped interventions that reinforce negative images of dominating mothers, and turns the attention of her client to some of the larger, socially defined gender imperatives motivating her behavior. This "re-referencing" is an essential ingredient in creating a context in which validation rather than critique is used to motivate change.

Betty Carter's case illustrates the ways in which a therapist committed to empowering her client can select and focus on information that will advance this clinical intention without needing to rely on contrivances of technique. When behaviors are understood in contexts larger than the individual, or the internal configurations of a system, the choice of material for therapeutic intervention becomes correspondingly larger and enriched, allowing us to draw from the experiences of others within our current social and cultural milieu.

So it is in the case I have chosen to discuss. Since my interventions focus on process within the session, using the *particular*—an interaction, comment, or behavior—to suggest generalizations, develop a theme, or create a new perspective, I have selected what might appear to be a minor, even obscure, bit of interaction within one session to illustrate the way in which a larger frame of reference can sensitize a therapist to the metamessages conveyed within a particular act or experience. In this case, the particular is an offhand comment that, given a feminist frame of reference, fairly shouts the message of poor self-image as a parent. In order to begin the process of helping a single parent to internalize positive self-images, the "particular" is turned into an event, an experience, and becomes a metaphor that can be used throughout the course of the therapy.

cases

Marianne Walters

Moving to the Front of the Bus

Sara brought her 14-year-old daughter, Tamara, to the Center amid an atmosphere of great urgency and crisis. Sara was intensely anxious and fearful about what she perceived to be a serious pattern of sexual promiscuity on the part of her daughter. In that first session it was difficult to connect Tamara to the sexually acting-out youngster being described by her mother. She looked more like a shy child, timid and soft-spoken, with braids wrapped tightly around her head. She seemed almost to fade into the woodwork as her mom spoke of her fears about Tamara's indiscriminate sexual behaviors. Sara was convinced that she would find herself on the way to becoming a grandmother any day now, and was terrified by the prospect. She was quite agitated, felt she had run out of any viable method for getting Tamara's behavior under control, and just felt angry and defeated with her most of the time. She believed she had "tried everything," and felt guilty and profoundly inadequate in raising this teenage daughter.

Background

Sara and Tamara had not lived together for 11 of Tamara's 14 years. When Tamara was 2 years old, Sara had placed her in a foster home, feeling unable to care and provide for her adequately. Sara has had a long-term drinking problem, has been on welfare in the past, and now works as a street vendor. In the past couple of years her vending business had been successful enough for her to become fully self-supporting for the first time in her life. When that happened, she obtained an apartment and petitioned the court to resume custody of her daughter. Tamara had been living with her mother for about a year when I first started seeing them.

Sara is black, has never been married, and has no family except for an uncle and his wife who live in Alabama. The only daughter of a dirt farmer who abandoned the family when she was 6, she lived alone with her mother until her mother's death when Sara was 17. After that she somehow found her way up north, soon became pregnant, and went on welfare. But clearly there was a fierce pride in this strong, attractive woman. She "could not," "would not" bring up her daughter in the slum conditions in which she was living at the time, and so she sought foster care for her child. Tamara had several sets of foster parents and a group home placement before she was settled into a long-term foster home not far from her mother—one that lasted for nine years. Sara kept in touch and had regular contact with Tamara throughout her foster placement, visited frequently, took her out, and had a good relationship with her daughter's foster parents, a relationship she worked hard to maintain. In fact, her life during this period pretty much centered around her visits with her daughter and contact with the foster parents.

Nonetheless, there was a sense of mystery that Sara projected as she tried to tell me something of Tamara's growing-up experiences. There were some allusions to her having been pregnant, or having thought she was pregnant, which at any rate had been terminated by a "spontaneous abortion." There were references to Tamara having been hospitalized for a mysterious ailment on several occasions. Despite the fact that clearly Sara was an exceptionally intelligent woman, although undereducated, and obviously quite articulate, her panic about her daughter's welfare and potential for getting into trouble obscured her descriptions and made her appear to be vague, and somewhat disoriented, whenever she talked about Tamara.

Despite this, Sara had already done some major structuring of Tamara's life in an effort to "protect her from herself." Tamara went to school on a special bus, and was returned home each day after school. She was not allowed off the school grounds and was under close supervision while at school. Sara had set up a regular system of reporting between the school and herself. But Tamara still found ways to elude and circumvent these structures, to act out, and thus to remain, in the view of her mother, greatly at risk. In a strange way, Sara explained everything and nothing to Tamara. She was full of warnings, admonitions, and cautionary tales—consumed by a foreboding that she freely communicated to her daughter. But, conversely, she expected practically nothing from Tamara except to "stay out of trouble." It was almost as if the beginning and end of their family rules were: "Don't get pregnant."

Alternative Interventions

Different methodological frameworks within family therapy might suggest some of the following approaches for intervention with this single parent and her daughter:

1. Frame the mother as extremely anxious about her daughter and thus overprotective, and help her to understand this dynamic by making connections with:
   (a) her own history of insecurity in her family of origin, early pregnancy, and the like;
   (b) real fears about the social consequences of teen pregnancy, as in fact she herself had experienced it;
   (c) her guilt about having placed Tamara in foster care, despite that having been a considered and realistic decision;
   (d) her lack of parental experience.
2. Redefine or relabel the mother as "working too hard," making some of the same connections listed above and adding a reframe that includes the reciprocal cycle between mother and daughter, the reactivity that exacerbates the problem.
3. Define the problem as a breach in parental hierarchy, relating this to the mother and daughter's having lived apart for so long. Suggest the need to restructure their living together by the implementation of clearer rules and expectations, and clarity about the consequences should Tamara's behavior continue or if, in fact, she should become pregnant.
4. Define the problem as having to do with poor generational boundaries resulting from
   (a) mother's drinking, or
   (b) mother's overinvolvement with Tamara because she lacks a life of her own, or
   (c) both. Suggest mother "back off" and begin to more actively pursue her own interests.

5. Suggest that Sara "watch over" Tamara even more than she is currently doing—perhaps even making regular visits to school, monitoring her telephone calls, and not permitting her out of the house unchaperoned.
6. Suggest Tamara's behavior serves the function of reducing her mother's social isolation—for instance, getting her involved with the school, with other parents, and so forth.

The therapist might ponder the dilemma for Sara—the advisability of de-escalating the focus on Tamara as against the possibility that she will become more isolated and depressed if she does so.

These approaches are, of course, presented here in an abbreviated fashion. Nonetheless, they do represent some of the major formulations that appear in the literature on family practice. Clearly all of these formulations have systemic ingredients and, indeed, each representation of the situation provides a useful perspective on the relationships in this family. Yet, all of the approaches outlined above implicitly highlight the mother's deficits; they focus on what is missing, what is not working well, particularly on the part of the parent. As such, they have the potential of bypassing, particularly at the outset of therapy, the crucial work of constructing a context—a corrective experience, if you will—that is explicitly directed at the amelioration, modification, or repair of those social messages and life experiences that surely will have served to diminish the self-esteem of the mother.

Using a Feminist Frame of Reference

Within a feminist frame of reference we anticipate that single mothers will enter therapy feeling invalidated, blamed, and disapproved of, and that such feelings, and the social and interpersonal messages that produce them, must be countered. As part of this context they will need to understand their situation as larger than themselves or their family, where it can be mistaken as solely their problem, regardless of systems interventions. Of course, it could be argued that if the mother begins to function in a more competent manner with her daughter, and if, by whatever means, Tamara's behavior is brought under control, self-esteem will be restored and a corrective experience will have been achieved. Clearly, I don't believe this to be necessarily true. I believe that change can occur in the context of therapy, with symptom remission and the improvement of dysfunctional behaviors, without changing the social and emotional context that engenders personal feelings of inadequacy, blame, guilt, and the like. In fact, therapy can exacerbate such feelings in the individual even while bringing about change in the system.

In this case, three areas for intervention seemed crucial to the construction of a therapeutic or remedial context: (1) the tenuous connection between mother and daughter would need to be strengthened, with some positive ties and emotional reciprocation developed; (2) the socially prescribed expectations for mother-daughter conflict, particularly in the area of sexuality, would need to be dispelled; and (3) the mother's guilt about having placed her daughter in foster care, and the social disapproval she would have experienced, exacerbating her feelings of inadequacy as a parent, would need to be addressed.

Here was a woman who had given up her child because she did not feel she could properly care for her; a never-married single parent who risked taking her child back only to find that her kid scared the hell out of her and made her feel de-skilled and bewildered. Her panic, and her very real lack of knowledge about what to expect from a teenager, compounded her poor self-image as a parent. Sara had no trust in her competence to handle this child, which Tamara reinforced by her acting out. I was less concerned about Tamara being in imminent danger of a pregnancy than I was about the erosion of any possibility for a good relationship between these two if some semblance of credibility for Sara as a competent and knowing parent was not pretty quickly established.

Creating a Therapeutic Context

In beginning our work together I compared the situation in which Sara and Tamara found themselves to what it is like to be a foreigner in a strange land: you don't know the rules, you can't read the signs, you lose your direction, you don't get the cues, things scare you that never would at home, in a place with which you are familiar. You share no history so that you're unsure how to use what you know from other experiences, and you're not sure whether what you know is relevant to these new conditions. I pointed out that, in fact, Sara and her daughter were in many ways strangers to each other—each something of a foreigner in the land of the other. I suggested that they needed to begin a process of informing each other, each about herself, so that they could begin to feel more comfortable and safe with each other; and maybe, later, even to discover a common language. While not denying the reality of Sara's panic about Tamara's sexual vulnerability, I suggested that it was exaggerated by her sense of not knowing, and thus not understanding, her own daughter, so that everything that seemed different from what she expected was frightening. Sara's lack of experience in being a full-time mother made her feel incompetent, so she did not fully use her own resources, her own knowing—just as an American arriving on the shores of France for the first time might be afraid to cross the street. And Tamara—frightened and confused, not knowing what exactly was expected of her—was clearly kind of thrashing around emotionally, experimenting. I agreed with Sara that this was a potentially dangerous situation.

I expressed my respect for the protective structures Sara had already established. I pointed out that she had done it again—responded to a problematic life situation by putting structures into place to protect her daughter and to create more manageable conditions— just as she had done in placing her daughter in foster care. And I asked her to consider if she could trust those structures for the next couple of weeks while we ventured along another path, one designed to help her and Tamara become more familiar with each other. Sara agreed and asked Tamara for her consent. Tamara was tentative; Sara explained what we would be doing, and she agreed.

We set up several sessions that would be devoted primarily to the detailed exchange of experiences, information, and memories between mother and daughter. This was also to be pursued at home with times scheduled for this activity. Even the process of negotiating times that would be suitable for both mother and daughter was an effort that produced some proximity between them. In the first session, we practiced this kind of conversation, with my coaching Sara on how to question, ways to elicit information on a subject, how to listen, and how to give feedback; then, coaching Tamara on how to expand an answer, how to decide what was appropriate to ask about, how to express interest, and the like. And each time Sara learned something new about her daughter (even something as small as her description of a school friend) I pressed her to figure out how this expanded her sense of "knowing" this daughter of hers, thus using content to expand a sense of familiarity.

Both Sara and Tamara warmed to the project, and began to understand how it fit their life situation and carried the potential to change things between them. During the next three weeks their life together improved dramatically as both of them really got into the experience of informing each other. Sara's panic subsided, and Tamara offered up no new behaviors to cause her mother concern.

Using Process

Sara arrived distraught and angry to our fourth session together. She began to speak of perhaps needing to place Tamara again. She was again in a panic. Tamara had left the school grounds at lunchtime on two occasions and had been found in a fast food place with a couple of boys. With things getting better between them, this was particularly disappointing.

SARA: Maybe it can't be repaired. It seems like so much disaster has already hit us—well, hit Tamara especially. She doesn't even know how harmful all this is to her. If she could just stop being so ignorant as to run off with every young man that walks up, puts his arm around her, and says, "Let's go"—under the bushes, or the staircase . . . (*Tamara softly demurs.*)

SARA: But, Tamara, *that* bothers me—it bothers me a lot. (*To me*) Because she's an attractive—she's my daughter, but she's still an attractive young lady, and . . .

MW: My goodness, Sara, do you hear what you're saying? What a way to think—what a way to think!

SARA: What do you mean, Marianne? What am I saying? Tamara is an attractive girl, even though she's my daughter, she is an attractive girl.

MW: "Even though" she's your daughter—even though! Heavens, Sara, have you looked in the mirror at yourself lately? Tamara, do you know you look a lot like your mom?

TAMARA: Thank you.

SARA: What did you say?

TAMARA: I said, thank you.

MW: Does that surprise you?

SARA: Well, yes—I'm her mother—I never thought she thought about how I looked, or thought I was pretty or anything like that.

TAMARA: (*Warming to the subject*) Well, you know when we were in the park the other day, those two boys I was talking to that were sitting on the bench—one of them said to me, "Tammy, your mother sure is a pretty lady!"

SARA: Well, I never—well, thanks.

MW: I think you're in for some surprises, Sara. You're so darned anxious about this kid of yours that you don't even let yourself know that she's pretty *because* she's your daughter—that's got to be part of the reason!

SARA: Well, yes, I see what you mean—I never, well I guess I never stopped to think about it like that.

MW: Look, Sara, I think in some ways you feel so down as a parent, as a mother—maybe because you're single, maybe because of needing to get alternative care for your daughter, or maybe because you drink too much—or whatever, anyway you find it so hard to even see the physical resemblance, the physical tie, between the two of you.

SARA: She is indeed a very pretty young lady, Marianne. (*Smiling at me*) Even though she's my daughter!

MW: (*Laughing*) And you're quite a lady! Stubborn to the end! Seriously, Sara, does it feel like boasting?

SARA: Maybe.

MW: Do you think you don't have a right to boast?

SARA: I guess, yes, I do feel that way, sometime. No, most of the time; maybe always.

MW: Because —?

SARA: Because, because—maybe because I've not done right by her.

TAMARA: Ma, momma—you've done lots that's right.

MW: Tamara, you know, it's hard to be a single mother with a teen daughter, a daughter you love a lot and have had to live separately from for so many years. (*To Sara*) You live in a disapproving world. The way you've lived your life is not how it's supposed to be. You can't help but feel disapproved of and so you begin to feel like you can do no right—and that it's probably in the cards that your kid will get into trouble and that you two will be in conflict.

SARA: (*Leaning over to Tamara and covering her hand with her own*) It's just that I've been so afraid. Concerned that Tamara was being a little bit freer than I'd like her to be.

MW: Oh, Sara—you're saying it so much better, so much better— bringing it down to size.

SARA: (*Smiling*) I am, aren't I. I see what you mean. I guess I am. But sometimes, Marianne, it feels so strange. Like we'll get on a bus together and Tamara goes and sits by herself in the back of the bus, away from me.

MW: In the back of the bus! I don't believe it! Don't you know about the back of the bus? (*Tamara looks bewildered. Sara starts to laugh.*)

SARA: I don't think she knows what you're talking about.

TAMARA: I don't get it—

MW: Sara, you think Tamara doesn't know about Rosa Parks, Montgomery—

SARA: (*Looking at Tamara who's shaking her head*) I don't guess she does. I wonder, hmmmm.

MW: Maybe you can tell her about it.

SARA: I think I should, it's important.

MW: You can start now, take some time now, if you like.

Over the next couple of months, while the panic about her daughter became less frequent and more controlled, such interventions needed to be repeated many times. Sara's sense of herself as a woman and as a mother had been so diminished that she needed a frequent "fix," one that challenged even the most innocuous-sounding, self-denigrating remark. Sometimes I would just need to remind her with the metaphor of "pretty like her mother."

As their relationship strengthened and Sara began to feel more sure as a parent, she began to expect more from Tamara, both in terms of their life together and behaving more responsibly outside. Soon Tamara began to make more demands on her mother to expand their home life, for example, wanting to have friends over. With my help she was able to confront her mother about her need to be sure that Sara would not get drunk in front of her friends. These sessions were among our most difficult, with tears, accusations, and recriminations flying back and forth between mother and daughter.

Four months into therapy, Sara signed herself into a detox program, arranging supervision for Tamara during her absence. While her mother was in the program, Tamara was allowed to travel to individual sessions with one of my colleagues at the Center, and to attend Al-Anon meetings. When Sara returned home, she and Tamara resumed therapy with me. These sessions focused on the dislocation engendered by Sara's absence and return. The earlier frame of "strangers" was replayed, but the content now was on the changes each of them had made, and the new sense of personal responsibility both felt in relation to this latest experience of separation and transition. Later, Sara came to see me alone over a period of about fourteen months on an as-needed basis.

In June, Tamara sent me a picture of herself in cap and gown at her graduation. Standing proudly at her side was Sara, holding her own GED certificate in one hand and Tamara's diploma in the other.

Betty Carter

"They Need a Strong Man in Their Lives"

This case presents many of the dilemmas and difficulties so common in single-parent families, especially the effects of the double message from the social system that says that a woman alone is not sufficient to raise boys but, on the other hand, only a "bad mother" gives up custody of her children. This two-edged message makes her "wrong," whichever way she moves. It also makes understandable, in spite of the self-invalidation involved, the frequent requests made by single mothers of sons for a male therapist. It is less understandable, however, that mental health services frequently take the same position.

The common practice of deliberately assigning a male therapist to a single mother with sons manages to invalidate *both* parents in a single stroke. To the single mother, the message that she probably can't raise her sons properly without the help of a man has the effect of a self-fulfilling prophecy. As in this case, the mother is probably experiencing difficulties with her sons *because* of her acceptance of the widely believed social myth that boys can't be satisfactorily raised by their mothers alone. If the therapy supports the myth, implicitly or explicitly, the mother will be further weakened in her functioning with her sons. At the same time, there is serious risk that the male therapist, unless he consciously works against the tide, will take the father's place with the boys and weaken, rather than strengthen, their relationship with their father.

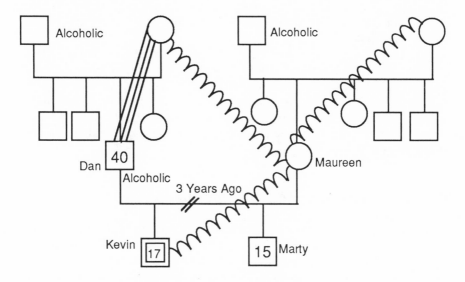

See page 96 for an extended definition of the genogram.

Presenting Problem: The "Catch-22" Position

Dan, a suburban police officer, and his wife, Maureen, a secretary, were divorced three years ago. Their sons, currently ages 17 and 15, are in Maureen's custody. Dan sees his sons frequently, though not on a regular schedule, and phones them frequently. Dan and Maureen have a conflictual relationship, which they handle by speaking as little as possible.

Maureen sought family therapy at a neighborhood clinic for herself and her two sons because Kevin had been failing in school and refused to "obey" her at home. She knew that he drank on weekends and she was afraid that he was involved in drugs.

Maureen expressed disappointment that she was assigned a female therapist, saying that she thought her sons needed a strong male influence in their lives. Her husband was a disruptive influence, she said. He was inconsistent with the boys, drank too much, punished them harshly one minute and lavished money on them the next, criticized her endlessly to them, and frequently disappointed them by changing and canceling visitation plans. Her ex-husband lived with his mother, Maureen said, who was "an old battle-axe."

Maureen's ex-husband had initiated the divorce, claiming it was because of her nagging, but Maureen thought he had been having an affair. She had not wanted the divorce—not because the marriage was that great—it wasn't—but because she felt she couldn't raise teenage boys alone. "Now," she said, "this proves it. I suppose I should let him and his blessed mother have custody of them, but what kind of mother would that make me?"

Maureen expresses the "Catch-22" position of the single mother. In this context, the appeal for a male therapist seems to provide a way out of the dilemma. Because of her sense of powerlessness with her sons, and her lack of connection with her own considerable strengths, phase I of the therapy (with the female therapist who had been assigned to the family) consisted of helping Maureen to realize that she could indeed raise teenage boys alone.

Phase I of Therapy: Empowering the Mother

Maureen took her mother-in-law to lunch and set some firm boundaries with her regarding the boys, while at the same time thanking her for being such a concerned grandmother. She talked to both her mother-in-law and her mother about their experiences in raising sons and elicited their support for her efforts to do the same.

This was a process that went far beyond the reaches of this one issue. In order to have meaningful personal conversations with both her mother-in-law and mother on this topic, Maureen had to take a look at her overall relationship with each of them, and sort out the reasons for her antagonistic feelings in each case. She had found her mother "too weak" and her mother-in-law "too hard," without ever fully examining what these women had been up against in their own lives, both with alcoholic husbands and many children. Before opening discussions with them, she spent many weeks examining the facts of their lives in response to the therapist's questions.

MAUREEN: She's a bitch-on-wheels, my mother-in-law. To tell the truth, I blame her for how my ex-husband turned out.

THERAPIST: In what way?

MAUREEN: Well, she was so strict—unreasonable really—when he was a teenager that it was like asking for him to rebel—and he did.

THERAPIST: Was he worse than your son, Kevin?

MAUREEN: I didn't really think he got bad till after she lowered the boom on him. And, in fact, that's one of the reasons I'm afraid to get too tough on Kevin.

THERAPIST: I wonder why she was so tough on him—Dan, I mean.

MAUREEN: I told you—she was a bitch-on-wheels.

THERAPIST: (*Laughing*) You mean she was born a bitch-on-wheels?

MAUREEN: (*Smiling*) Well, I guess she was afraid he'd turn out like his two older brothers. They both drank a lot, like the father, and the oldest one was always in trouble with the police.

THERAPIST: Boy, she must have been *worried* as hell. What a lot to deal with! Who did she have to help her?

MAUREEN: Well, no one, actually. The old man drank all night and day—in the end he didn't even work. And she was the only one in her family to come over. The rest stayed in Ireland.

THERAPIST: How isolated she was!

MAUREEN: (*With a flash of anger*) Well, at least her husband didn't walk out on her.

THERAPIST: Maybe she'd have been better off if he did.

MAUREEN: (*Smiling*) She'd have a fit if she heard you say that! She's made a regular saint out of him since he died. Still, I know what you mean. The father was a terrible influence on the boys, and there wasn't much she could do about that.

THERAPIST: She must have felt so helpless.

MAUREEN: Helpless? You should see her! You never met a louder, bossier, pushier person in your life!

THERAPIST: I guess she felt everything had to depend on her. She probably didn't feel able to do it all alone.

MAUREEN: No—now you're talking about my mother, not my mother-in-law. My mother felt helpless. (*Contemptuously*) You never met anyone so helpless. My sister and I had to raise the younger ones. My mother just dragged herself around in a trance and spent half her time in church.

THERAPIST: So she felt overwhelmed with your father's drinking— and so many kids.

MAUREEN: I guess so—but I don't think that's any reason to quit on your kids.

THERAPIST: Did she actually quit on you?

MAUREEN: Well, she cooked and cleaned and did laundry and all— but she had no *time* for anyone. She didn't listen to any of us.

THERAPIST: So that's why it's so important to you to listen to your kids.

MAUREEN: Yes—yes. But it's hard to know when to be sympathetic and when to be tough. You know?

THERAPIST: Yes—I can easily see that it would. You think it was your mother-in-law's toughness that ruined your husband after all.

MAUREEN: Yes—although it's true that she had a lot to deal with.

THERAPIST: Can you even think of that tough old bird as a worried, scared mother trying to do her best?

MAUREEN: It's hard. It's a stretch!

THERAPIST: Yeah, it is. Especially since you didn't know her then—only later when she was kind of hardened by it all. Who do you think is a more concerned, well-meaning mother—your mother, your mother-in-law, or you?

MAUREEN: (*Shocked*) What a question!

THERAPIST: You know what I suspect? I bet if you talk to each of them about those days when their kids were home, you'll find out they were dealing with a lot of the same stuff you are—including having an unreliable husband and thinking that there was no one to turn to or talk to about it.

MAUREEN: But we are three very different women!

THERAPIST: Yes—with a lot of similar things to deal with.

MAUREEN: But they'd never understand . . .

THERAPIST: That's what they thought, too.

MAUREEN: But they'd never listen to me, or take me seriously.

THERAPIST: That's up to you.

After several sessions like this, Maureen was willing to acknowledge some similarities in the lives of the three women. When she had developed a more compassionate and complex view of their lives, she began a series of talks with them, with coaching from the therapist, that moved these relationships from cold distance to personal, friendly exchanges. In the end, her mother provided support and encouragement and her mother-in-law at least stopped criticizing her and began making demands on Dan to "shape up or ship out."

Maureen's final resistance to the idea of taking full charge of her sons melted the day that the therapist told her how General MacArthur's mother had moved around the country to the various bases he was stationed to live near him. "That does it! No one could call him a 'momma's boy.'" And she decided that she could take charge of her sons.

Taking Charge of the Household: Strengthening Parent-Child Relationships

Then the therapist helped her to set and follow through on enforceable and age-appropriate rules with her sons. She was coached to insist that her ex-husband make a regular visitation schedule and stick to it. She started to talk to her sons about subjects other than their shortcomings and asked for their ideas on how to improve the quality of life in their household. She told them what help she needed from them to run the house.

It is extremely important to wait until a mother feels empowered with her children before giving her tasks related to disciplining them. If she doesn't feel able (or entitled) to be in charge, it is not helpful to set her up to fail or to push her into an authoritarian confrontation that she will surely lose. When she believes she can be in charge, she will be both more convincing and less authoritarian with them.

Exploring the Father's Relationship to the Children

After Maureen was in charge of her family and Kevin's symptoms had diminished, the therapist got Maureen's agreement on having her ex-husband invited to several sessions, alone and with his sons. Note that Maureen's ex-husband is not brought into the therapy until after Maureen has established control of her household, and the child's symptoms have abated. This eliminates the metamessage that father is being called in to "rescue" mother, or to take over for her, while it validates the importance of the children's separate relationship with their father. It is important to note also that this timing would have been adhered to even if father's relationship with his sons were not impaired by alcohol.

In these sessions, Dan acknowledged that he often picked fights with the kids or criticized his ex-wife because he'd had too much to drink. He denied that it was a serious problem, however, and refused to go to AA. After these sessions, the boys were better able to evaluate the role that alcohol had played in the family difficulties, and subsequently they agreed to go to Al-Anon to learn how to deal with their father when he had been drinking.

Resolving the Divorce and Moving On

Maureen was coached to contact her ex-husband only at times when he probably would not be drinking, and to postpone any discussions he might initiate while under the influence of alcohol. She was encouraged to give up the picture of herself as a "victim of divorce," and to embrace the propositions that her marriage hadn't been working and that she had a lot to gain from the divorce, even though she hadn't initiated it. She was coached to change her reactive and conflictual relationship with her ex-husband to a more distant, though friendly, form.

The final phase of treatment consisted of work with Maureen about her plans to return to school, her career goals, and her wish to resume dating. These issues now became central in the continuing conversations with members of her family of origin and in her own list of priorities.

Conclusions

In this case, the common presenting problem of an acting-out adolescent in a single-parent family was used as an opportunity to help the mother realize her competence; to give up the widespread notion that mothers alone can't raise boys satisfactorily; to reconnect her with the similarly invalidated older women in the family; and to help her to move on from the position of "abandoned wife" to a new lease on life.

The sequencing of the therapy was important and provides a general guideline: (1) empower the mother *before* inviting her ex-husband to the therapy; (2) empower the mother *before* giving her tasks relating to the disciplining of children, especially adolescents; (3) make issues of "discipline" secondary to the overall parent-child relationship—that is, work on the relationship in all its aspects, not just as an exercise in hierarchy, authority, and force that, in any case, doesn't suit the female style of being "in charge"; (4) pay specific attention to helping the woman to resolve the emotional issues of the divorce enough to move on with her own life.

Peggy Papp

The Right to Be a Mother

This case was a consciousness-raising experience for me because it forced me to examine some of my own biases. As therapists, we are seldom called upon to look at the basic assumptions under which we operate, even though they color everything we do, from the way in which we gather information to the way we intervene. When working from systemic concepts, it is easy to fool ourselves into thinking we are adopting a strictly neutral and nonjudgmental stance. Our values and judgments often go unnoticed because many of them are shared by the families we treat and by our colleagues. And yet they are everpresent and transcend any particular method or technique. It is only when they are challenged in some way that we are forced to come to grips with them.

This case represents a barometer of our changing times and involves an ethical as well as a therapeutic decision. It also reflects the way in which the ideas that were spawned by the women's movement have influenced the thinking of clients and therapists alike. Ten or fifteen years ago, the option that was taken here would not have been socially viable.

The Presenting Problem: Kim's Predicament

When Kim first brought up the idea of having a child without a husband and raising it herself, I tried to dissuade her. During the months she had been coming to see me, we had focused on many issues, one of them being her unsatisfactory relationships with men. She had first contacted me because she was having difficulty with her current live-in mate. She had just had an abortion because the man didn't want to commit himself to the relationship. This created a great deal of conflict between the two of them, and I saw them together for a few sessions. It was obvious that the man was not as invested as Kim in the relationship, and they soon separated.

During the next year, Kim dated several different men, but each time the relationship ended in disappointment and frustration. She didn't know if it was because there were no "decent" men available for a woman of 39 or if her expectations were unrealistic, but none of the relationships worked out. Each time she became involved, I tried to help her handle the situation differently and change whatever she was doing to contribute to the discord. If the relationship lasted long enough, I saw her together with the man, but eventually the relationship would end.

During this time we also worked on other issues in her life, and many positive changes took place. She was able to extricate herself from the emotional turmoil in her extended family and to set limits with them. She learned to look out for her own best interests at work and to advance in her profession. She no longer suffered from long lapses into depression, and her life generally was filled with less conflict and confusion. But she still had not been able to form a satisfactory relationship with a man. I did not realize at the time that this was more my goal for her than her own.

One day she said to me, "Listen, I want to have a baby and I have come to the conclusion I will have to do it without a husband. I am 39 years old. I can't wait until I form a good relationship with a man. Who knows when that will be, if ever. Maybe it's just not in the cards for me, for whatever reason. I can't take that chance. I want a child. I think it will enrich my life enormously.

"I know all the reasons why I shouldn't. All my friends and colleagues think I'm crazy. They say things like 'You'll become overly involved and turn the child into a schizophrenic,' 'You won't be able to manage and then you'll resent the child,' 'A child needs a father figure,' 'If it's a boy he'll become a homosexual'—or they blame you. They say things like 'How long have you been in therapy with Peggy? What has she been doing with you all this time? Maybe you should change therapists.'

"And all of these negative voices do get to me and undermine my confidence. Maybe this is very sick. Maybe it's an indication of how crazy I am. A psychiatrist I was seeing years ago told me I should never have a child because of my history." (Kim had perceived her mother as being abusive and neglectful and her father as being passive and distant. When she was four, her sister was born and Kim became her substitute mother. She felt needed by her sister, and this new job gave her life meaning.)

"But on the other hand something tells me not to listen to any of them, that it's right for me. Nobody knows what kind of a mother they're going to be. I think I have as good a chance as anyone else. I've had to deal with some difficult things in my life, and I think I can deal with this one. What do you think?"

Exploring a Radical Option

What did I think? In our work together I had supported her in trusting her own judgment and making her own decisions, but I was not prepared for the direction this had taken. She had raised this issue before, but never with such certainty and eloquence. In the past, although attempting to remain neutral, I had tried to dissuade her by raising all the practical stumbling blocks. How would she support the child, since she was just getting by on her present income? And when would she have time to take care of it? How would she cope with baby sitters and arrange for housing? Did she understand how much responsibility a child entailed? And wouldn't this drastically curtail her social life, further reducing her chances of ever having an intimate relationship with a man?

She had answered each of the questions in a way that indicated she had given a great deal of thought to the plan. She knew she would have to make major compromises and it would be difficult, but she thought it would be worth it in the long run.

Then, aside from these concrete reality factors, I had other concerns that I raised with her. Was she not repeating her earlier pattern of looking to be saved through mothering a child? She said she herself had thought about that, but added, "Maybe all that practice I had mothering my sister can be put to good use. It doesn't have to be all bad. Maybe it will serve the child well. Do you really think it's possible to predict ahead of time who will be a good mother?"

Confronting Conventional Assumptions

Confronted with this question, I was forced to examine anew my own ideas on marriage, motherhood, and the prerequisites for a happy family. In doing so I realized one of my guiding assumptions had been based on the popular rhyme, "First comes love, and then comes marriage, and then comes Mary with a baby carriage." My unacknowledged goal for Kim was to help her overcome whatever problem she was having with men so she could settle down and raise children in the confines of a financially secure and emotionally supportive marriage.

My first reaction to her challenge was, like a good mother, to ask myself where had I gone wrong in my therapy. My second reaction was to question the conventional assumption under which I had been operating—that a long-term, intimate involvement with a man was a mark of emotional maturity and a healthy personality. Why was this choice considered to be the only healthy one? While marriage may suit the needs of many women, why must I infer that Kim's failure to marry meant that I, as a therapist, had failed to resolve a personal problem? By trying to fit her into this traditional norm, I was perhaps depriving her of her own personal answer to her dilemma. Raising a child alone, although difficult, would undoubtedly produce less psychic distress for Kim than trying to raise one in an unhappy and conflictual relationship.

As for the child being raised without a father, hadn't many children been raised that way since the world began? The absent father syndrome is not a recent invention but a historical tradition, perpetrated by war, travel, work, and divorce. And despite the many social changes that have taken place, it remains to this day more the rule than the exception.

I then thought about all the intact families I saw in my everyday practice with seriously disturbed children. Certainly, bearing children in a traditional family was no guarantee of a child's health and happiness.

An Unconventional Decision

When Kim raised the question again in the next session, I replied, "You have convinced me that you should follow your inclination. Let's talk about how best to go about doing it." I then proceeded to help her anticipate the problems that would arise and to make concrete plans for dealing with them.

Six months later she made arrangements through a private attorney to adopt a baby at birth. It was a boy, and she named him Johnathan. He was born prematurely, weighed only 4 pounds at birth, and was in an incubator for seven days. She had the option of withdrawing the adoption, but she decided to go through with it. Despite some initial health problems, the child thrived.

Johnathan is now 5 years old. Kim brings him in to see me every so often. He is a delightful, lovable child, although highly active and difficult to manage. Kim has been through some trying periods, managing her own professional life, arranging for baby sitters, worrying about finances, and cutting down on her social life. At times she has felt overwhelmed and found Johnathan's constant demands wearing— much the same as every new mother. She has also experienced a profound pleasure and delight in being Johnathan's mother, and states that her life has been enormously enriched. Even when things are rough, she has never regretted her decision—nor have I regretted supporting it.

Summary

These days therapists are seldom called upon to deal with the optimum circumstances of two parents living together in harmony and taking equal responsibility for raising a family. Rather, we are asked to make decisions regarding deviations from this "norm," to weigh the various alternatives and consider the best compromises. In this case, when I recognized that my traditional goals and expectations were incongruent with those of my client, I made the decision to support her in an unconventional solution. Had I continued to try to dissuade her from her decision, I would have undermined her own intuitive understanding of what was right for her.

In the future, therapists are bound to be confronted with complex situations encompassing even greater deviations from the norm, such as test-tube babies, surrogate mothers, and gene splicing. If we are to help clients cope with these radical technological changes and the complex ethical decisions they provoke, we must revolutionize our thinking and amend our traditional values with the expanded options of a new age.

Olga Silverstein

Is It My Fault?

A woman, having been socialized to take responsibility for the emotional life of the family, has learned to accept blame for whatever goes wrong. It is not surprising, then, that when things are not going well, she will try harder to make things "right." Where the particular rules of her original family are added to the cultural injunctions, she is in double jeopardy. That was the case for Marcia.

The Problem

Marcia called for help with her 17-year-old son, Adam. She was worried because he and his father were getting into physical battles on the alternate weekends that they spent together. "I no longer know what to do," she told me tearfully on the phone, "Adam is getting big and I'm really afraid they'll hurt each other."

The First Interview

Marcia was a rather attractive but tense 37-year-old woman. Adam was a rather pale, shy, 17-year-old—a little overweight, soft, and anxious. I watched them as each waited for the other to sit down.

Finally, Adam sat down and Marcia positioned herself next to him. She glanced at me and then nervously pushed her chair a few inches away from him. She's either been in therapy, I thought, or someone has told her she's too close to him.

> **THERAPIST**: Okay, are you comfortable? Um—why don't you tell me what brings you here.
>
> **MARCIA**: Well, it's Adam and his father—they've been getting into these awful fights. Last weekend I had to call the police. It was terrible.
>
> **THERAPIST**: You called the police? How come? Where were you?
>
> **MARCIA**: I was home, but David called me—"You better get over here, things are getting out of hand." That happens almost every time Adams goes over there now.
>
> **THERAPIST**: How often is that?
>
> **MARCIA**: Every second weekend. But this time when I got there—
>
> **THERAPIST**: Hold it a moment. They call you every time, and every time you go?
>
> **MARCIA**: Well, not every time, but a lot, and I'm sick of it. I can't do anything for myself. I have to stay by the phone because I never know. Anyway, this time when I got over there, I could hear the noise from downstairs. They were hollering at each other and throwing things around. I called the police. I was scared, but I felt awful. The police!!
>
> **ADAM**: You didn't have to do that.
>
> **MARCIA**: I didn't know if you were going to kill each other.
>
> **THERAPIST**: Who were you most worried about?
>
> **MARCIA**: Both of them. David, I guess—Adam—I don't know.
>
> **THERAPIST**: Okay, let's back up a little. How long has this been going on?

History of the Problem

David and Marcia were divorced when Adam was 6 years old. It had been a fairly uneventful marriage, Marcia reported—no great romance. "David lived next door and we used to sit on the roof and talk. He, David, was unhappy and I guess I cheered him up." When Adam was born, David suffered an extreme depression. He was in bed for six months and didn't go back to work for a year or more. He never fully recovered but finally, Marcia said, "I couldn't stand it anymore and I asked him for a divorce." She took Adam and went to live with her father.

"I used to look forward to the weekends when Adam was with David," Marcia said, "because my father was getting old and cranky and I couldn't always keep Adam quiet. You know, he was just a little boy."

Marcia's father died a year ago and she began to look forward to the alternate weekends when finally her time might be her own. But six months ago David lost his job and started getting depressed again. Since then the fighting has become physical—the calls to Marcia for help more frequent, culminating in the call to the police and, finally, to the Institute asking for help.

It is not unusual to expect a woman to facilitate the relationships in a family, particularly between a father and his children. In this case the expectation, indeed the demand, by both her ex-husband and her son that she do so is very evident. That she complies to the extent that she does is often seen as her pathological need to serve, or to control, or to remain central. There are many—too many—blaming formulations possible. Since she is prepared to accept responsibility, in therapy she will appear to accept such labeling and try even harder to do the "right" thing.

The Family History

Marcia's mother died when Marcia was 3 years old, after a long and painful illness. Her maternal grandmother then came to live with the family. "My father couldn't cope," Marcia said. "My brother was 6 years old. He was not like Adam. He was wild. Anyway, my father couldn't manage. I don't think my grandmother wanted to be there, but what could she do?"

THERAPIST: Grandma must have been very sad. After all, she had lost her only daughter.

MARCIA: I guess she must have been. I don't know. She had her hands full. My father was very depressed so he wasn't much good. He went to work but that's about all.

THERAPIST: And you—how did you handle it?

MARCIA: I don't know. I guess I was a very good girl. But that didn't matter. My brother was the only thing that could make my father smile. After Grandma died and my brother had moved to Denver, I went back home with Adam because Daddy needed me.

THERAPIST: You also brought him another son. Did you manage finally to make him happy?

MARCIA: No, I guess not. My father was very cranky by then and Adam was young, so I spent a lot of time trying to keep Adam quiet.

In Marcia's case, the normative socialization of women was exponentially increased by her family story. She seemed caught in every conceivable bind, which put her in the position of constantly worrying about, and feeling responsible for, all of the family relationships. She was most particularly sensitized to the men and their relationships with each other. Role expectations are learned almost by osmosis, they are so pervasive. But for Marcia the added impact of her self-sacrificing grandmother, her demanding and unresponsive father, her depressed and dependent ex-husband, all converged and contributed to her overwhelming sense of responsibility for every male, separately, and for every relationship between them.

The Therapy

I asked Marcia and Adam to ask David to come to the next session. I don't necessarily include a divorced father in the therapy when a mother requests help for herself and/or her children. In this case the problem was defined in terms of the triangle. Father and son fight and mother becomes responsible, so his presence seemed logical.

David was happy to join the therapy; he came readily and joined in eagerly. He seemed genuinely concerned about Adam.

THERAPIST: You know I met with Marcia and Adam. I'd like to have your ideas about what's going on.

DAVID: I'm worried about Adam. He doesn't have any friends—he hangs around with his mother—or with me every second weekend. Don't get me wrong. I love having him. I don't know what I would do if he didn't want to keep coming.

MARCIA: Well, he isn't going to want to come soon—he has to grow up sometime.

DAVID: Well, yes. I was saying I think he shouldn't now. Want to, that is. I want him to come, but he shouldn't want to. And then his schoolwork is not good—not good. And I try to get him to do his homework at my house and he gets mad and I get mad.

THERAPIST: So how does Marcia get in the act?

DAVID: She's in the act. I say, "I'll call your mother and find out your grades," and then that starts a fight. She never sends me his grades.

MARCIA: Why should I? Do you ever go to school? I'm the one who goes to every meeting. I'm the one who talks to the headmaster. I do everything and you—

THERAPIST: How old are you, Adam—?

ADAM: (*Quietly*) Seventeen.

THERAPIST: (*To Adam*) If you start doing things for yourself, what will happen to these two guys? What will they have to talk about?

MARCIA: We were talking about Adam going on a tour this summer, but Adam got upset—"What's going to happen to my father if I'm gone for six weeks?" I was thinking about going away myself if Adam is away.

THERAPIST: So what would happen?

MARCIA: I don't know. (*Turning to David*) Will you be depressed? (*David doesn't answer, but looks miserable.*)

MARCIA: (*To Adam*) Well, you could go to camp again, instead. Then he could visit.

THERAPIST: You're still working very hard to take care of David. When was this divorce?

MARCIA: Eleven years ago. Well, I don't know what to do. If Adam goes away, do I have to stay home?

THERAPIST: I guess, if you've taken on the lifetime job of taking care of David. Between the two of you—you and Adam—it might not be so bad. You could take turns. But then if Adam is smart, he'll grow up, get married, have a life, and then it will be harder. But you'll manage.

MARCIA: No, that's not what I want. Why would I want to do that? (*Starting to cry*) I just want him to take care of himself and maybe help take care of Adam. He just complains about him but he doesn't do anything. I'm sick and tired of doing everything.

THERAPIST: What would happen if you stopped? Don't you think they could take care of themselves?

MARCIA: No, frankly, I don't.

THERAPIST: Maybe, but you're not very good at taking care of yourself either.

MARCIA: What do you mean? I take care of everything—everybody.

THERAPIST: That's true. Everybody but yourself.

A Feminist View

All therapists—individual, systems, whatever—would agree that Marcia is overresponsible. That her too helpful interference is not helpful to anyone is also obvious. Because her behavior is only a slight exaggeration of the woman we most frequently encounter in families, many therapeutic maneuvers have been devised to deal with her. An individual psychodynamic therapist might attempt to help her resolve "her narcissistic need" to remain central in her son's life. It is difficult, given the general precepts in the culture, not to blame her for the underfunctioning of her ex-husband and, particularly, of her son. The most sophisticated therapist might find herself/himself telling her to back off and leave them alone. It hardly matters the shape or form of that move. The covert message would be clear to her: "It's your fault. Your behavior is responsible for their difficulty." Since this message is congruent with her belief, it can only lead to an escalation in her efforts to do it right.

Validating her efforts on behalf of her son and ex-husband is necessary for the maintenance of her self-esteem. She can then be helped to assume more of that responsibility in her own behalf.

David asked to come again to the next session, and Marcia and Adam agreed.

DAVID: It took me ten years but I finally went to school and talked to the headmaster. It went well. I felt good.

THERAPIST: Do I hear you giving Marcia good news. Be careful—it might free her.

DAVID: To do what?

THERAPIST: To think of herself.

DAVID: No, no, I'm not saying I can do everything myself—no.

MARCIA: So I'm not free yet.

THERAPIST: (*To Adam*) Are you free?

ADAM: Are you saying I should live my own life and not care about them?

THERAPIST: Of course not. You'll always care about them, but taking care of someone is not the same as caring about them.

MARCIA: He should care about us, shouldn't he?

THERAPIST: Of course. But he should also care about himself. But right now, I'm thinking about what that would mean with a mother who has been trained to take care of everyone but herself. You do take super good care of these guys, you know.

MARCIA: They want me to.

THERAPIST: (*Laughing*) Well, that explains it. What do you think would happen to them if you let up a little?

MARCIA: I don't know. They don't let up on me. Adam comes home and tells me that David is depressed—he's lonely. He has no friends. David calls me and tells me that Adam is this or that. I don't know what to do. (*Crying again*)

THERAPIST: It's very hard, Marcia. It's always hard for women. We've been taught to take care of people—particularly of our men. It's doubly hard for you. You didn't have a mother to teach you how to care for yourself as well as others. I tell you what. Let's go easy. First see if you can start taking care of yourself before you stop taking care of them. Now what would you like to do on those weekends when Adam is with his father?

MARCIA: I've always wanted to go away but I'm afraid—

THERAPIST: You know if they're going to hurt each other—which I doubt—you can't stop them. Now where would you like to go?

The therapy focused on Marcia's learning to take care of herself. Of course, she consequently was not always available to take care of the other two. Not to the same degree as she had been. As she became more satisfied with her own life she demanded less from Adam. As Adam found himself alone and on his own more, he made some friends, joined a baseball team, did somewhat better in school. David appropriately dropped out of the therapy, and as Adam's behavior improved, their relationship improved.

The last two sessions were spent with Marcia alone. We talked about her plans for herself if and when Adam went away to school. She said that she would like to meet someone "but I'm afraid I would become a dishrag again," she confided. "Well," I told her, "it wouldn't be easy. You'll probably always be the caretaker, but there is nothing wrong with that. It's a nice part of being a woman. As long as you take care of yourself as well."

Conclusion: Defining the Problem

Every experienced therapist knows that it is possible to define a problem in many ways. We could define the problem in this family as that of an overfunctioning mother and an underfunctioning father. We would logically, then, work to decrease her functioning and so increase his. We could define the fighting between the men as an attempt to keep her engaged with her ex-husband. Logically, then, we might dismiss the son and see the couple in an attempt to work out their separation. We could define the problem as Marcia's unresolved grief at the early loss of her mother, which has caused her problems in separation. We would then work more historically, sending her back to work in her family of origin.

These are just a few of the most commonly used formulations. All of them, however subtly, however kindly, support Marcia's assumption that she ultimately is to blame if something goes wrong and she must fix it. Given the predetermined sensitivity of women to that injunction, the therapy then becomes isomorphic to the problem.

It is understandable that therapies embedded in a social system that emphasizes individualism as its highest value would stress differentiation and responsibility for the self. Recognition that such formulations are in direct opposition to the socialization of women has been the missing element in family therapy.

Feminist family therapy recognizes, validates, and appreciates the culturally supported role of women as family nurturers, mediators, and caretakers. Helping her and the family to recognize a woman's own needs as separate and legitimate constitutes a basic change in family organization.

8

Betty Carter

Remarried Families: Creating a New Paradigm

The Myth of Marriage

So strong is the American attachment to the idea of traditional marriage and family as the ideal context for the good life that when the escalating divorce rate threatened that ideal, we countered with the now widely held belief that second marriages generally work out better than the first. This belief, which is not at all supported by the statistics, allows us to reframe the failure of so many marriages as sort of "trial runs" or personal mistakes, which lead, when corrected, to the happily-ever-after dream we have been raised on. This belief allows us to avoid examining the economic, social, and political causes of the widespread marital instability in our culture and permits us, instead, to keep our dream of happy marriage and family intact by blaming individuals for the problem instead of examining and changing the fatal flaws in the original model and its social context. In this view, which I believe to be the prevalent one in our society, remarried families require only slight adjustments in order to become virtually the same as first families. It is as if the "broken home" could and should be "fixed," and business as usual would then proceed in the once-again-intact family of our dreams.

In fact, according to the United States Census Bureau, the divorce rate for second marriages is higher than for first marriages: 49 percent (as compared to 47.5 percent) and, for couples now in their thirties, is projected to rise to more than 60 percent by 1990 (Glick, 1984). The end of the marriage also comes more quickly—after an average of only four years, as opposed to seven years for first marriages.

333

This poor track record does not appear to deter many people, however, and the Census Bureau also reports that 65 percent of divorced women and 70 percent of divorced men do remarry (Norton and Moorman, 1987). There are hints that men and women may remarry for different reasons in such findings as the fact that women with low incomes and men with high incomes are among the first to remarry, while women with high incomes and advanced education are least likely to do so at all (Glick, 1984). Nevertheless, this usually unspoken, gender-related economic factor exists side by side with the belief of a majority of both women and men that marriage is a necessary life structure for fulfillment; that divorce represents a mistaken choice of partner or a personal or family emotional problem, not a flaw in the structure of marriage; and that remarriage offers an opportunity to have the "intact again" structure necessary to resume the traditional dream.

The New Family Paradigm

This set of beliefs prevents most people, including therapists, from recognizing the need for an entirely *new* paradigm of family to allow for the complex relationships and roles in remarried families (McGoldrick and Carter, 1980; Ahrons, 1980). In fact, attempts to replicate the "intact" nuclear family of first marriages lead to severe procrustean problems, most of which center around role conflict between members of the original and remarried families. For example, a tight loyalty boundary drawn around household members in remarried families excludes a biological parent or children who don't live in the new household, and thus is not functional. Although it is extremely hard to give up the idea of the "nuclear family household," in remarried systems "family" and "household" are no longer synonymous terms.

Furthermore, the fact that the parent-child bond predates the marital bond, often by many years, produces a tendency in the stepparent to compete with stepchildren for primacy with the spouse, as if the relationships were on the same hierarchical level. Further creating competition within the remarried family, traditional gender roles requiring women to take responsibility for the emotional well-being of the family pit stepmother and stepdaughter against each other, and place the ex-wife and the new wife in adversarial, competing positions, especially concerning the children.

The implied new paradigm for the remarried family would encourage an open, flexible family system in which rigid boundaries between old and new family members, roles, and relationships can be relaxed and finally revised. Within this new system, *permeable bound-*

aries around household memberships would permit children to come and go easily as agreed upon for visitation and custody, and would allow for open lines of communication between ex-spouses, and between children and their biological parents, grandparents, and other relatives. In addition, the new family model would encourage *acceptance of the parental responsibilities and feelings of one's spouse* without carrying out such responsibilities *for* the spouse, or trying to combat or compete with the parent-child attachment. Most important, the new model of the remarried family would allow for *revision of traditional family gender roles*. Such traditional roles, rigidly applied, are among the fatal flaws in the unstable structure of first marriages. And if the old rules that called for women to rear the children and men to earn and manage the finances are not working well in first-marriage families, they are even less applicable in a system where some of the children are strangers to the wife and where finances include sources of income and expenditures that are not in the husband's power to generate or control (for example, alimony, child support, or the earnings of one's ex-wife or current wife).

In a functional remarried system, then, the responsibilities of raising his and her children must be distributed in a way that does not exclude or combat the influence of biological parents. This really means that *each* spouse, in conjunction with his or her ex-spouse, takes primary responsibility for raising or disciplining his or her own biological children, especially in the early years of the new family. This principle rests on the thorny assumption that most ex-spouses are willing and able to cooperate in the raising of their children and thus requires a good bit of exploration before being acted on in any given family. Elkin (1987) lists several contraindications to post-divorce arrangements of joint or shared custody, among them the mental illness or addiction of one or both parents; a history of family violence and/or child abuse and neglect; or irreconcilable disagreement about child rearing. Ambert (1986) reminds us that when children are young there are special difficulties and disruptions pertaining to the degree of contact and communication necessary in a co-parenting partnership conducted more with one's ex-spouse than with the current one. And Chesler (1986) objects to the legal presumption of joint custody because of the power this puts in the hands of a vengeful ex-spouse. In short, no paradigm should lie outside the reach of good clinical judgment and common sense.

His and Her Children

Similarly, we need to clarify what is meant by holding the biological parent responsible for rearing and/or disciplining his or her own children. The intent of this suggestion is not to put the biological parent "in charge" in a rigid or authoritarian way, although that may be a necessary temporary measure in cases of severe adolescent acting out. In general, however, our intention is to encourage the biological parent to make major decisions and enforce general discipline and rules for his and her own children and *not* to delegate these crucial functions to a stepparent, even if such delegation feels familiar or seems convenient. A parent who is disinclined or feels unable to manage his or her children should not be encouraged to bully them (as the "put in charge" guideline is sometimes interpreted; but, rather, the entire parent-child relationship should be helped to progress to a more functional and cooperative level.

After the biological parent has taken responsibility for the day-to-day supervision of his or her children, the relationship of the children and stepparent remains to be defined and worked out by them in the light of factors such as the children's ages, the circumstances of the divorce, and the wishes of all concerned. Stepparents and stepchildren may thus work out a relationship that resembles parent (or godparent) and child, aunt or uncle, friends, or whatever other model of friendly relationship appeals to them.

This is a far cry from the assumptions of most people, women and men, that the stepmother, because she is a woman, will be responsible for the home, the children, and the emotional relationships throughout the family system. How she is to take charge of the children without wrangling with their biological mother is not considered until it happens, and then the conflict is labeled either her fault or the fault of the children's mother. Clashes between stepmothers and stepdaughters are common, since daughters feel a responsibility to protect their natural mother and get caught in this conflict over family roles. A recent study (Bray, 1986) revealed that girls in stepfamilies reported more negative stress than boys in stepfamilies or than girls in nuclear families.

Sometimes an attempt is made (by a husband or family therapist) to get the stepmother to "back off" and relinquish discipline of the stepchildren while supposedly remaining in charge of the home and the emotional tone of the family. When this happens, the situation worsens. The children make a mess of "her" house, come late to "her" meals, reflect badly on "her" at school, and she has no authority to intervene, no recourse except to nag her husband. This situation will improve only when therapy helps the family to see that it is also "his" house, "his" meals, and "his" province at school. The message that needs to be conveyed to the stepmother is *not* that her faulty wifing and mothering have created a problem in the new family that she can solve by "backing off," but rather that she has been sucked into a vacuum created by outworn social norms. And now, instead of fighting a losing battle with her husband's kids, she should support her husband's learning how to be more of a day-to-day parent to his children and how to participate more equally in household and family affairs.

The Issue of Managing Finances

Similarly, in the area of finances, only joint participation can resolve the complex and competing claims to the family's resources. Financial obligations to first families must be honored both through ongoing child support as well as in the provisions of one's will. Whether current income and expenses should be pooled, as they commonly are in first marriages, is very much open to question, depending on the sources, the nature, and the amounts of such income and expenses. Nevertheless, there is often tension and upset when a remarried wife decides to retain control of her own finances, or when a husband expects his second wife to let him manage their joint resources unilaterally, or when either of them wills "too much" to the biological children and "not enough" to the current spouse.

Like the issues of child care and household management, the issue of financial earning and management does not arise independently within each family system, awaiting that particular family's unique and creative solutions to the need for money, but rather is controlled by social norms and rules outside of the family that have for thousands of years dictated which gender, race, and social classes shall have access to the means of acquiring money, and to what degree. Against this background, it is premature to speak of *equal* financial participation by men and women in most cases, but *joint* production of income is already a fact in most American families and the age-old assumption of middle- and upper-class women that they would be financially supported throughout their lives by the men in their families is not only unfair, but unwarranted, unwise, and unsafe. This is all the more evident in remarried families, where each spouse usually has financial dependents and obligations that were incurred before the remarriage took place.

As post-divorce families change the old axiom of man-the-provider, often by default, certain sociological factors should be kept in mind by the therapist helping them: men make more money than women do, even in comparable jobs; most men expect and are trained to work and earn for life while most women to date are not; money is power, however benign, and men generally know how to act on that principle better than women do. In the area of "common sense," it should be noted that stepfamily integration and resolution of financial disputes can occur in very poor or very wealthy families, but will never occur in families where the spouses have vastly different financial resources unless equitable lifestyle and inheritance arrangements are made for the poorer spouse and her or his children.

Summary

To summarize, then, the additional phase of the family life cycle required for the formation of a functional remarried system has as its central emotional task the development of a new model of marriage and family. This new blueprint would replace the tightly boundaried nuclear family with several more loosely defined households, and several sets of extended kin, with open lines of access between them in a way that assures connectedness between all children and their biological relatives (McGoldrick and Carter, 1980; Ahrons, 1980). This model makes it more urgent and obvious than ever that the full joint participation of women and men is needed in both the emotional (child rearing) and instrumental (financial, organizational) aspects of family life. When traditional gender roles are *not* restructured in remarried systems, as they often are not, the result is the clash of different mothers trying to be emotionally responsible for the same set of children, and the roar of several fathers trying *not* to be solely financially responsible for several households. And the offices of family therapists resound with this clashing and roaring, as stepfamilies repeat the gendered problems that interfered in the first-marriage family, with even sooner and more dire consequences.

Restructuring Gender Function in the Family

Talking about a new model of family with restructured gender functioning is much easier said than done. Even granting good will and complete agreement on the ideal, the legacy of the past is hard to overcome. It's hard not to expect your new husband to support you and your children when he can earn so much more than you can and your child-support payments are so inadequate. It's hard not to expect your wife to take responsibility for your home and children when she has so many ideas about them and you're so busy at your work. In the short run, the old ways seem easier and more familiar; in the long run, the old ways don't work. But to add to the complexity, the new ways are not yet in place. This fact, that the social system does not support the restructuring of gender functioning in the family, becomes evident as soon as there is conflict. The decisions of the legal system in disputes over marital assets, alimony, child support, and even child custody (Weitzman, 1985) still favor men, and therapists must keep that fact in mind as we encourage specific families to take risks that challenge old norms.

Stepfamily Triangles

Let's look at some applications of the proposed new model to tease out predictable problems.

The Stepfather Triangle

The most common stepfamily household consists of a mother and her children living with mother's second husband. The gender issues in this constellation are subtle because it will feel quite natural to everyone for the woman to be central in the home and with her own children. Difficulties arise, however, if either she or her new husband think she can't manage her children, including adolescent sons, without his rescue operations. There also will be difficulty if everyone thinks it is *her* job to arrange a relationship between stepfather and stepchildren beyond the initial gatekeeper function of requiring her children to treat her new husband courteously and with respect. Another subtle gender issue arises if her ex-husband doesn't pay enough child support, or doesn't pay it regularly (which is a most common occurrence), and she is unable to earn enough to cover her children's expenses. It sometimes happens in this case that stepfathers may refuse to contribute even though they can easily afford to because of a competitive reaction to the failure or inability of the child's biological father to "support his own child."

In working with problems involving stepfathers, it is most helpful if the therapist supports the mother's ability to manage her children—both male and female—without "rescue" by the stepfather. De-emphasizing the stepfather's role in discipline and addressing financial issues in a direct and equitable way opens up the possibility of more positive modes of relating between the second husband and his stepchildren.

The Stepmother Triangle

The stepfamily triangle of father and his children relating to a stepmother is not the most common household composition, but this triangle nevertheless operates whenever father's children visit or phone, even if they don't live in full-time.

In this variation of the family triangle, it is father's gatekeeping responsibility to make an initial place in the existing relationship with his children for his new wife. She should not be left to fight her way in. Father needs to explain to his children that he expects them to render basic courtesy and respect to his new wife, but that she is not a replacement for their mother, or, for that matter, for him. *He* will lay down and enforce whatever rules are appropriate and necessary. Father should expect a certain amount of dismay on their part regarding his remarriage, the intensity of which will depend on the children's relationship with their mother and the relationship between the ex-spouses. He should expect the relationship between his children and his new wife to develop slowly and in accord with their own wishes about how to relate to each other, and not try to turn them over to her, or expect his wife and children to develop instant attachment.

The predictable problems in this triangle are almost entirely related to old assumptions about gender roles and are guaranteed to produce "wicked stepmothers," as reflected in the following examples:

1. Either father or his new wife, or both of them, may simply assume that *she* will be in charge of his children ("as mothers are supposed to be"), with endless resistance to that arrangement from the children *and* their mother.

2. Father's relationship with his children may be so distant or conflictual that his new wife intervenes to protect or help him and thereby gets caught in the middle.

3. Father and/or his new wife may feel that his "poor children" need a lot to make up for past unhappiness and think that such nurturance can come only from a woman. His children will resist his new wife's pressure for closeness; and she may also resent feeling that she has to provide "love" to "rude and ungrateful" children, especially if her husband criticizes her efforts instead of undertaking the nurturance himself.

4. Father may agree "in principle" to take responsibility for his children, but be so busy with work or business travel, or so inattentive or inexperienced with the children, that his new wife feels obliged to pick up the slack for him.

5. Father may deal conflictually or not at all with his ex-wife and thus require or lure his new wife into trying to do it for him "for the sake of the children."

6. The new wife may feel secondary to the children and end up competing with them for her husband's attention.

The Difficulty of Change

To counteract the problems stemming from conventional assumptions about gender role, the new model of family for remarried systems requires something like equal participation by husbands in family relationships and child rearing. The principle that women should generate income is already quite accepted by many men and women although there are fewer options regarding the amount of income women can earn, and there is frequent disagreement over the amount of female financial decision making that will be tolerated, regardless of who earns the money. Paradoxically, some men, whether from power orientation, from conditioning, or because it's woven into their identities, resist all attempts by their wives to work; and, if they can afford it, they will also support a nonworking ex-wife rather than accept drastic changes in their attitudes toward family finances. There is generally such widespread respect for men's attitudes about money that few men find their "right" to financial control challenged in family therapy.

Also paradoxically, the stepmother, who appears to have the most to gain from her husband's greater involvement in family life, will often resist his participation, fearing that it threatens the identity and expertise she has been taught to achieve at the center of the family. She is, nevertheless, universally challenged in family therapy to "back off." However, interventions that fail to validate her expertise and her concern with family relationships will probably *not* succeed. The change required is not simply *her* backing off, but rather that *both* spouses redefine and redistribute responsibilities so that she is no longer in the impossible position of trying to get *his* children to go along with the rules of "*her*" household. It will be necessary, therefore, not only to relieve the stepmother of her disciplinary role, but also to help her and her stepchildren to define and work toward a mutually satisfactory new relationship of some kind.

Stepfamily Formation Following Death

Although the vast majority of stepfamilies are formed following divorce, a word should be said about some of the different issues that arise in stepfamilies formed after the premature death of a parent. Again, there are gender issues: a stepfather may be perceived as rescuing a family from poverty following the death of the primary wage earner, whereas most children tend to view their mother as completely irreplaceable. However, when children are young, a stepparent, including a stepmother, will eventually be accepted as a "real" parent if the natural parent can help the children to grieve and then to accept the new person in his or her own right rather than collude with the children in wanting a "replacement" and continuation of the old family in every way.

Although there are certain advantages in stepfamilies formed following a death in that no ex-spouse is around to "interfere," still ghosts can be even more powerful, especially given the tendency to idealize someone who is lost prematurely. All of the family triangles will occur predictably but may be harder to recognize and deal with when one of the people in the triangle is a dead person. Talking, remembering, and acknowledging the dead person's human failings and foibles help to exorcize the ghost, but none of this can be done without the active leadership of the remaining natural parent. Children who are adolescent or older generally resist attempts to "replace" their dead parent, and the wise stepparent will honor that position.

The Couple

It is no accident that the relationship of the remarried couple comes last. The degree of adjustment, the difficulties, the complicated triangles, and the amount of disturbed behavior, acting out, or uproar is directly related to the number of children affected by the remarriage. Although they may have met, courted, and married with the idea that they were a "couple," they are soon inundated with so many "family" problems that their sense of identity as a couple is at serious risk, and, in fact, cannot be really separated from their relationships with children. Dahl, Cowgill, and Asmundsson (1987) found that marital satisfaction in stepfamilies correlated with the stepparents' good relationships with stepchildren. Booth and White (1985) found that remarried couples with children were more than twice as likely to redivorce.

The burden of conducting a satisfactory marriage in the presence of so many adjustments and complex relationships falls disproportionately on the wife, who is still held responsible by everyone, including herself, to make it all work. Although the problems presented to the therapist will almost always involve stepchildren, it is important for the clinician to give a great deal of attention and support throughout therapy to the couple bond, which, at least in the beginning, is the newest and weakest bond in the family.

The Challenge

The very high rates of divorce and redivorce in the United States have created an "alternate" family structure that is encountered in the office of family therapists as often, or more often, than the intact family structure that most of us were raised in and trained to work with. The challenge to us is this: Are we willing to reexamine our ideas about functional family structure to be helpful to these families, or will we continue to do what we know and to think of remarried family structures as "broken" and needing to be "fixed?"

If we open our minds to the possibilities in these new structures, we find that many of the changes that women have struggled to obtain in first-marriage families, but which were usually resisted as "too radical," suddenly make a lot of sense in a family system that just doesn't work when we try to polarize roles according to gender.

In remarried families, each spouse may bring to the system children and financial resources that were created independent of the new union. At the point of joining together to create a new family structure, each spouse is responsible for his and her own children and finances. Will their new marriage help each of them to continue to evolve in the direction of full participation in both the emotional and instrumental aspects of life, or will it be a reason for relapse to outworn patterns?

To the degree that either spouse enters the new marriage to be relieved of financial stress or to have child rearing managed by the new spouse, to that degree the new marriage will be burdened and eventually broken off if the burden is too great. Before that happens, "enlightened" family therapy can help husband and wife to continue to develop a family structure that works for all of its members.

The following cases illustrate several approaches to typical problems encountered in the complex transition to remarriage.

cases

Betty Carter

"I Don't Know Which of These Mothers Is Worse!"

This case exemplifies a rather frequent scenario in my teaching experience: a family therapist blaming the women in the remarried family for its difficulties and engaging in a frustrating struggle with the stepmother to get her to "back off." Several factors converge to produce this stalemate. In the family, the stepmother has "naturally" moved in to take care of the children, and has, of course, found herself in a competitive position vis-à-vis the children's mother. She gets angry and frustrated when she gets criticism instead of gratitude for her caretaking efforts, and is especially hurt when her husband joins the chorus of complainers. The final straw is added when the therapist echoes what her husband, his ex-wife, and the children have been saying: "Back off." Now it will be hard for her not to feel blamed by the therapist for doing a bad job. She will also wonder anxiously why the therapist can't see that the children need to be taken care of, and who else is to do it if she "backs off?"

The female family therapist is hampered in several ways. First, she herself has been socialized to defer to men and compete with women; second, she is tuned in to the welfare of children and holds the mother or "mother-figure" chiefly responsible for child care; third, she is reactive to the angry tone of the stepmother and misses the components of pain and anxiety in her complaints. Last but not least, her theory tells her that the "pursuer" must "back off" so that the "distancer" can enter. And so she creates a system of therapy exactly isomorphic to the family problem: one woman arguing with another about what's right for the children.

The Trainee's Presentation

The Brown family came to family therapy because the husband's young daughter, Karen, was doing poorly in school. Richard Brown shifted around uncomfortably while his wife, Phyllis, articulated a long list of angry complaints about her stepchildren, Richard's 16-year-old son, Richie, and 10-year-old daughter, Karen. Richard and Phyllis had been married 18 months ago, 6 months after Richard obtained a divorce from his former wife, Mary, which was precipitated by the affair between Richard and Phyllis. Phyllis had also been married previously, had been divorced for about 5 years, and had two young adult daughters who were on their own, sharing an apartment in New York City.

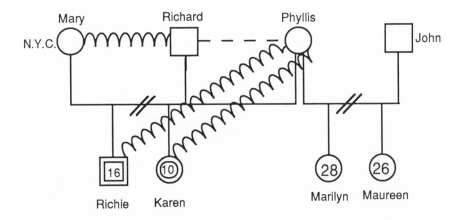

See page 96 for an extended definition of the genogram.

"I'm in the same spot again, only worse," said Phyllis angrily. "I left my first husband because I was tired of doing everything and then being criticized for it, which is just what's happening how, and they're not even my goddamned kids!" She then gave a detailed description of young Richie's lateness for dinner, sloppy room, late nights out, and rudeness to her. Karen, whom she sarcastically called "the princess," was "spoiled, lazy, and unhealthy," but her husband argued with everything that she (Phyllis) tried to do to help "these poor motherless children."

The children's mother, Mary, who had moved from the suburbs to New York City after Richard and Phyllis's marriage, retained joint custody of the children, saw them approximately every other weekend and during vacations, and felt they were better off living in the suburbs in their father's household while she tried to build a new career and resumed dating. Mary was furious at Richard and Phyllis, had not wanted the divorce, and spoke to them as briefly and infrequently as possible, never initiating contact herself. Richard said he couldn't deal with his ex-wife, who was "unhinged" by the divorce, even though they had had "a terrible marriage." Phyllis, who said Mary was a "heartless woman who never should have had children," felt she had to call Mary from time to time when Karen's health or school problems were "out of hand." Phyllis said, "Mary has always been a negligent mother and the children show it. I try not to blame these kids for their poor upbringing, but they drive me crazy, and I get no support from him."

Richard explained in a quiet, reasonable tone that Mary had not been a negligent mother but was now understandably angry at all of them. "She'll get over it, if Phyllis leaves her alone." He then said that he fully supported Phyllis's willingness to "be a mother" to his kids, but felt that her "standards of kid behavior and cleanliness" were much too rigid, and that she brought most of the tension on herself by trying to "reform" them all with her endless nagging and complaining.

The family therapy trainee, a woman of 34, turned off the videotape at this point and said: "You can see why I'm stuck—I don't know which of these mothers is worse, and the poor kids are really getting the brunt of it. The father is very devoted to the kids and does everything to keep his ex-wife involved with them and to keep Phyllis off their necks, but it's a losing battle, as you can see. She's a very controlling person and she just won't back off." The trainee had spent many sessions trying vainly to convince "the pursuer" (Phyllis) to "back off," and stop nagging Richard and his children, and she (the trainee) was feeling angry and defeated.

Redefining the Problem

As supervisor, I first addressed the impasse experienced by the trainee. This consisted first of challenging her idea that Mary was a "bad mother" because she had relinquished physical custody of her children and was pursuing her career and social life. In the supervision group, we counted seven current clinical cases and three personal

trainee divorces in which the fathers had relinquished physical custody, were pursuing their careers and dating, and were considered to
be "dedicated fathers."

We then listed all of Phyllis's complaints and found they could be
placed in two categories: (1) "worried about the children" and (2)
"trying to make this a real family and a nice home." The trainee agreed
that these were not the concerns of a bad wife or mother. We then
scrutinized Richard's role in all of this and discovered that he always
spoke calmly and reasonably, and that he expressed great understanding of his ex-wife, tolerance for his new wife, and concern for his
children. However, we had come to find out that he didn't deal with his
ex-wife at all; he criticized his new wife a lot; and he didn't take
responsibility for setting any rules for his children at home, nor did he
act on their behalf with the school, doctors, and the like. He had never
been given any tasks by the therapist or been engaged by her in any
discussion of his feelings about his divorce and whether he was satisfied with how he had ended that marriage.

Strategies in Therapy

When the therapist realized that she had indeed blamed Mary for
"abandoning" the children and Phyllis for "nagging" them, and had not
tried to engage Richard to any significant degree in dealing with his
family problems in therapy, she was able to pursue the different course
recommended in supervision.

Among her primary objectives, she set out to stop struggling with
Phyllis; to validate Phyllis's concerns for children and family; to redirect her efforts to integrate the new family away from rules such as
required attendance at family dinner every night and toward other
rituals that would be chosen by all family members; and to engage
Phyllis, Richie, and Karen in an exploration and reshaping of their
relationship in a way that didn't ignore the fact that they already had a
mother and father. The therapist also worked to engage Richard very
actively in his children's lives, in consultation with both Mary and
Phyllis. She sought to get him to stop criticizing Phyllis's efforts to
help his children. And she engaged Richard in an exploration of his
feelings of guilt toward Mary, and encouraged him to work at resolving
the divorce emotionally and learning how to negotiate with Mary
effectively about the children. The therapist contacted Mary and offered to meet with her if she wished to give advice or express concern
regarding her children. And she behaved in a manner that assumed
that Mary is a concerned, involved mother.

In addition, the therapist scheduled some meetings that included
Phyllis's daughters to see in what form they wished to pursue these

new stepfamily relationships. And she suggested therapeutic work with the families of origin of both Richard and Phyllis.

Summary

If therapists have to be taught slogans to work by, I'd like to suggest an important change. Let's get rid of "Get the pursuer to back off so the distancer can move in," and replace it with "*Validate the concerns of the more involved one and challenge the distance of the one less involved.*" This will aim the trainee therapist in the right direction without suggesting that the more involved spouse is to blame for the problem, or is blocking the less involved spouse, or that the less involved one will *automatically* move in if the involved one "backs off."

In this family, Phyllis was quite right to wonder who would take care of these children if she "backed off." Their mother lived elsewhere, and their father was a very busy businessman who expected her to handle the child care (although she also worked full time). Her "backing off" made no sense at all in the absence of an explicit plan to redistribute responsibilities in an unconventional way. As long as everyone, including the therapist, saw the problem as "Phyllis nagging her husband and his children," of course she would be urged to "back off." Then the problem was redefined as "Why on earth is Phyllis the only one in the family who is trying to establish new child-care routines and new family rituals to help you all to integrate?" This reframing of the problem, which challenged everyone's assumption that it is somehow the wife's job to create the new family, can lead to a redistribution of responsibilities and a sharing of goals that is much more complex and all-encompassing than one person's "backing off," although that too will occur along with the other necessary shifts in family structure, roles, and relationships.

Peggy Papp

". . . To Love Her Like a Mother"

This case deals with the mistaken notion, prevalent in remarried families, that a stepmother can and should love a stepchild like her own. This unreal expectation is part of a whole cluster of expectations centered around the shared illusion that the new wife will somehow magically pick up all the broken pieces and put them back together again. She is expected to assuage guilt, repair relationships, heal wounds, dissipate depression, and mediate conflicts. Since she has been conditioned to expect all this of herself, she automatically assumes this responsibility in her new family, only to find it an impossible job.

In this case, it is this whole cluster of unreal expectations that finally pushes the wife into wanting to leave the marriage. Having followed the dictates of a "good wife" while ignoring her own feelings and needs, she revolts when her husband brings his daughter into their home and expects the new wife to make up to the daughter for all her past hurts. At the time of this consultation, the wife can see no other solution than to leave the marriage. In the consultation, I focus on the impossible expectations that have been placed on the wife and suggest a ritual to change them.

The Presenting Problem

The therapist brought the couple into the auditorium where I had agreed to see them for a live consultation during a workshop. The therapist introduced me to Jim, a large, husky man with a very red face, and Flo, a small fragile woman with a reticent manner. The therapist had asked for the consultation because Jim was not able to "break through the wife's negative and pessimistic attitude" toward the marriage. The therapist described the husband as "highly motivated and desperate to preserve their relationship," but the wife remained "unresponsive and resistant" to the therapist's attempts to bring about a reconciliation. The therapist attributed the wife's intransigence to a "fear of closeness" and to her "overinvolvement with her family of origin."

The therapist presented the following synopsis: Jim, 50, and Flo, 36, had been married 12 years. This was the second marriage for Jim and the first for Flo. They had an 8-year-old son and a 6-year-old daughter, and the husband had two daughters, 17 and 19, who lived with his ex-wife after their divorce.

The couple initially came to therapy because of an impasse regarding financial matters but soon conceded that the problems were "much, much deeper," having to do with a "lack of communication." The therapist described Flo as having difficulty expressing her feelings; she kept them bottled up inside her and withdrew from the relationship with her husband. This served to escalate Jim's natural tendency toward jealousy and possessiveness, and he would fly into explosive rages. Recently Flo had become very pessimistic about the marriage, and in therapy sessions began saying she thought she wanted a divorce. Jim became frightened, and kept trying to persuade her to stay in the marriage.

The Consultation Session

I began the consultation by asking the couple what they hoped to get out of our meeting together. Flo said she didn't know if there was any reason for them to be there because she wasn't sure if she wanted to stay in the marriage. Initially, she had difficulty putting her thoughts and feelings into words but gradually, through my questioning, she became more articulate. She began to talk about how she felt her husband had a great need to control everyone, both at work and at home, and she felt suffocated by this control and all the demands he placed on her. She accused him of being overbearing and possessive, and said he had physically tried to stop her from seeing her friends and family. The husband claimed that was all in the past, and that he had reformed. The reason he objected to her seeing her family so much, he said, was that she was overly involved with them. He felt she preferred to be with them rather than with him, and that she spent too much time with them. Flo replied that she turned to them for support and understanding when it was not forthcoming from him.

The husband, looking frightened, made an eloquent plea to Flo to stay and to try and work things out. He begged, cajoled, apologized, promised, scolded, and ended with a long, patronizing lecture on the virtues of married life and the importance of sticking it out. "You can't just give up when the going gets tough. You have to find the courage and strength of character to hang in there. You can't just break up a home because you're unhappy." When I interrupted the lecture to ask why he thought Flo was so intent on leaving, he became teary-eyed and said in a shaky voice that he had done some very bad things in the past for which he was sorry and was willing to try and make amends.

When asked to be more specific about those "very bad things," he said he had been neglectful of his wife when they were first married and had imposed on her problems stemming from his old marriage. He had initiated a custody suit in an effort to obtain custody of his two daughters shortly after he and Flo were married. Flo broke in to say that he had been obsessed with obtaining custody of his children and thought about nothing else, day or night. He became embroiled in a bitter court battle that he eventually lost, after which he became profoundly depressed. Flo kept trying to bring him out of his depression, but he remained inconsolable, and she felt isolated and lonely. She had resented his complete absorption with winning the suit and thought it had something to do with his anger toward his former wife. At the time of the suit, Flo had never mentioned this opinion, nor had she ever complained, because she felt she was expected to go along with him. "I was trying hard to please my husband. It seemed so important to him. I thought if I complained he would leave me."

I asked Flo what finally made her decide to complain. She said the straw that broke the camel's back was Jim's 19-year-old daughter, Sharon, coming to live with them. Sharon had had a fight with her mother and asked her father if she could move in with them. Jim agreed without asking Flo, but Flo accepted it, knowing how much Jim's daughter meant to him. Jim then tried to make up to Sharon for what he considered to be his desertion of her by showering her with privileges and gifts, catering to her every whim, refusing to discipline her, and allowing her the complete run of the house. He expected his wife to do the same thing—"to handle her and love her like a mother and make up to her for everything her own mother didn't give her when she was growing up."

Sharon took advantage of her father's indulgences and became more and more antagonistic toward Flo, who was left with the unrewarding job of trying to discipline her and set rules. Sharon and Flo became embroiled in frequent arguments; Jim reacted to them by alternately placating and burying his head in the sand. Finally, Flo interrupted a heated battle with Sharon one day to lay down an ultimatum to both Sharon and Jim, saying, "This is the way it is going to be around here and anyone who doesn't like it can leave." Sharon left; Jim stayed but harbored resentment toward Flo and periodically accused her of throwing his daughter out.

When I asked Flo at what point she felt the most hopeless about the marriage working out, she said it was whenever Jim left the house to visit Sharon. This created enormous tension between them because she could feel Jim silently blaming her. Jim accused Flo of objecting to his having a close relationship with his daughter. Flo denied it, saying the only thing she objected to was his blaming her for the situation.

Reframing the Problem

At the end of the session, I excused the couple for a coffee break and elicited the workshop participants' reaction to the situation. The sympathies of most of the group members clearly lay with the husband, who had moved them with his poignant efforts to keep his wife from leaving. After all, he was contrite, had apologized, and was reaching out to his wife, who remained reserved and distant. Solutions to the problem were offered mainly in terms of what the wife needed to do. Some suggested she would have to make amends with Sharon in order to repair the rift between herself and Jim; some saw her as being jealous of Sharon and the attention Jim gave his daughter; others believed the therapist should explore the "overinvolvement" with her family of origin that prevented Flo from being close to Jim; and others suggested she must first forgive Jim for past grievances.

I had a different point of view, which I presented to the therapist and the group. I saw the major problem as Jim having expected Flo to do the impossible, which was to love his daughter "like a mother." Not only had Jim placed an unreal expectation on Flo, but he had then abdicated his role as parent by leaving up to her all the responsibility for disciplining Sharon. He then blamed Flo for not being able to get along with Sharon, which left her in a no-win situation.

Based on this evaluation of the problem, and with the consent of their therapist, I gave the couple the following feedback. I told the husband that by putting her foot down with Sharon, Flo had saved both Sharon and their marriage. She knew Sharon could never grow up and become an adult as long as her father treated her like a baby, so Flo made it possible for Sharon to leave and become independent. And Flo had saved their marriage because she knew it could never survive with Sharon in between them. Therefore, every time Jim left to visit Sharon, he ought to kiss his wife goodbye and say, "Thank you for helping Sharon to grow up and for saving our marriage."

The couple looked at one another in surprise and then smiled at the unexpected reframing. I then suggested that both Flo and Jim invite Sharon to visit them after the two of them had decided together on the specific conditions of the visit. They were to agree on the time, duration, and circumstances of the visit. Jim was to inform Sharon of these conditions, and Flo was then to join him in extending their welcome to Sharon.

The suggestion that Jim thank Flo rather than blame her removed the unreal expectation that had made it impossible for her to remain in the marriage. Having to agree on the conditions for Sharon's visit gave Flo joint authority and Jim joint responsibility for Sharon's behavior. Sharon would be expected to behave like a young adult rather than a child, and this might pave the way for a different relationship among all three.

Summary

This case exemplifies some of the typical processes that take place in remarried families when the husband and wife share unrealistic expectations regarding the wife's role. These expectations put an onerous burden on the wife, who is then blamed for not fulfilling them. The wife is often unaware that she is attempting the impossible, since repairing relationships has been part of her gender training. The therapeutic intervention reframed the wife's "failure" to love her stepdaughter like a mother as saving both the daughter and the marriage. It increased the wife's authority and the father's responsibility in such a way as to make it possible for the daughter to be included in their life together.

Olga Silverstein

Cinderella Revisited

Introduction

The mythology about stepmothers is so pervasive that it is often difficult for members of a family or, for that matter, a therapist, to distinguish between fact and fiction. If a child has been orphaned at an early age it can be particularly difficult for a new stepmother, her good intentions notwithstanding. The family issues that are at the root of the problem include the following:

1. The dyadic bond between a child and a surviving parent can seem impenetrable.
2. The expectation (by both child and father) of reparation for all the child has suffered is often unrealistic.
3. A woman too eager to prove that *she* will never be a wicked stepmother may try too hard and so, inadvertently, tighten the bond that excludes her.
4. A young woman, whether 10 or 20 years old, who has been the mistress in her father's house does not give up that role easily.
5. A father, who has felt inadequate to the task of raising a daughter, particularly if she presents problems, can be too

eager to turn her over to the stepmother with the false belief that she needs a "mother" to straighten her out.

6. The new wife's own children, struggling to incorporate a new spouse into their tight little circle, may find a stepsister one insult too many.

7. A guilty father may attempt to pay an unhappy child off by overindulging her—by false declarations of his devotion or by allowing himself to be manipulated into buying expensive presents.

All of these issues and dynamics were operating in this case, along with the usual difficulties that emerge following so great a change as the joining of two fragmented families.

The Family

Gilbert, the father, 49, was a big man, 50 pounds overweight. He had an air of authority. His wife, Judy, was attractive, well-dressed, and manicured. I estimated her age to be close to Gilbert's. Bringing up the rear was 20-year-old Leslie. I imagine that people seeing the young Marilyn Monroe might have had similar reactions of awe and pity. She was incredibly beautiful and looked extremely pathetic. Dressed in the costume of her generation—torn jeans, a big loose shirt, sneakers—she looked unkempt and uncaring. When I greeted this family at the door, Gilbert grasped my hand fervently and Judy shook hands cooly as if to say, "What am I doing here? It's not my problem." Leslie put her hand in mine limply, but kept her eyes on the floor.

Gilbert began by telling me the problem—Leslie. Leslie was breaking up his marriage. She was a slob—look at her. Her room was an utter mess. She couldn't keep a job. When he paused for breath, Judy would urge him on. "Tell her about that boy" or "Tell her about the time . . ." While he talked, Leslie kept her eyes down, but tears flowed silently down her cheeks. "Don't get sucked in by this beautiful child," I cautioned myself. She suddenly raised her head and looked at me. I caught my breath as she revealed huge violet tear-filled eyes. "She hates me," she confided in a small husky voice.

Gilbert jumped right in on cue. "She doesn't hate you, sweetheart. Nobody hates you." He looked at me helplessly. "I don't know," I said.

The Family Story

They then told me the following story. Leslie's mother died at her birth. Gilbert said that he didn't know she had a bad heart; had he known he never would have allowed her to become pregnant. Leslie's silent tears started again. Gilbert said, "Don't cry, honey."

He hired a succession of housekeepers for the child, and married again when Leslie was 4. When Gilbert's father died, leaving him (an only child) a large family business, he stopped working. "I think I was depressed. I know I was depressed. Anyway, that marriage lasted two years and then we were alone again. Leslie was a very good little girl, but she never got along with her housekeepers. I think I was a lousy father. I ran around a lot, was never home."

"When I met Judy," he continued, "I thought she was very attractive, but I fell in love with her when I saw her with her kids. Judy has four children, the youngest is Leslie's age. They are wonderful kids. They all live on their own now, but they're close—very close," he said, looking at Judy fondly. "I thought, 'Here's the mother Leslie deserves.' But it hasn't worked out that way. Leslie just won't cooperate. Don't you want me to be happy, sweetheart?" He looked at Leslie archly.

She never looked up. Judy said, "I told Gil that either she goes or I go. He never says no to her. He constantly makes excuses for her. No matter what she does, he tells me, 'She never had a mother.' Well, I'm not her mother. If I treat her as I did my own kids, she locks herself in her room and cries. I'm fed up."

Leslie finally looked up, straight at her stepmother. "She sits in the kitchen talking to her daughter for hours. If I walk in, they stop talking and just look at me till I walk out again. How do you think that makes me feel? I had to move out of my room, into the maid's room because—I don't know why." Gil whispered, "It was too close to our bedroom, it made Judy uncomfortable. You know."

On and on, the list of mutual gripes seemed endless. I tried to shift focus but it was very difficult. I'd get a short answer, and then back to Leslie, her hair, her manners, her clothes, her joblessness, et cetera, et cetera.

The Family Dilemma

Gilbert was obviously caught between the two women. He jumped from side to side in response to their behavior. When Judy complained about Leslie he not only joined her, but outdid her. If Leslie was then upset, he reassured and comforted her, and often rewarded her by giving her money or gifts.

Leslie was equally caught between her father and her stepmother. Although she obviously admired the older woman and longed for a friendship with her, she could not relinquish her role as "poor little orphan" as long as her father pandered to it and her stepmother objected to it.

Judy was caught by maintaining her parental role as the setter of rules and standards for both Gil and his daughter, who joined covertly to defy her, thus keeping her in the outside position. Gilbert's very determination to put Judy at the center of his daughter's life paradoxically kept her out.

Family therapy has tended to elevate the parental relationship above the parent-child relationship, perhaps in reaction to the child-centered families of the fifties and sixties. I felt that a therapeutic move in that direction would further alienate the two women to the loss and detriment of both. A primary protection of the marital relationship could lead to precipitously propelling Leslie out of the house into an illusion of "independent" living, a move too often applauded by a culture fixated on autonomy. More information was needed.

THERAPIST: (*To Gil*) Tell me a little bit about yourself. Are you working?

GIL: (*A little embarrassed*) No. I should be, but I just can't seem to get going. When my Dad died I think I had a little breakdown. I drank a lot. Anyway, I didn't really have to work, the business took care of itself. I think I was afraid to go in. Nobody liked me there.

THERAPIST: So what did you do?

GIL: Well, till I met Judy I hung around the house a lot. When you're depressed you don't care much where you are. I watched television.

THERAPIST: And now?

GIL: Now it's different. Judy and I spend our time together. She's a wonderful woman. We shop. We play cards. Go out to eat.

THERAPIST: How old are you, Gil?

GIL: (*Looking embarrassed*) Forty-nine. You think I should work, don't you? Well, so do I, but I can't go in there. They look at me like some snot-nosed kid. They don't want me there, that's for sure. What can I do, sell shoes? That would be stupid.

THERAPIST: (*To Judy*) What do you think?

JUDY: Well, it's hard to have a man around the house all day, but it's up to him.

THERAPIST: Gil tells me you're a wonderful mother.

JUDY: Well, I've raised my kids alone. They're terrific kids.

THERAPIST: How old are they now?

JUDY: Twenty-six, 24, 23, and 20. Their father died ten years ago.

THERAPIST: That had to be pretty tough.

JUDY: You better believe it.

THERAPIST: How did you manage?

JUDY: I had a little money, not much. But the kids worked, I worked. We did fine.

THERAPIST: And now?

JUDY: Now I hang out with Gil and wait for something to happen. (*She laughed.*) You know, he's like a big kid. No, I mean a little kid. He wants to play. (*She shook her head.*) He wants to play all the time. I sometimes feel like a camp counselor. (*She then told me that she's seven years older than Gil, that they met in a bar where she had gone for the first time.*) Would you believe—the very first time? He was there for the first time and so was I. But he was just bored. So was I. He just never knew what to do with himself. Now I keep him pretty busy.

THERAPIST: How is that for you?

JUDY: Well, it beats working and going home alone at night. Right?

THERAPIST: I don't know. You didn't answer my question.

JUDY: It's not easy. I'm not used to a man who is always around. Mind you, he's sweet and good-natured enough, if you keep things moving. I get a little tired. I'm fed up with his darling daughter.

THERAPIST: We were talking about you and Gil.

JUDY: Never mind. We would be fine. It's Leslie. She hangs around the house all day with that long face. Gil can't take his eyes off her. One tear and he reaches for his wallet. With me, it's different. The money—I have to ask and wheedle. Leslie just looks with those moon eyes. She drives me crazy. If she were my kid—

THERAPIST: What would you do if she was your kid?

JUDY: I'd lay down the law. I'd see that she went to school, or to work. Imagine, a 20-year-old slob around the house all day?

LESLIE: *They* don't do anything, but she expects me to do everything—

THERAPIST: Like what?

LESLIE: Go to work. Clean. I hate her. I walk in the kitchen and she says, "What do you want?" It's my house, isn't it? She's almost as mean to him. I think she would be, but he just walks away. Or he goes out and buys her something. I hate her.

Evaluation and Strategy

Between sessions I wrote down the following facts.

1. Gil behaves like one of the children—looking to Judy for support and leadership, then joining his daughter in subverting Judy's attempts to impose some structure on their lives.

2. Judy treats Gil as if he were a retarded child—affectionately. But she patronizes him. She confronts him only about Leslie, although she has many issues that concern him directly.
3. Both Gil and Judy are afraid to jeopardize the new marriage. Both have suffered loss and are overly careful with each other.
4. Leslie behaves like a spoiled child, but she too has suffered loss. The early loss of her mother was compounded by the emotional absence of her father.

Then I asked myself, what's my task and in what order? I came up with the following goals, listed in the order of their importance:

1. To find a way to unite the two women in a common cause. At this point, that focus can be only around Gil's welfare.
2. To elevate and empower both women without patronizing or decentering Gil.
3. To help Gil assume a more parental role with his daughter— for example, setting limits and expectations for more mature behavior.
4. To help Leslie on the way to a more mature and self-motivated level of functioning, first by joining her stepmother as another woman and, second, by joining with her stepsiblings as young people who are members of the same household. (The latter turned out to be the easiest part. It was accomplished by seeing all five young people several times without their parents. They shared stories and experiences and finally joined in some good-natured complaints about the parents. As Judy's children expressed some negative feelings about their mother, Leslie was able to share some concerns about her father. They all agreed that it was a relief that the two parents could now depend more on each other, and not so much on the children.)
5. To help Gil face his fear of loss, and consequently ease up his inertia and paralysis, so that he could move toward evaluating his own life and goals for himself.

Subsequent Sessions

THERAPIST: (*Addressing Judy and Leslie*) It's becoming quite clear how the two of you collude to take care of Gil. You, Leslie, refuse to get on with your own young life in order to act as a stand-in for your dad in his marriage. You know very well that if you were out of the house, Judy might be a bit impatient with having a demanding 49-year-old man around the house all the time. And you, Judy, you put aside everything you know about good mothering (and anyone who has raised four good kids knows a lot) to join Leslie in protecting Gil from the things you find difficult in his behavior.

THERAPIST: (*To Gil*) It's hard for me to understand why they are so protective of you. In a way it seems disrespectful, as though they think you couldn't take a little conflict. I don't know.

In subsequent sessions Judy talked about her unhappiness, and Gil admitted that he was afraid to leave her alone—she might disappear. Leslie joined him by saying, "That would be a disaster!" She and Judy exchanged a knowing look.

In the following session I encouraged Judy to exercise her relationship skills with Leslie, pointing out that they had made such a good team in Gil's behalf, maybe they could do something for each other. Leslie was defying Judy, who was trying too hard to be a mother. Maybe they could settle for being distant relatives, or good friends, or maybe just friends.

In the final session Judy was urging Gil to go down to the store and take his rightful place there, and he was considering how and when to do it. Leslie had enrolled in a cooking school, planning to be a chef. Judy suggested that she get a job in a restaurant first. Gil protested. "What? Wait on tables. That's ridiculous." Leslie said quietly, "No, Dad, I think she's right."

Summary

This case was difficult work, and stretched over a period of a year and a half. There is no way to avoid some conflict around the integration of two family systems, each with its own center, each with its set of rules both overt and covert, each determined to maintain its own integrity and stability. By the time a remarried family comes to a therapist's office, they have generally reorganized around a central problem, frequently around a problem with a child. Since the assumption is that it's the woman's job to manage children (hers as well as his), by implication she has failed if there's a problem in this area and is perforce the wicked stepmother. In addition to the unique family dynamics, a therapist needs to recognize the complex social factors, including prescriptive gender role functions and the impasse they create, which have such powerful impact on the family.

Marianne Walters

Is What You Need
What You Want?

Typically when men and women enter therapy together they present themselves in quite different ways. Women will make "we" statements and men will make "I" statements; women will ask, "What did I do wrong?" and men will ask, "What went wrong?"; women will seek interpersonal transformation and men will seek problem resolution. Such patterns seem to be even more pronounced in remarried couples, perhaps because they will have taken root and settled in during their previous marriage(s). Indeed, these broad, gendered patterns of behavior are at the very foundation of most couple systems, and will be entrenched in the behavioral repertoire of each partner as they enter a new couple or marital relationship. Often even the effort to "make things different" in the new marriage serves only to exacerbate this coupling paradigm. In her discussion, Betty Carter has described many of the complexities and pitfalls for the remarried family that tend to polarize the habits and interactional patterns each spouse brings into the new marriage. Mothers and stepmothers will continue to compete with each other around the care of the children so long as child rearing remains their primary source of social approval; and fathers and step-fathers will continue to distance themselves from the family fray so long as their power remains associated with the belief that this is not their domain.

Despite the increasing number of remarried couples and blended families there remains a social ambiguity surrounding the relationships both within, and between, these couples or families. Of course, this is particularly true where children are involved. Images of wicked stepmothers and bumbling stepfathers haven't changed that much. And when either partner has children the reasons for the remarriage itself are shrouded in cultural myths and social mores. Perhaps you remember those long-running, ever popular films *The Sound of Music* and *Mary Poppins*? Oh, how I loved those movies. So much so that I hardly noticed the message they were transmitting to all of us romantic souls: that a good man, with children, finds love in the arms of a woman who will be a good mother to his children!

In my therapy I work for a reconstruction of the presenting scenario, offering the family a new set of "cues" by using their content as counterpoint to feedback on their process. The struggle to incorporate a feminist perspective in my therapy suggested new ways to offer clients a conceptual revision of their dilemma, ways that retain some of our systemic analysis while correcting for the inevitable biases of the larger systems of thought within which it is embedded. So, for instance, as in the case description below, a reframing that uses the concept of the "function of the symptom" is expanded to make the connection between function and socially prescribed behaviors, gender development, and the collective experience of women. This does not have to be "heavy-handed," nor does it mean lecturing on equality or shared power in the family! Quite the opposite. Concepts of gendered behavior, socially constructed and common to many, contain a "truth," a collective consciousness, that enables people to experience an immediate "Aha!"—an attachment to an idea that is at once depathologizing and humanizing.

In working with remarried families my initial interventions are focused on the *current* couple and/or family relationships, not on the preconditions of their marriage, such as previously divorced, multiple marriages, single, widowed, children from previous marriages, and so forth. Remarried couples, and their children from previous marriages, often focus on what has gone on before, on previous conflicts and failures, or on unresolved issues from those previous relationships. I work initially to redirect their energy toward strengthening their new relationships and building new family patterns, arrangements, and routines. In family sessions my effort is to focus the family on their current interactional process. Often this renders the new family more competent to deal themselves with the complexities of previous marriages, several sets of grandparents, more than one family raising the children, child support, child custody issues, and the like. At any rate, with the new family strengthened, ongoing therapy, where needed, can utilize their new behaviors, individually and as a family, to confront the complex issues involved in constructing multiple families within the same generation.

My case is based on a consultation session which—since the purpose of such sessions is to redirect the therapy—I structure much as I would an initial session, within a framework that is discussed below.

Consultations

As part of a workshop I was doing in a southern state, I was asked to have a consultation interview with a recently remarried couple who were having a great deal of difficulty in adjusting to their new (eight-month) marriage. The interview was done "live," closed-circuited to the workshop participants. The therapist had been working with the couple for about a year prior to their marriage and was seeing them through their early months of adjustment. The quality of his work was evident in the readiness of this couple to "hear" new information. He had requested the consultation because he felt therapy had plateaued and had become a series of "putting out fires." The most serious of these "fires" had occurred about six weeks before I saw the couple: The husband, Pete, who is in Alcoholics Anonymous and had been sober for over a year, went on a binge following a fight with his wife, Sara Jean. Sara Jean, also a member of AA, who has maintained sobriety for over three years, asked him to leave the house. They were separated for five weeks and Pete returned to their home just a few days before our interview.

A word about consultations. Whenever I do a consultation, the therapist joins me with the family so that I can get his or her feedback about ongoing directions and can turn to him or her for confirmation or disagreement about my observations and perception of family members and family processes. The therapist's prior and more substantial knowledge of the family is always affirmed. Our agreements before the consultation are that I will conduct the interview, will ask for his or her feedback, and that he or she should be cautious about entering into the interview process. If the therapist has a substantive disagreement or concern, we might absent ourselves from the session and discuss it. The consultation is always about seeking a new direction in the therapy. It can demonstrate some therapy techniques but is never about "doing therapy." Doing therapy requires an ongoing commitment and relationship, and, most important, accountability. When one does a consultation, particularly outside of one's own place of practice, these absolutely necessary parameters of any therapy are absent.

The Family

Sara Jean and Pete live in a small town and traveled for several hours for the consultation session. Both husband and wife have a history of alcoholism, and both have had previous marriages. Pete's two adolescent children, a boy and a girl, live with their mother in another state and he, regrettably, has minimal contact with them. Sara Jean has two sons, ages 6 and 10, who live with the couple. Both spouses come from families in which there was abuse and alcoholism and continual fighting. They dated, and then lived together for three years before their marriage. Sara Jean is a bridal consultant in a department store and probably wonderful at it. She has a soft, gracious quality with a tough, no-nonsense edge to it. Pete manages a fast-food restaurant. He is big and strong, with a kind of gentle clumsiness. And these two fight and argue interminably. Perhaps their saving grace is a shared sense of the ironic.

Earlier in their relationship they had fought over his drinking and her previous marriage. Since their marriage they fight and argue mostly about the children—rules, expectations, and who's to set them. Pete feels Sara Jean is too easy on the kids and overprotects them. He complains that they are undisciplined and out of control. Sara Jean thinks Pete goes about his efforts to discipline the kids in the wrong way, that he doesn't understand them. Pete feels she doesn't appreciate all he does for the kids. Their life together is chaotic; both want some order, but claim they don't know how to achieve it.

This state of affairs was exacerbated by Sara Jean's ex-husband who resents Pete, interferes in Sara Jean's care of the children, and threatens them with court action to regain custody. He and Pete several times have come close to blows. However, the therapist had clearly helped them to stabilize their relations with Sara Jean's ex-husband, to begin to manage the children somewhat more successfully, and to decrease the violence of their confrontations. Yet their life together remains volatile. The therapist believes that Pete, unhappy about his relationship with his own children, had "rushed headlong" into trying to be parent to Sara Jean's kids, only to be faced with stiff resistence on her part. Sara Jean, by her own description, was becoming increasingly more irritable and argumentative with Pete. Both were in doubt about their ability to have anything approaching a harmonious family life with the children. Our session together, after the introductions and amenities, began in the following way:

The Scenario

MW: I understand you've been having some rough times. Yet I see a handsome couple, who've come a long distance to meet a stranger in front of cameras, and with cameramen, and mikes, and a whole bunch of my colleagues watching, so I know you care about each other and want to straighten things out between you—so what's wrong?

SARA JEAN: Just everyday problems; you know, like with our communication, the kids—everyday things, irritations . . . I get jumpy, bent out of shape . . .

MW: You've been married only a short time?

PETE: We lived together before . . .

MW: Oh, right. But you're married only seven months . . . settling in . . .

PETE: We're still not settled into our marriage.

MW: What do you mean, not settled in?

PETE: I see our marriage as a whole as a disaster

MW: (*Jokingly*) Terrific!

PETE: But I wouldn't get out of it if I had the opportunity.

MW: So, you like disasters?

PETE: No, but I'm comfortable in a negative atmosphere because I've never been in a positive one. So it's bad—but it makes me comfortable because it's a way I can live and fight on a daily basis—all right? Because I'm used to fighting instead of feeling good. We both come from backgrounds that are negative and we have learned how to live with this on a day-to-day basis. That's what makes us comfortable . . . well, me anyway. I'm comfortable with the bad things, but I don't like the bad feelings and thoughts that go along with it . . . and we both want to be comfortable with the happy things when they do come along for us, but we don't know how.

MW: Pete—you're a wise man. You understand a lot about yourself and your relationships. How did you get so wise?

PETE: (*Blushing*) I don't know if it's wise . . . it's just the way it is.

MW: It think it is wise. (*Turning to the therapist*) So, Donald, did you help Pete to be so wise, or is he . . .

THERAPIST: No, Marianne . . . I taught him all he knows! Seriously, I agree that Pete has a lot of insight—they both do—they've been struggling with this stuff for quite a while.

MW: (*To Sara Jean*) It sounds like what's been happening is that you've been providing for Pete that negative atmosphere . . . that negative energy . . . that you believe he needs, in order to feel comfortable . . . in order to relate to you.

SARA JEAN: I never thought of it that way . . . never that way . . . I . . . I surely don't do it on purpose.

MW: No, not on purpose, definitely not on purpose. It's just that you know him so well; and you do . . . almost instinctively . . . you do what you feel will make him comfortable.

SARA JEAN: (*Smiling*) Well . . . I guess you could look at it that way . . . it's kind of . . . different . . .

MW: Well, Sara Jean . . . in fact I think it's quite nice of you to be so "ornery" and argumentative in order to provide this guy with a home atmosphere that will be familiar and comfortable to him.

PETE: Well, yes, that's what I'm comfortable with . . . I don't know how to be in a situation without it. But it's not what I *want*.

MW: You don't want what you're comfortable with? I don't get it, Pete.

PETE: Well, I don't like the arguing all the time—and her being so angry and stuff—I don't want it, even though I don't know how to be in a situation without it.

MW: Ah . . . so . . . there's the dilemma. What you need is not what you want! But you see, Pete, you have a woman who loves you and is willing to be mean, or argumentative . . . or even a "stinker"—in order to make the man in her life comfortable. That's lovely—even self-sacrificing.

SARA JEAN: But I don't mean to be mean—I don't mean to, Marianne. I guess I just get irritated . . . you know, coming home after work, the kids—all that . . .

MW: Yes, all that, all that and more. I know you don't mean to be mean, Sara Jean. It's just that Pete has convinced himself—and you—that he doesn't know how to live in a positive atmosphere. So, like the good wife, you're the bad guy! That's how it is for lots of couples. Women learn early on how they're supposed to find ways to make their menfolk comfortable. So you just—well, just intuitively do what you think he needs you to do.

SARA JEAN: Well, I never, I never . . . I sure didn't think of it like that! (*She looks down, a slow grin crossing her face. As she looks up at Pete his face is a mixture of disbelief and delight. They grin at each other.*)

PETE: Well, well, well—well now . . .

MW: (*To the therapist*) So, Donald, I think somehow Pete is going to need to convince Sara Jean that even though he's not sure he can handle a positive atmosphere he doesn't want Sara Jean to keep on providing a negative one even though that's what makes him comfortable.

THERAPIST: I agree with you, but he's convinced Sara Jean he can't, so she protects him from feeling failed by giving him what he knows how to deal with—lots of fights!

PETE: Well, I sure know the fighting's not what I want.

MW: Yes, but Pete, Sara Jean believes what you've been telling her all this time . . . that you know how to fight but not how to enjoy life. So she thinks—like you—that you need the fighting in order to feel competent in the relationship. I think you're going to need to convince her that she doesn't need to protect you from yourself—that you can deal with this yourself—like learn to handle positive as well as negative situations. Donald can help you with this. I guess, Pete, like so many guys, you've learned how to say what you need, never realizing that your wife would think it's also what you want.

PETE: Well, yeah . . . I guess I see what you're getting at. I tell you it's not what I want—but I'm not sure I know how . . .

MW: Let's start just with trying to find a way to convince Sara Jean it's not what you *want* . . . convincing her it's not what you *need* will be harder. You'll have to convince yourself of that first . . . that you can manage things you hadn't thought you could manage. You've got your work cut out for you!

Reframing the Scenario

The scenario presented by this couple has several familiar themes: the difficulty for stepfathers in entering a new family that includes children from a previous marriage; the natural mother gathering her wagons 'round her to fight off the intruders; the reciprocal cycle of conflict and misunderstanding; the reproduction of dysfunctional interpersonal patterns; the polarizing of father, who wants to set rules and expectations for the kids, and mother, who wants a better understanding among all of them. Therapists sometimes pursue these themes directly—for instance, encouraging mom to "back off" so dad can enter the family in more positive ways; working with the parents to negotiate mutually agreed-on goals for the children; blocking the cycle of reciprocal conflictual transactions; or directing the couple to fight in prescribed ways.

From a feminist perspective, the issue is how to offer this couple a new vision of their situation that is as enlightened by their respective gender roles and expectations as it is by their marital or family system. Reframing Sara Jean's combative behaviors as accommodation to the needs of her husband, rather than as conflictual, reduces the possibility of any message of blame. But it also describes a socially prescribed expectation for women's behavior in marriage and in families. It is important that this be made explicit and the reframe not left as merely a "positive connotation" within the context of this particular family system. If the woman's behavior is understood as merely serving a function within the system, a function that has become the problem, the tendency will be for the therapy to be directed solely at the woman for change. Moreover, any development of the reframe, regardless of its positive intention, can become sexist. For instance, suggesting a woman is "self-sacrificing" could easily be experienced as mocking, or a put-down, if there is not a mutual understanding between the therapist and the woman client that this is one of the many behaviors and roles she will experience in family life that are socially constructed. So the reframe is expanded to include the idea that women learn to protect their husbands from the challenge to change, even while furiously wishing they would do so. Pete, on the other hand, is deeply unsure of his capacity to be emotional and has learned to relate to "what is" rather than "what could be." Sara Jean, despite her arguing and fussing, doesn't really believe that Pete can change. And neither does Pete. These are characteristics that are as profoundly cultural and gender-based as they are structured by the family system. By creating for this couple a heightened awareness of the larger context that organizes their behaviors with each other, the arena for continued effort to improve their relationship is, it is hoped, expanded.

One of the ways in which Pete sought to convince Sara Jean that he didn't want the chaos and acrimony that had characterized the first months of their married life was in relation to his stepchildren. For instance, later in the session there was the following interchange:

PETE: Soooo—if the kids would just be able to sit through a meal . . .

SARA JEAN: But, Pete—you get them all excited, egg them on, and then, when they get out of hand, you want them to settle down right away, to suddenly obey rules.

PETE: Well, I want them to have a good time, but I also want them to learn when to stop.

MW: So, Pete, you want to be an instant father to these kids—I don't blame you—it seems they're a pretty dynamic duo . . .

PETE: No, that's not what I want.

MW: Oh—well, maybe it's like what we've been talking about—it's what you think you "need"—that is, to be their dad, right now, even if it's not what you "want." And maybe, like their mom, these kids are trying to find a way to be with you. It must mean a lot to them, just as it does to you and Sara Jean.

PETE: Yup, it does. They need a father.

MW: And now they have two! And don't forget, one pretty terrific mother.

PETE: Yeah, but a soft touch.

SARA JEAN: Oh, I don't know about that . . .

MW: Maybe Sara Jean is especially a soft touch when she sees you being so tough . . . trying to balance it out.

SARA JEAN: That's exactly what happens.

MW: Sara Jean, how do you think Pete could enjoy your children while you're becoming a new family? Because, you see, I think it's going to take some time and he's impatient—maybe you're both impatient, because maybe you both think the kids haven't had enough fathering. I think, Sara Jean, you need to trust your mothering more so you can help Pete to take his time about finding his place in his new family.

When a mother has been a single parent for a time before remarrying, as was the case with Sara Jean, she will often feel that the children have been deprived of fathering and will be anxious that her new husband begin to parent right away, even as she feels the need to protect her parenting "rights" and expertise. Interestingly, such a remarried couple will share a belief system—that the children have been deprived of a consistent father figure—even while they are in conflict over issues of management and control. This shared belief system needs to be acknowledged and challenged as part of the process of redistributing responsibility and power.

Finally, it should be noted that the issue of inclusion of the children in the therapy was discussed with the therapist as part of the consultation. I recommended that they not be included in the ongoing therapy. Unless young children are the symptom-bearers, I see no reason to include them in the therapy and thus risk making patients of them.

part four

Single Women

Dedicated to my sister Margaret, who taught me that women can lead single lives with courage, dignity, and joy.

9

Peggy Papp

Single Women:
Early and Middle Years

THE FOLLOWING ANNOUNCEMENT was sent to 200 friends and business associates by Susan Hesse, a 38-year-old creative director, when she moved into her new house:

> *Alice and Carl Hesse*
> *of Washington, D.C.*
> *are pleased to announce*
> *that their daughter*
> *Susan A. Hesse*
> *of Piedmont, California,*
> *is settling into*
> *Joyous Old Maidhood*
> *at bedtime on*
> *Saturday, June 23, 1984,*
> *after which she will cease*
> *looking for Mr. Right*
> *and begin giving*
> *scintillating dinner*
> *parties and soirées.*
> *To help celebrate this*
> *wonderful occasion,*
> *gift place-settings*
> *of Newport Scroll Sterling*
> *by Gorham*
> *are available at*
> *Macy's Department Store.*
> *Thanking you in advance,*
> *Carl and Alice.*

Dinner dates to be announced
when Susan acquires a dining table.*

This notice is one woman's way of rejoicing in her single state and celebrating it as a rite of independence. With this proud announcement, she declares her intention of living a full and happy life without a man.

This is a far cry from the humbled status of unmarried women in 1862 that prompted the English journalist W. R. Gregg to suggest that 750,000 single women be exported to countries with better marriage markets. Unmarried women were deemed social pariahs and were hidden away within the confines of the family.

The percentage of never-married women between the ages of 25 and 34 has more than doubled in the last ten years as more and more women all over the country are delaying marriage or deliberately choosing not to marry at all. This dramatic increase in the single female population has coincided with the women's movement, which has opened up an array of new alternatives for women. Rapid changes in sexual mores and a greater flexibility in personal relationships have produced new options that need no longer be based on long-term, exclusive heterosexual relationships. These new arrangements embody a resistance to the idea that marriage and maternity are the primary sources of fulfillment for women. Establishing a woman's own separate and independent home confirms her independence and asks for recognition of her single status.

The Rewards and Deficits of Being Single

Many single people favor a social pattern that pivots around a variety of relationships with a number of people rather than being centered on an exclusive and intense involvement with one specific individual. They opt for occasional loneliness rather than sacrificing privacy, and cherish their social and geographical mobility, which permits them to travel on their job or relocate should the opportunity present itself.

A solitary life of independence involves the cultivation of personality traits that are opposite from those that marriage requires. Traditional marriage encourages women to become compliant, dependent, and selfless, and to put the emotional needs of others before their own; single women, on the other hand, are free to put their own needs first, become self-sufficient, make independent decisions, enjoy their privacy, and act in their own behalf.

These traits are in direct opposition to the conventionally accepted idea of what constitutes a desirable female. The psychiatric

*Reprinted with permission of Susan Hesse.

fraternity might label these characteristics in women as narcissistic, neurotic, egocentric, and indicative of an inability to form close emotional relationships. Most people in the mental-health field believe that the ability to make a long-term interpersonal commitment is a mark of emotional maturity, and that to subscribe to a different set of values is to demonstrate personal inadequacy and maladjustment. Single women are thought to be repressed, frustrated women with unresolved conflicts regarding their sexuality. Thus, they are stigmatized by these psychological theories of normality.

But as Margaret Adams points out ironically in *Single Blessedness*, whatever problems these women may have, they should be congratulated for staying single because their decision indicates that they have sufficient insight into their problems and sense to stay with a way of life that suits them better. "Eschewing marriage under these circumstances could be interpreted as healthy evidence of self-awareness, self-determination, and a measure of personal strength, which is necessary to face an existence that is often fraught with economic vulnerability, loneliness, personal devaluation and social stigma. . . . A glance at rising divorce rates would suggest that many individuals who venture unwittingly into this combat zone (of marriage) have as serious deficits in personal relationships as those imputed to their single peers and perhaps less awareness of their limitations" (1976).

She goes on to point out that the increases in divorce, unhappy marriage, and reported child neglect and abuse suggest that, in some cases, what society has deemed as the primary aspirations of women are socially imposed rather than based on natural instinct. Under the best of circumstances, a single life can provide for a woman a very strong sense of psychological self-sufficiency and personal integrity. For some women, privacy and independence are essential to their happiness and well-being, and they are willing to pay for it with occasional loneliness, financial vulnerability, and social ostracism.

This social ostracism has an economic as well as psychological base. The economic independence of women threatens the social fabric in a profound way. In the traditional organization of life, women take care of the family and leave men free to develop economically and to carry on the work of the world. Women who can make it on their own are no longer available to take care of men. As the women of Lysistrata brought an end to men's adventures in war by withholding sex, so economically independent women could eventually threaten the foundations of patriarchy, which is based on the unpaid labor of women.

Despite this social context, innovative schemes for experimental living, which reconcile the need for freedom and privacy, on the one hand, and social interchange, on the other, have been burgeoning at a rapid pace during the past decade. In some instances, men and women live together in a purely practical business arrangement for home sharing that does not entail sexual involvement. Some form groups of women who buy apartments or homes and work out living arrangements. These are cooperative ventures that save the group members money, energy, and time while simultaneously accommodating their common need for separateness and sharing. Social and financial commitments are made to a group of people rather than to separate individuals, and interdependence is therefore much less intense.

Social and Sexual Hazards

There are inevitable disadvantages and hazards that single women face. Because single living is untraditional, it lacks the institutional definition and support of marriage. Single women must create their own guidelines for living and depend on their own resources to organize a social framework. One of the major disadvantages is the lack of availability of one particular partner with whom to talk over the events of daily life or share a regular social and sexual life. For example, planning a social life takes a high degree of discipline and sustained effort when one is going it alone. The United States is a country in which social life is organized mainly in "pairs," and it can be awkward to be without a partner. This is more true for women than for men since single women are considered a social liability.

Most single women need and want social exchange with the opposite sex, mutual enjoyment, companionship, and support. But there is a shortage of facilities for genuine heterosocial exchange outside of marriage. Existing avenues do not provide an authentic forum for meeting the needs of the unattached. Those activities that are commercially promoted are generally sexually exploitive, such as cruise ships, singles' weekend vacations, special parties, newspaper ads, computer dating, and singles' clubs and bars; they are exploitive in nature and generally fraught with disappointment if not outright danger. These formats, referred to as "meat markets," share some of the characteristics of pornography in their humiliation and use of women as sex objects.

Thus, the desire for male companionship and simple human exchange can be filled with complex ramifications. In our sexually oriented society, an unnaturally high premium is placed on sexual activity. It is difficult for the unattached woman to meet men socially without making herself vulnerable to sexual harassment or even rape. The woman's awareness that men are more interested in her sexual skills than her other accomplishments often leads her into obligatory sexual liaisons at the expense of her genuine needs or feelings. This undermines her self-esteem and diminishes her integrity as a whole person. If she capitulates against her own inclinations, she sacrifices her precarious sense of independence; but if she doesn't, she, too, often finds herself without the companionship of a male. The cult of obligatory sex ends up being as oppressive as the repressive mores of the Victorian era.

It is no wonder, then, that some unattached women regard sexual skills as the ultimate gauge of their feminine identity and personal success. Their own life experience is augmented with messages from the mass media placing high value on a woman's sexual attractiveness and limited value on her intellectual achievements. This does not hold true for men, whose sexual attractiveness is often based almost solely on their status or high income. Despite the many changes in sexual mores that have taken place during the last decade, women have limited control over the sexual relationship and often end up subordinating their needs to those of men.

Identity Conflicts

Because the singles' scene is fraught with perils, many women center their lives around finding Mr. Right. As they reach the "Age Thirty Crisis," this search becomes more and more of an obsession. The thought of their identity and fulfillment coming from other than marriage and motherhood is incomprehensible to them. They think of themselves as being "uncoupled" or "half a person" when they are not partnered by a man. They play down their own initiative and aspirations, fearing that if they become too successful and self-sufficient they may lose their sex appeal. For these women, independence and freedom are synonymous with loneliness and exclusion. In therapy, they present a wide variety of symptoms ranging from loss of self-esteem to depression, anxiety, work problems, and physical illnesses. They regard friendships with other women as second best and become phobic about being called a lesbian.

There is another category of women who are engaged in a valiant struggle between the old and the new. They alternate between forging ahead independently to develop their own lives and getting caught up in ideas and dreams from the past. The more traditional values they learned at an earlier age rise up to haunt them and displace their newer attainments of the present. They are plagued by the deeply embedded dicta they received from their mothers especially, and from other women and men who strongly influenced them regarding love, marriage, and the pursuit of happiness.

New Options

These sexual culs-de-sac and plaguing dilemmas account for the increasing number of women who are deciding to have children without being married. In the past, when a woman forfeited marriage, she automatically gave up motherhood. This is no longer necessary. Some women have changed the words "unwed mother" to "elective parent" or "single mother by choice." These are not "accidental" pregnancies, as with many unwed teenagers, but are deliberately and carefully planned. The woman either chooses a consenting male, adopts a child, or goes to a fertility clinic for artificial insemination. Fertility clinics, which in the past were used only by married couples, are now opening their doors to single women. Roxanne Feldschuh, co-director of Idant Laboratories, says of the women who apply for their services: "Our single recipients are bright, talented superwomen who refuse to settle for just any man in order to get married and have a baby."

These are women who want to experience the joys of childbirth on their own. They are willing to face the many difficulties and hardships involved in assuming responsibility for a child on their own, including worrying about paying the bills, hiring baby-sitters, arranging for schools, and enduring the inevitable social stigma connected with this unconventional enterprise.

Many criticisms are leveled at these elective mothers, one of the most prevalent being that they are damaging the child's natural development by depriving it of a father. This ignores the fact that most children are traditionally raised primarily by mothers.

Dr. Martin V. Cohen, a clinical psychologist on the faculty of New York Hospital–Cornell Medical Center, has something positive to say about this new social development. "Fifty percent of kids in grade school come from divorced couples, so it's practically the norm for children to only have one parent . . . in a way, it might even be easier for out-of-wedlock kids. They don't have to suffer the rejection of having a father move away or remarry. I don't think it's a bad thing at all."

Another harsh accusation leveled at elective mothers is that they will be unfit mothers because of their inability to commit themselves to an intimate relationship with a man. However, statistics show that many mothers of abused and neglected children are involved in a conflictual and overly dependent relationship with a man and that the extreme distress involved in this relationship is most often a factor in the abuse or neglect. The pernicious triangle that results when a child is caught between two warring parents can be far more damaging to a child than an exclusive involvement with one parent.

The qualities involved in sustaining a relationship with a man and those needed to raise a child are indeed quite opposite. One requires a narcissistic involvement with one's physical attractiveness, with sexual pleasure, compromise, and depending on another for one's emotional needs. The other requires maturity, self-reliance, taking charge, trusting one's own judgment, and making independent decisions.

Up to this point, the discussion of singleness has focused primarily on the options it offers middle-class white women. I am acutely aware that these same options often do not exist for black women and other minority groups. Psychological liberation is dependent on social and economic liberation. Ntozake Shange sums up the plight of black women in her play *For Colored Girls Who Have Considered Suicide When the Rainbow Is Enuf*, with the definitive statement that to be black and a woman is redundant.

Therapeutic Implications

One of the most common problems that single women bring to therapy involves their relationship with a man. They believe something is wrong with them if either they haven't been able to find one or haven't been able to form a satisfactory relationship with one. Many therapists share the women's belief that either of the above conditions indicates a neurotic problem and that when the woman has overcome this neurotic problem through therapy, love will automatically come her way.

In a recent article on single women in the *New York Times*, the reporter describes a 44-year-old therapist who becomes convinced she is single because of her personal problems and enters analysis. "Women are in this situation because of neurotic conflicts," she said. "I see it in my friends. I see it in myself. And I see it in my patients." On the same page is a census bureau chart showing the growing disparity between the number of available women in New York City as opposed to the number of available men: 154,815 unmarried women as compared with 95,058 unmarried men. In order to cure the "neuroses" of all the single women in New York City, it seems it would be necessary to either import 59,727 available men, or legalize bigamy. Personal neurosis is an easy dumping ground for all the complex social, cultural, demographic, and political problems that exist. It can be found anywhere that one cares to look for it.

In working with single women it is especially important not to pathologize their singleness by searching for causes of it deep within their psyches or past lives. Rather, the therapist can help them to examine the way in which cultural attitudes are influencing their personal experiences and choices, to differentiate socially imposed ideas from those that are valuable and appropriate for them, and to replace old expectations with new options and ideas. Women's need for relatedness and nurturance can be fostered by helping them to obtain it from sources other than sexual relationships, such as family and life-sustaining friendships that offer consistent comfort and stability. Their concentration and energies can be turned away from yearning after what they don't have to concentrating on what they do have—their own talent and creativity—so they can discover that life can have meaning and purpose with or without a man.

Cases

When a woman seeks therapy because of a relationship in which she is currently involved, I prefer to see her and the man together. However, if the man is married and intent on keeping the relationship a secret, which is often the case, I work with the woman alone. In these instances, the woman's goal in therapy is usually to find a way of holding onto the man, as we see in my case, "Scaling the Heights of Life."

In Walters's case, "Drowning in a Sea of Success," although the woman initially requests therapy for herself, Walters involves the man in the second session. The woman presents her psychosomatic symptom as being related to her "fear of success" and her "competitive relationship" with her mother. Walters redefines the symptom as her protectiveness toward her male friend, who feels needed and helpful when she behaves in incompetent and dependent ways. Walters then links this reframing to the social premise that women intuitively try to protect men and make them feel strong and important even at great cost to themselves. Therapy focuses on helping both the woman and her male friend find ways of sustaining their relationship without the woman's symptomatic behavior.

These two cases demonstrate different ways of increasing the options for single women: one by letting go of a destructive relationship with a man, the other by letting go of playing a traditional woman's role in a relationship with a man. Although the situations and therapeutic approaches differ vastly, both involve altering the women's attitudes toward some basic issues and providing them with alternatives.

cases

Peggy Papp

"Scaling the Heights of Life"

History is replete with the tales of women who center their lives around brilliant, creative men, living vicariously through their talent and achievements. These women are often willing to endure all the exigencies of stormy moods and unpredictable temperaments for the privilege of basking in the reflected glory of these charismatic men. It is not surprising that women have a tendency to seek power and glory through men, since men have easier access to them than women.

In her best-selling book, *Women Who Love Too Much*, Robin Norwood vividly describes women who neglect their own best interests in the pursuit of distant, unavailable, and often emotionally unstable men. Norwood credits the self-destructive behavior of these women to neurotic tendencies due to rejecting parents and childhood traumas, without taking into account the cultural norms that encourage women to fulfill themselves through men. Despite some movement in the opposite direction, our basic cultural dicta still condition women to seek their social destiny through men rather than themselves.

This case deals with a woman who, because she was not able to compete with the man openly, built him up into outrageous proportions and became obsessed with winning his love. In my therapy with her, I helped her to evaluate the meaning of her adoration and the price she was paying for it in terms of her own potential. By focusing on developing her own talents she was released from her obsession.

Holly's Obsession

Holly was a bright young woman of 24, who first consulted me because of difficulties with a married man, Oscar, with whom she was having an affair at her place of work. She was Oscar's research assistant on an important project at a prestigious institution. She described him as a "genius" who had won much acclaim for his achievements, and she had developed an all-consuming passion for him. She felt alive only when she was with him because he was all the things she admired. Besides being "brilliant," he was "cultured and artistic" and "knows about everything in the world." Holly felt like a "country girl" in comparison, "still wet behind the ears." She had come from a small town where she had received a scholarship to do graduate work at a large university.

On the basis of her exceptional work during graduate school she had been offered the current position where she had made rapid advances.

Three months before seeking therapy, she had broken off a relationship with her fiancé, Bill, because, although he was solid and dependable, he was boring in comparison with Oscar. Bill loved her, was attentive and supportive, but lacked ambition and drive and was not "exciting." He was satisfied to settle for a mundane existence while she wanted to "scale the heights of life."

Her dream was to scale these heights with Oscar. He was to lead the way and she was to follow him into this exciting new world of science, art, literature, and philosophy to which he had introduced her. Her problem was that there was a very high price to pay for this adventure. Oscar was moody and temperamental. He would fly into rages when things didn't go his way. He was extremely critical of Holly, never gave her credit for her accomplishments, and often belittled her in front of her colleagues. But she overlooked all of this because of his "extraordinary mind" and his "prodigious accomplishments." She found his complete dedication to his work inspiring and brought me articles and newspaper clippings describing his most recent honors and awards.

Holly's agenda when she first consulted me was to find a way to make Oscar love her more so that he would leave his wife. At times he seemed about to do this but would then waver in his decision. Oscar's affection for her ran hot and cold, and Holly felt she was on a yo-yo. There were frequent agonizing scenes of jealousy in which Holly found herself losing control of herself, screaming, crying, and threatening. Oscar reacted to her hysteria with contempt and further withdrawal.

Before consulting me she had seen a psychiatrist for several sessions. She had stopped her visits to him because he focused on her "masochistic personality." Although she thought he was correct in his diagnosis, she did not want "deep analysis" because she was in a crisis and didn't know how to handle it.

Reframing the Issue

After hearing her story, I told her I had a different point of view than the psychiatrist. I didn't see her as being masochistic but rather as being quite the opposite. It was not that she was in love with suffering and self-abnegation, but with the power, fame, and prestige that came from productive creativity. It was not so much Oscar himself who enthralled her but his energy, knowledge, and talent. She wanted to absorb all of that through osmosis rather than through her own efforts. She felt inadequate and incompetent in relation to him and hoped to come alive through his creativity and brilliance, rather than through her own.

Some therapists at this point might have suggested that she overcome her infatuation by becoming involved in another romantic relationship with someone more attainable and suitable. The rationale behind this way of thinking is that the best way to get over one love affair is to start another one. Other therapists might plan distancing maneuvers for her on the theory that this would incite Oscar to move toward her rather than away from her, as he was now doing. Both of these interventions are based on the idea that the best thing for a woman to do in an unhappy relationship with a man is either to begin a new one or to try, by hook or by crook, to salvage the one she already has. Both perpetuate the idea that a woman's life should revolve around a man.

My belief is that one of the most effective ways for a woman to extricate herself from a destructive relationship with a man is to develop the qualities in herself that she is trying to live through in the man. As long as those qualities and attributes are outside rather than inside herself, she will always feel insecure and inadequate. This doesn't mean that a certain kind of complementarity is not desirable and indeed necessary in any satisfying relationship. Everyone at some level is attracted to others who have certain qualities they admire and lack in themselves. However, there is a difference between a workable complementarity in which both partners feel they make different but equal contributions and a relationship in which one lives vicariously through another.

My therapy with Holly focused on *her* brilliant mind and what she wanted to do with it, the direction of *her own* career, and ways of exploring the exciting world of science, art, and philosophy *on her own*.

As we pursued this course I learned more about her own exceptional talents, which became evident early in her life. She was considered something of a child prodigy by her family and teachers because she so far outdistanced her classmates. She skipped two grades before high school and won a scholarship on the basis of her high scores in math and chemistry. While growing up she had cherished a dream that one day she might "contribute something important to society."

That dream was now being eclipsed by her tumultuous involvement with Oscar, which sapped her time and energy. When things were rocky between them she found it difficult to concentrate on her work in the lab and, instead of spending her free time at home keeping up with the current literature in the field, she waited by the telephone for him to call. After a fight he would punish her by not visiting her lab, and she would be so devastated that she would find it difficult to function properly.

Therapeutic Moves

In order to lessen Holly's intense preoccupation with Oscar, I suggested she take the phone off the hook every night as soon as she arrived home so that she would not spend the evening waiting for his call. After dinner she was to spend her time reading all the literature in the field pertinent to her own research, and the more she missed him the longer she was to read. She was to take time out every now and then to practice her violin, which she had been neglecting. Holly was an accomplished musician who had played in a string quartet for several years; she had dropped out when she became involved with Oscar, and the quartet had disbanded. I used Holly's love of music to break into her obsession by connecting her with her musical colleagues, suggesting she reassemble the quartet and practice in the evenings or on weekends now that she wasn't seeing so much of Oscar.

When Holly told me she had a habit of sitting and staring at Oscar's picture for hours as though in a trance, I prescribed a humorous ritual aimed at satirizing her reverence for him. Before she went into her trance, she was to cover her head with a scarf as though in church, light candles around the picture, and kneel down in front of it in a prayerful position. In the middle of carrying out this absurd instruction, Holly started to laugh, and her reverential attitude was dispelled.

At Christmas, I encouraged her to make a trip home and discuss her situation with her parents, who were very supportive of her. She found her long talks with them comforting and returned feeling less lonely and desperate. However, despite the fact that she followed through on all the suggestions, Holly still clung to the secret hope that she might work out a relationship with Oscar.

Then one day she reported that their research team had made a presentation at an annual conference and that she had presented a paper on the results of her particular phase of the research. It aroused a great deal of interest, and she was encouraged by a number of people at the conference to publish her findings. When she suggested this to Oscar, he became enraged and said he was to decide what aspect of the project would be written up by whom and when. He seemed to be jealous of the attention she was getting and reluctant to give her any credit for the results of her experiment. From then on he began to minimize the work of her lab as "unpromising," and finally one day told her he was thinking of discontinuing it and assigning her to another project. She was stunned and came to the session distraught and in tears. She believed that the work she was doing was yielding fascinating and valuable findings, and it would break her heart to give it up. On the other hand, she knew that if she contested Oscar's decision it would mean the end of their relationship. From time to time he still gave her indications that he would leave his wife, and she continued to hope he would marry her.

With my encouragement, Holly decided to discuss his decision further and state her case for continuing her work. When she did so, Oscar became violently angry and accused her of being ungrateful and arrogant. A fight ensued, which escalated to the point where he struck her and pushed her to the floor. She came to the next session in shock and expressed feelings of tremendous humiliation and rage. She was confused and distraught as she discussed what she felt were her various options: She could apologize to Oscar, give up the project, and try and patch up their relationship; she could resign from the job and seek work elsewhere; she could report his behavior to the president of the Institute and make a case out of it; or she could continue to try and persuade him to change his mind. None of the alternatives seemed satisfactory to her. I suggested another one. Would it be possible for her to apply for a grant of her own, set up her own lab, and continue with the work she had been doing? That idea had not occurred to her. We discussed the technicalities and whether or not such a move would be ethical. She said she could write up the grant proposal from a different angle but one that would still permit her to retain the advances she had made.

Changing Course

This was the course she followed. She received the grant and set up her lab in a different state. From time to time I receive letters filled with enthusiasm and excitement over the progress of her work. In one letter she included an article from a scientific journal with a picture of her and her lab team. She describes the town where she lives as beautiful and peaceful, not as exciting as New York City but with as many cultural events as she has time for. She also has difficulty finding time to date the two men in her life, but has decided definitely not to become involved with her lab assistant, who has been making amorous advances.

Holly was able to leave her destructive relationship with Oscar only when she found the courage to challenge his authority and assert her own. By putting her own creativity and imagination to work, she no longer needed to live vicariously through his.

Marianne Walters

Drowning in a Sea of Success

When I work with a younger woman who is living alone, that is, not with her family of origin, in a new family, or with a significant other, my intention is to find a way of helping her to feel in charge of her own life, and comfortable with it, without either resorting to an exploration of problems within her past living situations or focusing on internalized conflicts as origins of her current life circumstances. In most situations, my initial effort is to engage my client in redefining and rethinking the nature of her current reality, and motivating her to participate actively in restructuring that part of it that is interfering with successful functioning.

Women in many different life conditions will need to reference themselves in new ways. For instance, even the language surrounding "women alone" is misleading. Usually these women are not alone; they just live alone. But women are generally so family-oriented, and so identified by their family roles, that when they are not living with others they refer to themselves, and others refer to them, as "alone."

Women living alone often seek therapy around issues of identity and self-esteem, their sense of self-worth diminished by the social stigma surrounding the unmarried state for women. They also often present with psychosomatic symptoms, as is illustrated in the case of a young woman with a successful career who sought help for a symptom that was endangering her career. This young woman is involved with a man; she has a pleasant social life, good health, and reasonable relations with her family. She has seen a number of therapists and tried a number of cures. So what accounts for the symptom?

Margaret called for an appointment, saying she really hoped this was going to help because she was close to despair about her problem, had seen a number of therapists, and so far nothing "had worked." Margaret is a 34-year-old marine biologist who works for a large Washington-based research center. She has had a brilliant career, having received her PhD when she was 28, with a dissertation that was immediately accepted for publication. Her research in her field is highly regarded, she publishes regularly, has made some breakthrough discoveries concerning the ecological chain in a species of fresh-water fish, is extremely well-paid, and has a good deal of autonomy in her daily work life. She told me all this quite matter-of-factly, but not without pride. The problem in this "sea of success" is that the Institute for which she works requires her to make presentations both to groups of colleagues who come to the Institute and at professional gatherings around the country. This is a requirement not only for continued career advancement but also for maintaining the position she already holds in this prestigious research center.

Such public presentations have always been difficult for Margaret, creating a lot of anxiety accompanied by physical symptoms that played havoc with her performance once she could get herself out there. Dry mouth impeded her speech, light-headedness her concentration, and muscle spasms her ability to read her notes. But in the last year it had gotten much worse; the anxiety before the presentation has become sheer agony and the physical symptoms greater and longer in duration. She is so worried about all of this that it is affecting her entire job performance. "I don't think I've had a good work day for the past ten months, I'm so obsessed with trying to conquer this problem. As fast as my career blossomed—just that fast it's going to crash if this keeps up. I don't want that to happen. I love my work—or at least I used to. I can't let this destroy all I've accomplished. I'll do anything . . ."

And indeed she had. She'd been to one therapist who was supportive and "really terrific with me," and who explored with her "my fears of success and how like so many women I was afraid of being too out-front, exposed; how if I was successful I feared I might not get my dependency needs met—and all that—and even that maybe I had gotten into all this crazy stuff so I wouldn't have to compete with my mother. I don't know. It sure seemed to make sense and I learned a lot about myself—but this damned problem keeps getting worse, it's gotten to be like . . . a phobia or an obsession . . . the more I worry about it the worse it gets." Margaret also had sought help at a behavior modification clinic and from an acupuncturist; she had used relaxation tapes and sought advice from her close network of friends. People told her not to worry so much, or that maybe the price of success was too high, or that everyone got anxious before public presentations.

THERAPIST: I don't see why some of the explanations didn't help. Some of them are really good.

MARGARET: They are. And they all fit too. They really fit. And the behavioral exercises did help for a while . . . they really did. When I first got into it, it gave me some relief. But only for a while.

THERAPIST: Well, I can see your dilemma. Yet this whole business about the fear of success seems to fit, to be right on. Have you . . . ?

MARGARET: Oh, sure . . . of course. It fits . . . it's good stuff. I just can't seem to budge on this thing.

THERAPIST: What thing?

MARGARET: The anxiety about public speaking.

THERAPIST: Oh yes. Right. Well, let me get some sense of what's going on for you apart from your anxiety about public speaking. Do you live right in the city? . . .

Margaret has a great apartment in town, a few close friends, a lot of professional acquaintances, a warm family life, and a pretty solid relationship with her boyfriend of two years, a junior partner in a struggling architectural firm. Her parents, married nearly forty years, live in Baltimore where her father is a chemistry professor and her mother a housewife and ceramicist.

Margaret and her mother have a close but conflictual relationship. Margaret feels she is always seeking, and never quite getting, her mother's approval. On the other hand, she feels her father accepts her as she is. Margaret is the middle of three siblings. Her older sister teaches high school, married in her mid-twenties, and is raising a family. Her younger brother is married and is a labor lawyer. The family members enjoy each other's company, although Margaret and her mother clash frequently. Margaret feels her mother is competitive with her, both admiring and critical of her way of life. Her sister and mother enjoy a much more comfortable relationship, and her brother is the "apple of her eye." David, her boyfriend, lives in Baltimore and so sees Margaret's family sometimes more than she does.

THERAPIST: What do you and David do for relaxation?

MARGARET: Concerts, music, drives in the country, evenings with friends.

THERAPIST: What do you two talk about?

MARGARET: Well, David is a pretty quiet guy, into himself a lot. Thoughtful. We don't talk a whole lot. Lately, we talk more, but it's mostly about my problem. He really can be quite helpful. He really tries hard to understand, explain, reassure me . . . We talk about it a lot.

THERAPIST: Do you think David enjoys helping you in this way?

MARGARET: Well, yes . . . I guess he does.

THERAPIST: What other ways does he help you?

MARGARET: Well . . . well . . . you know, I'm not sure there's a lot else I need help with . . . except maybe like some mechanical things . . . like the hi-fi set . . . but otherwise there's nothing else . . . I'm not very needy.

THERAPIST: You're not very needy! You sure could have fooled me, Margaret! Do you think you've fooled David?

MARGARET: What? I'm not sure what you mean.

THERAPIST: Well, I mean—do you think David needs you to be needy in order to have a place he can be of help to you—to feel "up"—to do for you—even to have a subject he can really talk about. Do you think you need to make sure he knows you can't take care of yourself in all ways—that there's a big chunk that needs to be taken care of—so he'll feel more important in your relationship? Or more competent?

Margaret sat back, started to speak, and the tears came.

THERAPIST: (*Passing the tissues*) What's that about, Margaret?

MARGARET: Ohhh, Marianne . . . you know, I really love David . . . but he seems so—well, disapproving, sometimes—or maybe dissatisfied, and he gets, well, morose—or so it seems to me. He's proud of me and loves me, I'm sure. But I know he wishes something were different. And yet, he can really be wonderful, supportive, comforting—really helpful when I'm a wreck over these damn public appearances. So maybe, Oh Lord, I don't know—maybe that is when I get the best he has to give—but, he must know I need him.

THERAPIST: Isn't it something the way women just intuit when something's missing and try to fill in the spaces? No matter what else women do, that is expected of them.

MARGARET: (*Laughing through the tears*) And all men have to do is look sad!

Margaret really wanted to tackle her behavior and to explore ways of understanding it, but I suggested we not go into it further, that in fact she should just let it sit for now. She should consider the ideas we had talked about by herself, not discuss them with David, and not try and do anything about it. Just let it settle in. We agreed that she would not talk with David about her problem this week and would ask him to join us for a few sessions.

I saw Margaret and David together for three sessions. The first time they came in as a couple I told David what I thought Margaret's public-speaking problem was about and asked him if he could think of any ways he got her to believe that he needed her to be needy. He articulated some behaviors on his part that might have conveyed this message—but basically expressed annoyance and concern that Margaret thought so little of him. I pushed him to explain this to her:

DAVID: Well, really, Marg, it just seems strange to me that you could think I'd need you to give me a problem to help with—or like you think you should be more dependent so I can feel needed. That stuff sounds more like something your mother would be into. I know you need me, honey, we need each other.

MARGARET: David, that sounds good, I agree with you. But, darling, how about those nights when you get into yourself, when nothing seems to get to you and we sort of act like strangers with each other? Or when you get so angry with me because I ask you to make some of the decisions, arrange some of our social life. David, remember last Tuesday . . . I just couldn't get you to tell me what . . .

DAVID: Marg, baby—you're just gonna need to get off my back. Nothing is wrong—it's just your imagination.

MARGARET: That's not true. (*There followed a long, deep, uncomfortable silence. Finally, tremulously, breaking the impasse*) Well, ah . . . David, I wonder . . . ah . . . if what's happening is we're just suffering from a very different style of relating or of communicating. I'm not sure what is happening. I begin to think you're unhappy or distant with me . . . but maybe you're just distracted. Anyway, I get concerned and—do you understand what I'm saying?

DAVID: Not really, because I think you're just creating problems that don't exist between us.

THERAPIST: Well, David, I think I see how you get Margaret to believe you need her to be needy.

MARGARET: I'm confused.

THERAPIST: Well, there it is. David, you shut down. And then Margaret begins to feel that the only way to engage you is to be less than her articulate self, to get kind of fuzzy and anxious. And when you do that, Margaret, David does come through, he is there and helpful. But when you try to articulate your differences and concerns, David, like I said, I think you shut down. So these are ways you let each other know what is expected of the other. And some of this is not just of your own making—it is what men and women have learned to expect of each other in intimate relationships.

During the next couple of sessions, I worked with David to find ways of reassuring Margaret that he really didn't need her to be "down" for him to feel functional with her; interrupting and interpreting his process of avoidance; and framing it as an invitation to Margaret to behave in less competent, more dependent ways.

Margaret continued to see me for several months. She began to handle her public speaking problem on her own, and as it receded in significance, we hardly spoke of it. Our sessions focused more directly on her concerns about how to establish a relationship with David and still maintain her own sense of identity and autonomy. Again, this dilemma was framed in the terms of a socially constructed dilemma for women, and certainly one shared by women in her situation. It thus began to be experienced as less her particular problem and so not as debilitating. Then we could work on defining Margaret's life conditions—her goals, her options, her needs—and how she could conceptualize fitting a relationship into these conditions, rather than fitting herself into a relationship.

Obviously, this case illustrates the use of a functional interpretation of Margaret's symptoms: that it served the purpose of engaging David in more intimate interaction, and of enhancing his self-esteem by making him feel more needed. If we stop there, we have a positive reframe that can be linked to formulations such as: Margaret is working too hard; she needs to find other ways to engage David; or she is applying for sainthood in her willingness to give up her success to make David feel needed. Or the symptom could be linked to familial behaviors, competition with her siblings, or not wanting to outdo her mother. But none of these formulations link the function of her symptom with the larger social context that *in fact constructs that function*. For me, the latter is an absolutely vital ingredient in both depathologizing women and in helping them to reference themselves in terms of the experience of other women. I believe this is a necessary first step toward individuation and self-directed functioning for women.

10   *Olga Silverstein*

Single Women: Later Years

The Basic Needs of Older Women

Of the two major forces in the lives of older women, the most pressing is, of course, economic. More than 21 percent of women over 55 live alone, and at least a quarter of these women have incomes that fall below the poverty line. Single older women are the most likely to be poor.

Traditional social expectations that shape the female life cycle often prevent women from preparing to be economically self-sufficient in the last third of their lives. As a result, when a woman finds herself suddenly alone, she is apt to be lacking in adequate work skills, and she may also feel resentment at being pressured to fulfill a role that has always been delegated to the husbands or fathers in her family. Failure to be self-supporting leads not only to the obvious material deprivations that many older women suffer, but also to a profound sense of inadequacy. What is more, the inability to work denies an older woman access to a new and potentially rich social network, in which successful performance can make a person feel both needed and useful. Economic failure in the life of an older woman is a double-edged blade. It deprives her of material as well as emotional well-being.

The second major force in a woman's life is more purely emotional and thus falls more clearly within the domain of therapy; however, it too hinges on issues of self-sufficiency. It is the older woman's need to function on an emotional and interactional level in a society that makes few accommodations for the special needs of being female, single, and old.

390

The Search for Autonomy

In the past several decades the traditional family bonds that guaranteed a haven for grandmothers and "maiden aunts" have been loosened. The number of households containing three generations has diminished greatly since World War II. It is difficult to know whether the mental health professions have increasingly stressed autonomy as a value for all family members in order to accommodate these changes— or whether the emphasis on autonomy has contributed to the loosening of family ties.

Women who have spent most of their lives defining themselves by their importance to husbands, children, or parents often experience the plunge into single living that frequently comes later in life as a period of great discontinuity and uncertainty. Many of the personal and social qualities that afforded them a sense of self-worth in the past are now suddenly recast as faults by the new social context in which they find themselves. This sudden shift in social and self-definition is rarely faced head on by the therapist. Yet older women who seek therapy continue to do so primarily because they have begun to devalue their "unhealthy dependence" on others.

There are three major groups of older women seen in the therapist's office, and although each group faces a particular set of problems, all of these problems are focused around the same issue: a perceived need to develop a capacity for autonomy.

The Unmarried Older Woman

The first type of woman who comes to see a therapist is one who has never married. In many cases, a single life may have led her to develop job and survival skills and a capacity to function well independently. Now, perhaps the time for retirement has come and she is wondering how to fill the years ahead. In other instances, a therapist may encounter a single woman who has spent her life in intimate relationship to a parent or sibling, and, now, because of the loss of that significant other, feels confused and despairing.

Whatever the particular details of her situation, a single older woman will usually come to a therapist with the assumption that the task at hand is to look for an explanation for a perceived character defect. Underscoring all her thoughts about herself is a sense of failure at not having achieved what is perceived to be woman's most fulfilling role, marriage and motherhood.

Older unmarried women often come to therapy as a last-ditch attempt at making themselves more acceptable for a potential "mature relationship." Such a self-improvement "campaign" is sometimes accompanied by a series of physical reconstructions, such as a face lift, a diet, or a new wardrobe. There is a reawakened concern about the nature of appropriate female behavior and anxiety about behavior in the presence of males. The greatest therapeutic error in treating such a woman is inadvertently to join her in blaming herself for being single by letting the therapeutic process question what is wrong with her.

Therapists who base their clinical practice on models of mental health that stress autonomy often approach the single older woman with the assumption that her situation has been determined by "over-involvement" with her family of origin. Whether she has spent her life alone or living with a parent, the focus of therapy becomes an attempt to discover the reason that she has failed to develop any permanent male relationships outside the family of origin. In the course of this process of self-examination, she is being encouraged to devalue her relational skills only because they have not been directed toward conventional objects, that is, toward husband and children. A woman who has spent the first two-thirds of her life caring for a parent or sibling will often come out of therapy feeling that her caretaking behavior was misdirected or neurotic because it did not occur in a conjugal context. If, however, the therapist focuses on her primary relationships as positive and productive, her self-image will be validated and enhanced.

A Clinical Example

A 72-year-old woman came to see me because she had for the first time in her life begun to experience anxiety attacks that made it difficult for her to leave her apartment. She had been retired at age 70 from her job as a social science professor at a local university. The retirement had been mandatory and she had been in intellectual agreement with it. "We have to make way for the young," she told me. She had even prepared herself emotionally for the retirement by planning to write a long-deferred book as soon as she stopped teaching. Two years later the book had still not been written, and there were no goals to replace it. "The walls are closing in on me," she confessed, "but I can't go out because I have no place to go. What's wrong with me?"

Her constant self-questioning never addressed her need to exercise her relational skills. She was the youngest of four siblings, the last survivor of a close-knit family. Her family history had given her the capacity for empathetic, intimate behavior. Now the two contexts that had given her a chance to exhibit her prodigious interactional skills—work and family—were eclipsed. Rather than encouragement to become more autonomous, she needed fresh opportunities to use her relational skills.

I reassured her that there was nothing abnormal in the anguish and anger she felt about the prospect of losing some of her physical and mental powers as she grew older, but I also stressed the fact that the primary cause of her anxiety was the loss of her network of relationships. As a result, she decided to go back to her university as a student in a different department. She formed a small study group that met in her apartment weekly. Her anxiety lifted, then returned for a while as I urged her to plan ahead for some form of group living in the future. After she had visited some of the communities designed for the well-aged, the anxiety abated again. "Maybe when I'm 80," she told me. I agreed that might be a good time.

The therapeutic process for this patient consisted of encouraging her to gradually reapply the skills she had developed in a lifetime within a new social context. It would have been unproductive to frame her problem as a need to become more self-sufficient or autonomous. Taking such an approach would have devalued her strengths, plunged her into self-doubt, and decreased her ability to function still further.

The Widowed Older Woman

Another type of older woman who becomes involved in therapy is the newly widowed who has never worked or who has not made her career a central focus of her life. The average widow is 59 years old and can expect to live an additional thirty years (Aging America, 1982). Because she has been abruptly placed in a context of singlehood that demands self-sufficiency, she may be exhibiting an aura of ineffectuality. Tasks such as home repair management, financial matters, or the logistics of transportation may have always been the domain of her husband. The prospect of having to handle these situations herself may cause great anxiety. This woman's functional problems are not caused by a lack of motivation. Neither is her fear of handling situations that may seem commonplace to others a manifestation of phobia. She simply lacks the experience to utilize her own talents and the resources of her community. She is apt to hide in terminal widowhood, and the social structure she lives in will tend to reinforce her behavior.

Older women typically find themselves on the devalued end of the social scale. Their fear of coping with experiences for which they lack the skills is often escalated by this social devaluation. Therapy is most effective for these women when it encourages them to creatively value the skills they already possess rather than when it counsels them to begin work on wholly undeveloped skills. A lack of aggression or single-mindedness can be compensated for by a gift for intimacy, attention to the needs of others, and emotional sensitivity.

I saw a 67-year-old woman who had been in therapy for the past three years because of a debilitating depression that began with the death of her husband. Her previous therapist had told her that she needed to concentrate more on herself. Claiming that she had spent her entire life "hiding" in relationships, he had tried to encourage her to shift to an emphasis on self-development. Since she was the type of person who was always eager to please and accommodate, she tried to follow his suggestions. She cut herself off from many of her friends and spent hours poring over her supposed inability to face who she really was. By the time she came to me, she was obsessively recounting her failure to "make something of herself." "My whole life has been taking care of others' feelings," she recited. "That's why I don't even know my own." Her former therapist had taught her to conceptualize her relational abilities as dependency. My approach was to reframe them as a basic human need for significant others. This reframing was done through a reexamination of the woman's family history and recent past with a goal toward defining her caretaking positively. Afterward, the woman was able to face her future more realistically and reestablish a sense of continuity with her past life. In a sense, the therapeutic process was a reclamation and reaffirmation of her original identity.

The Newly Divorced Older Woman

The third category of older woman who enters therapy is the newly divorced. This group can be divided into subgroups: those whose husbands have left them, and those who have left their husbands.

The Abandoned Divorcée

The abandoned divorcée has often been left by her husband for a younger woman, though this is not always the case. At any rate, there is bound to be a period of rage directed against the husband, the other woman, or fate in general, followed by a later period of self-recrimination. Working therapeutically with the abandoned wife has its pitfalls. She is different from the widow who has experienced a successful marriage because the divorced woman's relational skills have already been seriously devalued by the very man to whom they were directed, that is, by her husband.

Betty was 62 when she discovered that her husband was having an affair with his secretary. Her first response was rage and righteous indignation. She insisted that he choose between them, and he left her to move in with the other woman. A period of self-blame and castigation followed. Her sessions were spent cataloguing her failures. When questioned about what there was about her marriage that she now missed, Betty was hard put to answer. Instead, she shifted her focus to her husband's chronic faults, going into great detail about his unavailability, his temper, his insensitivity, and his poor sexual performance. After it was pointed out to her that she didn't seem to be missing much, she described her embarrassment and shame when she imagined herself in the eyes of her friends. Eventually she admitted that the major issue at hand was her pride. Betty was missing the marriage role, not the man.

The second stage of Betty's therapy was to reappraise those qualities in herself that she saw as the cause of her husband's leaving. These included her need for intimacy, both emotional and sexual, and an intolerance for bullying or insensitive behavior. Betty's personality traits were slowly reframed as positive social skills, and her self-blame subsided.

The Woman Who Initiates Divorce

Older women who take the initiative to leave their husbands have usually suffered a long, unhappy marriage. Divorce represents an act of liberation and is attended by fantasies of realizing yet undiscovered potential. Such a woman comes into therapy only after these expectations for self-realization have been squelched by the pain of loneliness. As a single woman, she may find herself in disturbingly unfamiliar social territory. The reactions of family and friends to her late-in-life rebellion may be very discouraging. Suddenly she may realize how much she has always depended on the convention of marriage as a social crutch.

In therapy, this type of divorced woman may insist on focusing primarily on developing a new set of social skills. There is no reason to discourage this attitude, but a respect for the relational skills she already has demonstrated in her life should also be encouraged.

In every case, the well-functioning woman in her later years is the woman who has maintained a network of relationships in which she feels most useful and appreciated. Whether the form that such a network takes is wholly conventional or purely experimental is of little importance. Her relational skills can flourish in the workplace, the family, or in any type of romantic or platonic liaison. The principal task of therapy is to help such a person affirm her relational skills so that they can be further developed and enhanced.

I do not mean to suggest that all women are born with God-given relational skills. Those women who, for whatever reason, fall outside the cultural norm and have developed neither relational nor occupational skills are, in their later years, in serious trouble. This is as true for men as it is for women—except that men are at least three times as likely to have an opportunity for marriage as a solution.

The facts are that the majority of people who live alone are women (11 million versus 6.8 million men), and that women who live alone tend to be widowed and/or divorced elderly (the men tend to be young and never married) (*Current Population Reports*, October 1981). It is imperative that the social context which makes life so problematic at this stage of life for women be changed.

If a woman is defined only in relationship to others, when those others are no longer an active part of her life, the last years cannot be seen as other than empty and meaningless. Other cultures, and certainly more agrarian societies, extended the period of connectedness to family by extending a woman's years of service through grandparenting and continued functional attention to the needs of extended kin. This nostalgic romanticizing of a hard and often bitter past in the lives of women only serves to impede the search for new solutions. The pendulum swing from service to autonomy leaves out the whole range of those attributes that make connectedness a positive force in humanity above and beyond its exploitation potential.

It goes without saying that old men when alone are not necessarily better off. They suffer more from the diminution of power and potency, both physical and social. The solution of finding a spouse (preferably a woman young enough to take care of him) is, of course, considerably more available for men at any age than for older women. However, that's a *non*solution, or perpetuation of the status quo, both for the man and for the woman he marries in his later years.

I do not pretend to offer new solutions to centuries-old social problems. But I want to suggest that as systems therapists we must recognize the power of the social system in defining and constraining individual life. Long after the functional role is over, the vestigial attitudes remain.

A conventional therapist confronted by a woman past her middle years (with or without grandchildren) might try to reinvolve her in service to others with the assumption that she needs to feel useful. A feminist view would help her to see herself and her life as worthwhile whether she is still "useful" to others or not.

Conclusion

It is significant that the following two cases deal with older women struggling to redefine themselves as women alone.

The term "women alone" is commonly meant to assume women without men, which implicitly carries a stigma, a sense of failure, and above all an aura of loneliness. A "woman alone" is still seen by society, and often by herself, as isolated, vulnerable, and unprotected.

This is paradoxically most true for women who have successfully and competently cared for husbands, children, and aged parents.

It is important for therapists to distinguish between the real vulnerability of old age and physical debility and the ascribed and felt vulnerability of the still healthy and vigorous woman in her early old age who is caught in the cultural stereotyping of her generation.

cases

Olga Silverstein

The Faded Flower

A culture that objectifies women will put exaggerated value on her looks and, by definition, then, on her youth. A woman who has been successful in exploiting her physical assets will often find herself without available resources when those assets are no longer working for her. Dependent on male admiration and attention, she sees women as competitors. She has few female friends and describes herself as a "man's woman." As her looks fade she may attempt to maintain herself by being "a good sport." She can often be found in the local bar, drinking with "the boys." Alcoholism in older women is a serious and often neglected problem.

Lillian was 59 years old when I first saw her. She came to therapy on the advice of her physician, who was concerned about her drinking. She said she was here because her drinking was ruining her looks. "The booze is ruining my figure," she told me, pointing to a small potbelly on her too thin frame.

In a tight dress, heavily but expertly made up, her hair blonde and well-styled, she appeared considerably younger from a distance. Close up, her face was puffy and her eyes bloodshot. She retained the aura of a former beauty by her coquettish walk and mannerisms.

The Story

Lillian was the youngest of six children, born seven years after the cluster of her five siblings. She described her mother as "worn out" and "over the hill" when she was born. "For her I was not a happy surprise," she told me. "My father was different. I was the apple of his eye. I guess I was the proof that he could still do it. He took me everywhere. He bought me dresses when my sisters were making their own. They were very jealous of me, but I didn't care. I knew I was prettier than they were." She pulled a picture of a startlingly pretty teenager dressed in a prom gown out of her purse. "That's me at 16," she said, looking at the picture admiringly. "I really was something else, a little wild but, oh, I had fun. I was a good-time kid," she laughed.

"My father died a year after this picture was taken." She started to cry, but dabbed carefully at her makeup. "A year later I was married. All the others were gone and I wasn't going to get stuck taking care of my mother. She was no fun, let me tell you."

"I married a man ten years my senior. When he went into the army in 1940 I lived near the base till he went overseas. Then I joined the USO and it was party time! Oh, I had fun." Again her eyes filled with tears. "When the war was over and John came home I hardly knew him. He worked very hard and I had two kids just like that, two kids in three years. No more fun. John hardly looked at me. I gained a lot of weight and I guess I was not much to look at."

When her children were 8 and 10, Lillian went into therapy, and two years later she divorced her husband. She moved from the suburbs into a small apartment in the West Village of Manhattan, enrolled in courses at New York University, and started what she called "my new life." Always gregarious, she made friends easily. Between the ages of 30 and 40, she had many affairs. She emphasized "many"—"I don't remember how many." She worked at several low-paid jobs sporadically, and continued to live in "splendid poverty" on alimony and child-support money and "help" from her male friends.

When the children left home, Lillian was still a young woman in her early 40s. "I got scared," she told me. "The day my daughter got married I looked in the mirror and I cried. Then I knew I'd better get moving while there was still time. I married Elliot. He drank some, but not so anyone would know it. We had a good time but he died six years ago from lung cancer. Wouldn't you know it. I always had rotten luck. Well, not always, because Elliot left me a little money, not much, but I don't have to work." She started to cry again. "I don't know what's the matter with me. I'm not poor. I have a nice little apartment. My children are healthy. And I'm not fat."

The Therapy

It was very difficult to find a point of entry with this woman. She could have easily been characterized in individual therapy as a narcissistic character disorder—in which case she might have been told that she was too old to expect much change. Or a therapist could embark on a long-term project of self-exploration, implying thereby that she could, by discovering what was wrong with her, potentiate some change.

I explored her current social network and noted its impoverishment. She had an occasional date with an old lover, now married, a sparse, spread-out group of casual women friends, and, of course, "the boys" at the bar where she spent most of her evenings. She had twice-a-year contact with her children. Thanksgiving they came to her. Christmas she went to them. "I don't want to be a burden," she told me. "My sisters took care of my mother, but they resented it. I know I would have resented it."

"Why would they need to take care of you?" I asked her. "Is that the only way a mother can relate to her children, or they to her?"

"I don't know," she answered. "If there is another way, I don't know it." She laughed. "I'm not the grandmother type." "What type is that?" I asked her. "Oh, you know, the fat little person who makes chicken soup." "Oh, like your mother." "Yes, like my poor mother." For Lillian, it was one or the other: either depend on others or have others depend on you.

Exploring Women's Issues

We talked a lot about what it means to be a woman, to grow up female in a world that seems to offer two options for women—family drudge or sex object and playmate. Given those two choices, the choice she made was clarified. "You must have been very aware of your mother's unhappiness to be so resolved to live your life differently."

"Oh, I was, I was," she said, "but I could never be nice to her because I thought she was jealous of me."

"Well, why wouldn't she be?" I asked.

We talked at length about her mother's life, and finally Lillian wept for her. "I really missed having a mother like a friend. She and my sisters were always buzzing together."

"I guess," she admitted, "maybe I was jealous of them." She cried for a long time.

I suggested that she visit the sisters she had long written off as jealous of her. "They won't want to see me," she worried. "Maybe not. Certainly not if you go in with the old defensive chip on your shoulder."

She reluctantly went to see her oldest sister. She hadn't seen her in six years. She was not greeted with open arms. There were a great many unsettled old scores in this family. But gradually with consistent encouragement and coaching from me, the two sisters began to talk about their common history. Finally, Lillian asked if she could bring her sister Anna to a session.

Lillian's sister Anna was a woman in her late sixties, no beauty like her sister. Still, it was clear that she had been and still was a good-looking woman. Alone now, like Lillian, she was a widow. She felt lonely and unfocused in her own life. "My husband was everything to me," she confided. Lillian laughed, "We're not that different, are we?" Her sister bristled at that and said, "I always wanted to be like you. Papa gave you everything. He never even looked at me. 'Help your mother' was all he ever said to me. And that's what I did all my life, that's what I did."

"That's what you both did," I said, "You tried to live your lives to please your father and, later, the men in your lives. Now it's not so easy, even if you have the freedom to live to please yourself. However, I think you have a good resource in each other. Perhaps Lillian can share with you her capacity for having a good time and you can begin to join her in that. And you [to her sister] can share with Lillian your capacity for caring so that you can both see it doesn't have to be one or the other."

"First she has to stop drinking," Anna said. "I don't want anything to do with her when she's drinking. That's her idea of a good time. I don't want any part of her good time."

Beginning of Change

Two weeks later Lillian told me that Anna had convinced her to join AA. "She cares," she told me, "she really cares." Six months later, in a follow-up session, Lillian told me that she had persuaded Anna to join her on a cruise. "It wasn't easy but I reminded her about what you said."

It might be argued that Lillian's drinking problem could have been addressed directly. She might have found in AA a substitute social hall. Many have. Her physician had suggested, first bluntly, that she stop drinking and then later that she join AA. Both times she told him indignantly that she was not a drunk. Her drinking was part of her perception of herself as different from the hard-working "serious" women in her family. She was a man's woman. Her lifelong loneliness and perceived exclusion from the sorority of women in her growing up was covered over by her rationalization of their jealousy and by the male admiration and attention she learned to substitute for intimacy. In her mind, caring and unhappy drudgery were very closely connected.

As she began to accept caring from me, a woman contemporary, she was able to look back at herself not only as the beautiful doll child but also as the lonely little girl. In sharing with her sister her own feelings of jealousy, she joined her in a mutual recognition of the price both had paid growing up in a father-centered home. "We all competed for his attention," they told me, "Mama most of all."

"I never saw that," Lillian said. "I always knew it," Anna told her. "She was the best cook, the house was so clean. And if he said, 'Dinner was good,' she'd blush and smile. I used to get furious with her. Crumbs, she always settled for crumbs. But you, you always got everything." "No," Lillian said sadly, "No, I didn't, did I?"

Lillian's drinking was not the problem. It was her attempted solution. Her lifelong loneliness and feelings of emptiness could not be alleviated by a few simple moves in therapy. However, she and Anna maintained a relationship that, although stormy at times, never lacked in intimacy.

When Lillian called me a year after we terminated and asked if she could come in with her daughter, I felt very encouraged.

Betty Carter

"I May Never Find Another Man"

The following case illustrates one of the most pervasive and enduring themes in the lives of women: the feeling that being without a man reflects badly on a woman and somehow precludes the possibility of a rich and satisfactory life. As women grow older, they are more and more likely to find themselves without a man, either because they have never married, have divorced, or have been widowed. An older man in these circumstances can still expect to date or remarry a younger woman, but after "a certain age" most women who find themselves without a man will remain without a man. At age 65 to 75, only 49 percent of women are married as opposed to 81 percent of men. Over age 75, 70 percent of men remain married, while only 22 percent of women still have husbands. Since the prospect for women is to find themselves without a man as they grow older, it is important that therapists find ways to help women of all ages to counteract the strongly held myth that a woman without a man must lead a lonely and unfulfilled life. This is best accomplished by validating the importance of women's other relationships of all kinds, including those with family, friends, and colleagues.

Sara's Predicament

Sara was an attractive, well-dressed woman of 60 who looked quite a bit younger than her years. She worked long hours as a psychologist at a mental health clinic and maintained a private practice in her suburban apartment as well.

Sara's husband, an incipient alcoholic, had left her twenty years ago to marry his secretary. She had three children who were then ages 7, 10, and 15, and no profession or particular skills. With little money, no support from her family (who disapproved of the divorce), and much struggle, she had put herself through a doctoral program in psychology and helped all three children through college and graduate school. She was proud of her accomplishments and of her relationship with her children, who were all well established in productive lives. She had a large network of women friends with whom she traveled or went to concerts and theater. She radiated confidence, competence, warmth, intelligence, and humor.

I was beginning to think that perhaps I should go into therapy with *her* when she finally told me why she had come: "It's men," she said. "I can't live with them and I can't live without them." Specifically, she was concerned that her relationship with Robert, a 65-year-old lawyer, was often frustrating and depressing, but she was afraid to break off the relationship because, she said, "I may never find another man." She wasn't living with Robert, a divorced father of two grown sons, but had maintained an exclusive relationship with him for over five years.

Sara had had three or four intense long-term relationships in the twenty years since her divorce, but had never seriously entertained the idea of remarrying. "In the early days, they didn't want to marry a middle-aged woman with three young children, and then I finally realized that I didn't have to and didn't really want to marry again. But I love men, I love sex, and I've never been without a steady relationship for long." Now, however, she was afraid that at her age it might be Robert or no one.

Sara's sense of aging had been heightened by the relatively recent death of her elderly mother and the birth of her third grandchild. Her only remaining family member was a younger brother with whom she maintained a friendly but rather distant relationship.

Defining the Problem

This was the kind of case that used to fill me with feelings of helplessness. Who should come to treatment? What should we work on? How should we define the problem—"getting old"? Should I, after all, refer her to an individual therapist?

Sara was clear about certain aspects of her situation: She did not want conjoint therapy with Robert because she was quite sure she would be better off apart from him, *if* she had the courage to leave him. He was distant, noncommunicative, and depressed. She agreed with my ideas about the importance of family connections and had worked on them all of her life. Her parents were dead, and she felt that she had resolved "adequately" her relationships with them before they died, and had since done her grieving over their loss. She was clear about not wanting individual therapy because she had had enough of it, including enough personal "insight" to fill three autobiographies. "I'm not *personally* disturbed," she said, "but I need some help to leave him."

I thought about Sara and how best to help her. That final comment of hers made me think about the limits of therapy, which can't change the problem of the social response to aging women. The trap for the therapist here would be to assume that Sara would be better off with Robert, or anyone, rather than being alone. I took seriously her statement that she needed help to leave him, even though, at her age, her fears of remaining without a man were realistic.

Clinical Strategy

I thought of several other single women that I was currently seeing individually, and the fact that they weren't "personally disturbed" either. "They're trying to figure out their relationships with men," I thought, "and how to wade through all of the social messages about women and men to find out what they really want." It had bothered me for some time that many of the problems that women struggled with in my office were considered "personal" problems when they so clearly arose from the social system. "Men have lots of problems in their relationships with women," I thought, "but most men don't take such problems personally, they usually aren't devastated by the problems, and they're not turning to the mental health establishment for help— maybe to a dating service." For some time I had had the uneasy feeling that by seeing single women "in therapy" with "the problem" defined by them as "needing" a man (whether to break up with a man, how much to give up for a man, et cetera), I was contributing to the idea that difficulties with men indicated personal emotional disturbance, and that a course of therapy would eliminate such difficulties and help the women to stop "sabotaging" their relationships with men. I found myself repeating many of the same ideas in session after session as I tried to help these single women factor in the role played by their socialization as women, a socialization that clearly defined them as failures if they found themselves without a man for any reason except widowhood in later life.

I finally decided to try an experimental group of single women to see if their universality of experience would provide a more "objective" view of their circumstances and socialization and thereby shift their view, permitting them to see that it is the socially prescribed gender arrangements that are "disturbed," not them "personally."

Clinical Method

A word about my use of terms like *individual* and *group*. I don't do "individual therapy" with individuals, and I did not now propose to do "group therapy." I don't focus on intrapsychic process with individuals, but rather work with them within a family systems framework; that is, I evaluate the difficulty in the emotional process of the individual's family (husband, children, parents, siblings), decide what role the individual is playing in the dysfunction, and help them (my clients) to change their relationships as well as their participation in the problem. The individual is thus thought of and evaluated in the context of the three-generation family. And, as I have indicated, the family is also seen in its context, as the social, cultural (ethnic, religious), political, and economic factors that bear on the problem are included in the evaluation of the problem and in the plan for change.

By deciding to see several clients in a group, I did not propose to shift the focus to the relationships among the women in the group, as is done in group therapy, but rather I decided to continue the "individual" focus on each woman in her own family system, with the women, in effect, listening in on each other's work with me. They were not to interrupt each other's discussion with me, but were given an opportunity to express their ideas and reactions to each woman at the close of that woman's "turn."

The Group

In addition to Sara, then, there was Annette, 49, a businesswoman whose husband had left her and filed for divorce "out of the blue" because he had fallen in love with his secretary; Joan, 32, a jewelry designer, who was trying to decide whether to marry a particular man or not; Susan, 50, a nonpracticing lawyer, whose wealthy husband was having an affair and refused to come with her to therapy; and Marianne, 36, who didn't work outside the home, and who saw me with her husband for marital problems. (Marianne and her husband agreed that Marianne's lack of assertiveness was a problem for both of them, as was his bossiness. I therefore invited her to join the women's group for extra help with that problem.)

As I had expected, through all of the ethnic, economic, and age differences, what stood out in the group as each woman talked about her difficulties was the woman's belief that she could not be happy or whole without a man; her belief that if she did "the right thing" and worked on her "personal problems," the difficulties with finding a man, or keeping a man, would end. Each woman felt responsible for the problem, and responsible to solve it through changing herself. Each feared being without a man and seemed willing to tolerate almost anything in the relationship rather than risk losing it.

Although each woman felt overwhelmed by her own situation, they were all able to view each other's situations more objectively, and to challenge each other's positions of helplessness. A great deal of empathy and understanding were expressed, and everyone had had experiences or feelings that were the same or similar to those of the others.

Sara, particularly, because of her longer experience of life, underscored and amplified the tentative expressions of the other women. With her humor and intelligence, she soon gained a position of prestige in the group, due also to the imposing credentials of having lived for 25 years without a husband while she raised three children and pursued a successful career. This experience—what the others most feared, but felt they might well have to face—lent weight to her comments to the other women. She refused to accept their helplessness; she didn't join the occasional "man-bashing"; but she resolutely located the problem in the "myths and expectations we've been raised on."

As the months went on, the focus of the women's concerns slowly shifted to taking charge of their own lives, making decisions that were advantageous to themselves (rather than procrastinating and martyring their way along), and focusing on what they could arrange for their lives instead of what they wished others would "let them" do.

Eventually, Annette decided she would survive, and perhaps thrive on, her divorce; Joan decided to marry her boyfriend after letting him know what she did and did not expect from wifing and husbanding; Susan returned to the practice of law with the idea that when she had organized her own life more effectively she would refuse to continue tolerating her husband's affair; and Marianne's experience in the group helped her to stand up to her husband in a way she hadn't before, and which dramatically shifted the balance of power in their marriage.

The Outcome for Sara

Sara, who stayed in that "trial" group for two years, eventually broke off with Robert. As she had feared, she didn't meet anyone else, but when she left the group she was still deeply involved with several peer groups, remained closely attached to her children's families, and was about to organize a "travel club." "I'd like to meet a new man," she said, "but I wouldn't give up any of my activities for him—he'd have to be willing to fit into my life as much as I would accommodate to his. And if I don't meet anyone—it's not that big a deal anymore. I'm not alone in life—I just live alone."

She said that she had known before she joined the group that she'd be better off without Robert, but had been unable to give him up without feeling she had "failed" somehow. "The main thing that changed for me," she said, "is not feeling like a failure without Robert or anyone else. I was always able to leave other men, or to recover from their leaving me, because I knew I'd find someone else. Now I know I probably won't and it's okay."

Conclusion

The format of a women's group for working on the difficulties experienced by women who are alone has been a useful one. Women of all ages find their commonality of experience an immediate bond. There is empathy and validation of experience while, at the same time, the women challenge each other to acknowledge and use the strengths and coping skills that underlie the tears and feelings of dependency. Younger women's experience in a radically different world helps to inform their elders, and within this group format the older woman's wisdom finally gets a receptive response.

Marianne Walters

Epilogue

In the end, it feels very much as if we are just beginning. The process of seeking to identify a feminist perspective in family therapy, and to connect clinical interventions to that perspective, has been a stimulating and provocative journey for all of us. But it *is* just a beginning. A feminist frame of reference will continue to create a dialectic within family therapy, and among family therapists—an arena for critique and self-criticism, for proposition and counterproposition, for point and counterpoint. There will be a period of self-consciousness, and many will tire of the effort and cast it aside as but another "issue" in the field that has seen the light of day and can now be assigned a place in our history. But there will be those who will persist because they have come to believe, as we do, that gender is a crucial and a critical variable in all human systems.

The interface between feminist thinking and family therapy is often obscured by issues of clinical expediency and methodological preference. In our work together, coming as we did from different, indeed distinct, clinical perspectives, this was often the case. It was necessary for us to establish a method that, for the purposes of this book, would give precedence to the process of correcting every intervention, regardless of its theoretical framework, for sexism and gender bias. Then we could proceed to the business of evolving alternative techniques and new interventions, which, in turn, had to be measured against sexist constructions. This process has been something akin to affirmative action—a deliberate effort to counteract the negative effects for women of gender stereotyping. It has been a deliberate effort to identify those experiences of women that could be generalized as socially constructed; to listen to the voices of women; and to hear, in our work, the echo of messages that devalue or objectify women.

The Women's Project in Family Therapy began in 1977. Our efforts were supported by an environment in which an awareness of women's issues had already been stimulated by feminists and a broad-based women's movement. We hope that in our field we will have provided some of this consciousness raising so that our colleagues seeking a feminist perspective in their work will enjoy an environment that nurtures their efforts.

There have already been a number of encouraging developments. On two occasions a group of fifty women active in the field of family therapy met together for several days at an inn in Connecticut. We shared ideas, experiences, research projects, work in progress, clinical anecdotes. We set up informal networks and expanded our friendships. We argued theory and strategy and agreed on the need to raise women's issues in our professional meetings, journals, workshops, conferences. And this is happening. Few, if any, conference agendas of our national professional associations do not contain some theoretical or clinical discussion around women's issues in family therapy. There is a women's task force. A number of journal articles have been devoted to the subject. Several books are in progress or have been published recently. A new journal of feminist family therapy is being organized.

Yet, of course, it still remains difficult for women to challenge sexist practices or clinical descriptions, particularly when these are presented in open forums. And a feminist perspective has not yet been integrated into the training curricula of most of our professional training programs, so we often fail to notice the biased, stereotyped, or denigrating message conveyed in an intervention that seems to work. There is still much to be done before gender and system can comfortably coexist. For this is just a beginning.

References

Chapter 1 Toward a Feminist Family Therapy

Pollak, S., and Gilligan, C. "Images of Violence in Thematic Apperception Test Stories." *Journal of Personality and Social Psychology*,
vol. 42 (1982): 159–167.

Chapter 2 Mothers and Daughters

Bateson, G. *Steps to an Ecology of Mind*. New York: Jason Aronson,
1972.
Bruner, J. S. *The Process of Education*. New York: Vintage, 1960.
Caplan, P. J., and Hall-McCorquodale, I. "Mother Blaming in Major
Clinical Journals." *American Journal of Orthopsychiatry*, vol. 55,
no. 3 (July 1985): 345–353.
Friday, N. *My Mother, Myself*. New York: Dell, 1977.
Fromm, Erich. *The Art of Loving*. New York: Harper & Row, 1956.
Gilligan, C. *In a Different Voice*. Cambridge, Mass.: Harvard Univer-
sity Press, 1982.
Rich, A. *Of Woman Born*. New York: Bantam Books, 1977.
Smith-Rosenberg, C. "The Female World of Love and Ritual: Relations
between Women in Nineteenth-Century America." *Signs: Journal
of Women in Culture and Society*, vol. 1, no. 1 (1975): 1–29.

Chapter 3 Fathers and Daughters

Appleton, W. *Fathers and Daughters*. New York: Doubleday, 1981.
Bowen, M. *Family Therapy in Clinical Practice*. New York: Jason Aron-
son, 1978.
Broverman, J. K., Broverman, D. M., and Clarkson, F. E. "Sex Role
Stereotypes and Clinical Judgments of Mental Health." *Journal of
Consulting and Clinical Psychology*, vol. 34 (1970): 1–7.
Carter, E., and Orfanidis, M. "Family Therapy with One Person and
the Family Therapist's Own Family." In P. J. Guerin (Ed.), *Fam-
ily Therapy: Theory and Practice*. New York: Gardner Press,
1976.

Cohen, T. "The Incestuous Family." *Social Casework*, vol. 62, no. 8 (October 1981).

Cohen, T. "The Incestuous Family Revisited." *Social Casework*, vol. 64, no. 3 (March 1983).

Conte, J. R. "Progress in Treating the Sexual Abuse of Children." *Social Work*, vol. 29, no. 3 (May-June 1984).

Freud, A. *A General Introduction to Psychoanalysis.* New York: Washington Square Press, 1967.

Hammer, S. *Passionate Attachments.* New York: Rawson Associates, 1982.

Hennig, M., and Jardim, A. *The Managerial Woman.* New York: Pocket Books, 1978.

Herman, J. *Father-Daughter Incest.* Cambridge, Mass.: Harvard University Press, 1981.

Herman, J., and Hirschman, L. "Father-Daughter Incest." *Signs: Journal of Women in Culture and Society*, vol. 2, no. 4 (Summer 1977).

Janeway, E. *Cross Sections from a Decade of Change.* New York: William Morrow, 1982.

Lozoss, M. M. "Fathers and Autonomy in Women." In R. B. Knudsin (Ed.), *Women and Success.* New York: New York Academy of Sciences.

McGoldrick, M. Commencement Address, Smith College School of Social Work, August 1984.

McIntyre, K. "Role of Mothers in Father-Daughter Incest: A Feminist Analysis." *Social Work*, vol. 26, no. 6 (November 1981).

Social Work, vol. 23, no. 1 (January 1978).

Chapter 4 Mothers and Sons

Arcana, J. *Every Mother's Son.* Garden City, N.Y.: Anchor Press/Doubleday, 1983.

Chodorow, N. *Reproduction of Mothering: Psychoanalysis and the Sociology of Gender.* Berkeley: University of California Press, 1978.

Goldner, V. "Feminism in Family Therapy." *Family Process*, vol. 24, no. 1 (March 1985).

Hare-Mustin, R. T. "A Feminist Approach to Family Therapy." *Family Process*, vol. 17, no. 2 (June 1978).

Hare-Mustin, R. T. "Focusing on Relationships in the Family," *Harvard Educational Review*, vol. 53, no. 2 (1983): 203–209.

Klein, C. *Mothers and Sons*, Boston: Houghton Mifflin, 1984.

Milgram, S. *Obedience to Authority.* New York: Harper & Row, 1973.

Weiss, J. S. *Raising a Son.* New York: Summit Books, 1984.

Chapter 5 Couples

Bernard, J. *The Future of Marriage.* New York: World Publishing, 1972.

Blumstein, P., and Schwartz, P. New York: William Morrow, 1983.

Ehrenreich, B. *Remaking Love.* New York: Anchor/Doubleday, 1986.

Hite, S. *The Hite Report.* New York: Macmillan, 1976.

Hite, S. *The Hite Report on Male Sexuality.* New York: Knopf, 1981.

Kimball, G. *The Fifty-Fifty Marriage.* Boston: Beacon Press, 1983.

Lerner, H. *The Dance of Anger.* New York: Harper and Row, 1986.

Miller, J. "The Construction of Anger in Women and Men." Wellesley, Mass: Stone Center for Developmental Services and Studies, Wellesley College, work in progress.

Miller, J. B. *Toward a New Psychology of Women.* Boston: Beacon Press, 1976.

Pollak, S., and Gilligan, C. "Images of Violence in Thematic Apperception Test Stories." *Journal of Personality and Social Psychology,* vol. 42 (1982): 159-167.

Prochaska, J. O. "Restriction of Range on Date and Mate Selection in College Students." University of Rhode Island, 1977, unpublished manuscript.

Slater, P. "What Hath Sock Wrought?—Freed Children, Chained Moms." *Washington Post,* March 1, 1970.

Stiver, I. "The Meanings of 'Dependency' in Female-Male Relationships." Wellesley, Mass: Stone Center for Developmental Services and Studies, Wellesley College, work in progress.

Veroff, J., and Feld, S. *Marriage and Work in America.* New York: Van Nostrand-Reinhold, 1970.

Chapter 6 Divorce: His and Hers

Carter, E., and McGoldrick, M. "Overview." In E. Carter and M. McGoldrick (Eds.), *The Family Life Cycle: A Framework for Family Therapy.* New York: Gardner Press, 1980 (2nd edition, in press).

Glick, Paul C. "Marriage, Divorce and Living Arrangements," *Journal of Family Issues,* vol. 5, no. 1 (March 1984).

Hopps, J. "Is No-Fault without Fault?" *Social Work,* vol. 32, no. 1 (January–February 1987): 3.

McGoldrick, M., and Carter, E. "Forming a Remarried Family." In E. Carter and M. McGoldrick (Eds.), *The Family Life Cycle: A Framework for Family Therapy.* New York: Gardner Press, 1980 (2nd edition, in press).

Norton, A. J., and Moorman, J. E. "Marriage and Divorce Patterns of U.S. Women" (Population Division, Bureau of Census). *Journal of Marriage and the Family* (February 1987).

Rubin, L. *Intimate Strangers*. New York: Harper & Row, 1983.

Weitzman, L. *The Divorce Revolution: The Unexpected Social and Economic Consequences for Women and Children in America.* New York: Free Press, 1985.

Chapter 7   Single-Parent, Female-Headed Families

Hope, K., and Young, N. *MOMMA, The Sourcebook for Single Mothers*. New York: New American Library, 1976.

Marotz-Baden, B., Adams, G. R., Bueche, N., Munro, B., and Munro, G. "Family Form or Family Process? Reconsidering the Deficit Family Model Approach." *The Family Coordinator*, 1979.

Peterson, G., and Cleminshaw, H. K. "The Strength of Single-Parent Families During the Divorce Crisis: An Integrative Review with Clinical Implications." In N. Stinnett *et al.* (Eds.), *Family Strengths: Positive Models for Family Life.* Lincoln: University of Nebraska Press, 1980.

Rix, Sara E. (Ed.). The Women's Research and Education Institute of the Congressional Caucus for Women's Issues. *The American Woman, 1987-88: A Report in Depth.* New York: W. W. Norton, 1988.

Wallerstein, J. S., and Kelly, J. B. *Surviving the Breakup: How Children Actually Cope with Divorce.* New York: Basic Books, 1980.

Weiss, R. S. "Growing Up a Little Faster: The Experience of Growing Up in a Single-Parent Household." *Journal of Social Issues*, vol. 35, no. 4 (1979).

Weitzman, L. J. *The Divorce Revolution: The Unexpected Social and Economic Consequences for Women and Children in America.* New York: Free Press, 1985.

Chapter 8   Remarried Families: Creating a New Paradigm

Ahrons, C. H. "Redefining the Divorced Family: A Conceptual Framework for Postdivorce Family Systems Reorganization." *Social Work*, vol. 25 (1980): 437–441.

Amber, A. M. "Being a Stepparent: Live-in and Visiting Stepchildren." *Journal of Marriage and the Family*, vol. 48, no. 4 (1986): 795–804.

Booth, A., and White, L. "The Quality and Stability of Remarriages: The Role of Stepchildren." *American Sociological Review* (1985).

Chesler, P. *Mothers on Trial: The Battle for Children and Custody.* New York: McGraw-Hill, 1986.

Dahl, A. S., Cowgill, K. M., and Admundsson, R. "Life in Remarriage Families." *Social Work*, vol. 32, no. 1 (1987): 40–44.

Elkin, M. "Joint Custody: Affirming That Parents and Families Are Forever." *Social Work*, vol. 32, no. 1 (1987).

Glick, P. C. "Marriage, Divorce, and Living Arrangements: Prospective Changes." *Journal of Family Issues*, vol. 46 (1984): 563–576.

Marriage and Divorce Today, vol. 12, no. 9 (1986).

McGoldrick, M., and Carter, E. "Forming a Remarried Family." In E. Carter and M. McGoldrick (Eds.), *The Family Life Cycle: A Framework for Family Therapy*. New York: Gardner Press, 1980 (2nd edition, in press).

Norton, A. J., and Moorman, J. E. "Current Trends in Marriage and Divorce among American Women." *Journal of Marriage and Family*, vol. 49, no. 1 (1987): 3–14.

Weitzman, L. *The Divorce Revolution: The Unexpected Social and Economic Consequences for Women and Children in America*. New York: Free Press, 1985.

Chapter 9   Single Women: Early and Middle Years

Adams, M. *Single Blessedness*. New York: Basic Books, 1976.

Norwood, R. *Women Who Love Too Much*. New York: Simon and Schuster, 1985.

Index